Assessing Child Survival Programs in Developing Countries

Testing Lot Quality Assurance Sampling

Joseph J. Valadez, Ph.D., M.P.H., S.D.

Department of Population and International Health
Harvard School of Public Health
Boston, Massachusetts

December 1991
Distributed by Harvard University Press

ISBN 0-674-04995-0

Library of Congress Cataloging-in-Publication Data

Valadez, Joseph J.
   Assessing child survival programs in developing countries: testing lot quality
assurance sampling / Joseph J. Valadez
      p.   cm. -- (Harvard series on population and international health)
      "December 1991."
      Includes bibliographical references and index.
      ISBN 0-674-04995-0 (pbk.) : $10.95
      1. Child health services--Developing countries--Evaluation.
   I. Title.   II. Series.
      [DNLM: 1. Child Health Services. 2. Developing Countries.
   3. Primary Health Care. 4. Quality Assurance, Health Care.
   5. Sampling Studies. WA 395 V136a]
   RJ103. D44V35   1991
   362. 1 '9892' 0091724--dc20
   DNLM/DLC
   for Library of Congress   92-1433
                                                           CIP

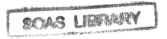

Funding provided by:
African Medical and Research Foundation
Danish International Development Association (DANIDA)
PRICOR Project*
United Nations Children Fund (UNICEF-Costa Rica) (UNICEF-ESARO)

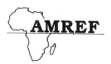 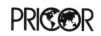

* The PRICOR Project is implemented by the Center for Human Services, Bethesda, Md., in
cooperation with the United States Agency for International Development under Cooperative
Agreement DPE-5920-A-00-5056-00.

Dedication

*To HMV, and the Community Health Workers of the
Primary Health Care System of Costa Rica and Latin
America*

Principal Collaborators:

Ministry of Health of Costa Rica and Local Project Team

Dr. Carlos Valerín Arias, Costa Rica, Former Director General of Health

Dr. Carlos Muñoz, Costa Rica, Director of the Department of Primary Health
Care

Lic. William Vargas Vargas, Costa Rica, Director of the Office of Quality
Control

Enf. Zoila Rosa Ajiuro Rivera, Costa Rica, Department of Nursing

Enf. Rosibel Méndez Briceño, Costa Rica, Department of Nursing

Lic. Silvia Boada-Martinez, Spain, Project Assistant, Harvard University

Pan American Health Organization

Dr. Hugo Villegas, Peru, Former Country Representative to Costa Rica

Dr. Carlos Ferrero, Argentina, Former Regional Advisor for Information
Systems

Dr. Raúl Penna, Argentina, Country Representative to Costa Rica

Contents

Tables

Figures

Preface

This book presents the development and field test of a rapid method for assessing the quality of routine primary health care activities (PHC) aimed at enhancing child survival. The results of this work have applications far beyond the context of the Costa Rican Primary Health Care Program from which the findings reported here were developed. I have applied the method successfully in Guatemala and Trinidad and I have helped health professionals in Haiti, Uganda, Kenya, El Salvador and Bolivia adapt this approach to the programs in their countries. Others have applied the method independently in Peru and Indonesia. All work presented here was a collaborative effort of the Ministry of Health, the Pan American Health Organization, and Harvard University, so that principles and procedures presented here would be relevant to other developing countries.

The population included in this work consists of children under three years of age and their mothers. Three criteria of quality were used for program assessment. The first one was "service adequacy," which determines whether risk groups in a community are receiving services at the appropriate age as defined by Ministry of Health norms. This criterion was important for assessing the Expanded Programme on Immunization (EPI) since the Ministry norms required, for example, that infants be vaccinated for polio beginning at two months of age with a minimum of a one-month interval between doses until three doses and two boosters have been received.

The second criterion was "coverage," which measures whether a sufficiently high proportion of individuals in a community have received services regardless of the age in which they received them. This criterion was pertinent to all services included in the assessment since the mothers of all children under three years should have been, for example, educated in the preparation of oral rehydration therapy, or had their vaccination status up to date even if doses were received at ages older than specified by Ministry norms.

The third criterion was "quality of the technique" of community health workers (CHWs). This consideration was included to ensure that critical components of the health system (e.g., maintaining the cold chain, the availability of oral rehydration salts, CHW hygiene, education of mothers) were performed by health workers at sufficiently high levels of quality to result in the intended health impacts.

Up to now, the standard method of evaluating coverage of health interventions has been limited to sampling designs that measure coverage throughout an entire region or nation using observations of children representing the whole population. This book describes and reports on the field test of a comprehensive approach, which assesses service adequacy, coverage, and CHW technique in the communities served by local health facilities within a region or nation. With a small investment beyond those typically used, this method enables program directors to identify those particular health facilities with inadequate services, and which therefore require special attention.

This book was written in response to an invitation from the Minister of Health of Costa Rica, Dr. Juan Jaramillo Antillón, in 1985, requesting a system of monitoring and evaluating the Costa Rican Primary Health Care (PHC) Program. The request was to the Harvard School of Public Health and specifically to me to assist them in the development of this system. At once we started to establish priorities, always having it in mind to produce work that could be used by other countries.

The PHC system extends services from the Ministry of Health in San José to hundreds of asistentes de salud (community health workers) stationed at community based health posts. The priority question was how regularly and effectively were health assistants providing prescribed services. Each worker was assigned roughly 500 families. Obtaining a measure of average performance of these health workers at the national scale would have been inadequate to identify individual health posts or regions where the work was substandard. For example, a community may be at risk of a measles epidemic if the health worker vaccinates less than 80% of susceptible children against measles. The Minister agreed that his program staff needed a rapid and inexpensive method of measuring the adequacy of the health service delivery provided by each health worker. Lot Quality Assurance Sampling (LQAS), adapted from industry, provided a promising method to achieve that limited goal.

This book presents the theory, procedures, analyses, reporting systems, and an economic assessment of LQAS. It describes all preparatory tasks as well as those performed in this field test.

Other chapters discuss methodological principles for data collection in international public health projects. The basic precepts of program monitoring and evaluation, and of field research presented in general terms here, were used in the LQAS work carried out in Costa Rica.

These presentations respond to Dr. Jaramillo Antillón's request for a practical and rapid tool to control the quality of primary health care at the level where it either succeeds or fails, namely, in the community. It is also a general statement of principles of monitoring and evaluation activities, of which LQAS is a useful and powerful technique.

As an international public health practitioner, my first obligation is to address the needs of my client's clients. My client is the Ministry of Health and their asistentes de salud. Their clients are the mothers and children of Costa

Rica. However, I also have obligations to my academic and scientific associates. I have tried to address both commitments. While the limitations of this volume are mine alone, I owe much to others and wish to acknowledge their support and advice.

Acknowledgements

This work would have been impossible without the support of Dr. Juan Jaramillo Antillón, Minister of Health of Costa Rica from 1982 through 1986, and then the continuing support of Dr. Edgar Mohs, who became Minister of Health in May 1986. Dr. Carlos Muñoz, Director of the Rural Health Program through 1986, formulated the formal invitation from Dr. Jaramillo through the Harvard School of Public Health to request my participation.

As to the day-to-day affairs of the project, the influence of two individuals has been fundamental: Dr. Carlos Valerín Arias, Director General of Health, and Dr. Hugo Villegas, the former National Representative of the Pan American Health Organization in Costa Rica. Both were intimately involved in the establishment of the Rural Health Program in Costa Rica in 1972, and have continued their involvement since then. They supported this project from beginning to end. My deepest thanks to them.

Dr. Carlos Ferrero, the Regional Advisor in Health Information Systems at the Pan American Health Organization in Washington, supported my research through a consultancy during 1986 in which I developed LQAS theory. This critical consultancy provided by Dr. Ferrero through PAHO furnished the crucial seed money leading to the award of three grant proposals. The first one was to the National Research Council/Ford Minority Fellowship Program for which I was appointed Senior Ford Fellow during 1986-1987. The second proposal resulted in the Harvard Institute for International Development receiving a subcontract from PRICOR under a cooperative agreement from the Office of Science and Technology of the Agency for International Development.[1] Dr. James Heiby of the Office of Health at AID discovered our proposal and encouraged our application to PRICOR for funding. Dr. Heiby's prescience and understanding of the potential use of LQAS for managing community-based public health programs were among the most essential ingredients that led to this project. Dr. David Nicholas and Dr. Stu Blumenfeld at PRICOR made numerous valuable comments and provided help in shaping the proposal that PRICOR eventually funded.

The third proposal was from the Board on Science and Technology for International Development at the National Academy of Sciences (NAS) (CRG Grant No. RGA-CR-1-87-71). I wrote the proposal that resulted in the awarding of a grant to the INISA (Instituto Nacional para Investigaciones en Salud) Foundation at the University of Costa Rica to fund part of this project. Ms. Karen Bell, the then BOSTID Program Officer for Rapid Epidemiological Assessment, was instrumental in having the project receive helpful suggestions from two NAS reviewers, Dr. George Stroh and Dr. Stan Lemeshow. Through her support we arranged with INISA that they would manage the BOSTID funds.

I should like to express my gratitude to several colleagues closer to home, at the Harvard Institute for International Development, which has been the base of operations for this project: Dwight Perkins, Al Henn, Chris Hale, Dzvinia Orlowsky, Drew Factor, and Flo Chien. Special thanks is due Leisa Weld, my associate and partner in operations research at HIID beginning in 1990. Her comments and clarity were greatly appreciated. Also, I thank Dr. David Marsh and Ms. Lori DiPrete for their careful reading of an early version of the manuscript and their many helpful suggestions. Don Shepard shared many of the critical early decisions with me in this project. Don pointed me towards LQAS in the first place by sharing with me Centers for Disease Control (CDC) memos and internal papers written mostly by George Stroh about potential applications of LQAS to public health. From that point I found the original Dodge and Romig papers from the 1920s in Massachusetts Institute of Technology's Dewey Library. The potential contribution of LQAS to public health became steadily clearer.

At the Harvard School of Public Health I thank Dr. John Wyon whose consistent questioning and incomparable experience in community public health has guided my thinking as a public health scientist and practitioner. Drs. Guillermo Herrera, Walter Mertens, and John Orav have also given critical and timely comments. Dr. Ana Contromitros provided valuable assistance in organizing the economic data on which Chapter 7 is based. I am especially grateful to Drs. Lincoln Chen and Michael Reich, without whose support this book would not have been published.

In Costa Rica, I want to thank our team. They are the only ones who really know what we shared to bring this project to life: the diarrhea, the inspections by military personnel at the Nicaraguan border, the months of beds shared with cockroaches, and the camaraderie and the loyalty that those experiences bred. Firstly, I thank Silvia Boada Martinez, formerly my student and now my colleague, who traveled from Argentina to Costa Rica to work during the entire data collection period (January through August 1987). No job was too difficult nor too menial for her to perform; she was the consummate field investigator. Secondly, I thank William Vargas Vargas, appointed by the Director General of Health as the Ministry's counterpart. His wisdom was demonstrated by his desire to learn every detail of the project and to participate in every phase of the data collection. Vargas participated in all phases of field work from 1987 through 1990. Our goal was to produce a functioning assessment system for Costa Rica and to produce a careful critical field test of LQAS. My deep thanks to a loyal friend, colleague, and since May 1990, first director of the newly formed Office of Quality Control of Peripheral Health Services. Thirdly, I should like to thank our drivers from the Ministry who knew every back road of Costa Rica: Yamil, Rodrigo, Victor and Guido.

There are numerous others who, alas, must be acknowledged as a group. The asistentes de salud, the auxiliares de salud, the supervisores del campo, the nurses, and the Regional Directors. On a day-to-day basis we depended on them for access to all of the information the project collected, and their collaboration was magnificent. I wish to thank the interviewers organized by Boada and Vargas with the help of Luis Rosero of INISA. Mr. Rosero also helped develop and pretest the questionnaire, managed the BOSTID funds, and organized the actual data entry into a computer database. The data were cleaned by myself, Boada, Vargas, and members of the INISA staff.

At Harvard University Press, I am grateful to Howard Boyer who guided me through the preparations. The comments he obtained on earlier drafts of the manuscript from Dr. George Silver and Dr. Rashi Fein were essential for structuring the final version. Dr. Remi Clignet of the Institut Francais de Recherche Scientifique pour le Developpement en Cooperation (ORSTOM) kept me focused on the broader issues of applied research. Patrick Santana of Desktop Publishing & Design, of Boston, MA, designed the book and Marc Kaufman managed production. In all activities they went much more than an extra mile. Thank you all.

In conclusion, I thank U.N.I.C.E.F., D.A.N.I.D.A., and the African Medical and Research Foundation / East African Flying Doctor Service for their support. They were prescient in recognizing the application of LQAS to assessing the quality of   child survival services in difficult conditions found throughout the developing world. With U.N.I.C.E.F./E.S.A.R.O.'s support ministries throughout East and South Africa are now informed on how to use LQAS to monitor child survival, mother care, and AIDS prevention programs. At D.A.N.I.D.A. Henning Frøtlund and Dr. Kirsten Havermann recognized that controlling the quality of service delivery in East Africa may eliminate one of the region's most important factors that place people's health at risk. This insight led to D.A.N.I.D.A.'s support for this book. Through AMREF, LQAS is now being applied in Uganda by Ministry of Health district medical teams, and is planned for use among nomadic, rural, and periurban communities of Kenya. I would like to give special thanks to Dr. Basil King, Director of AMREF's Nomadic Health Unit; his insightful reading of the manuscript led to several changes that greatly improved the clarity of important passages. I also thank very much the Costa Rica office of U.N.I.C.E.F. for supporting the production of this book. Lic. Athenia Montejo and her associates came to my rescue in the eleventh hour of this publication with essential assistance.

J. J. Valadez
Cambridge 1991

1. *The work upon which this presentation is based was performed in part under a subagreement with the Center for Human Services under its Cooperative Subagreement No. DPE-5920-00-A-5056-00 with the U.S. Agency for International Development.*

Assessing Health Services

General Definition of Lot Quality Assurance Sampling

The principal goal of this book is to demonstrate how a quality control technique that was developed originally for industry has been adapted to assess the quality of services provided by health workers in developing nations. The technique, Lot Quality Assurance Sampling (LQAS), is explained in detail so that managers of international health programs can understand and apply this exceptionally rapid, precise, and inexpensive method to their own work both in theory and practice.

Like other sampling approaches developed for applications in industry, LQAS is oriented toward practical action. Its potential for application in developing nations is based on its use of small sample sizes to provide useful management information. A typical health system has hundreds of service providers, each carrying out dozens of distinct activities. Currently, managers have few tools available to know how these activities have been performed, and therefore, they have minimal influence on them. Any realistic strategy for collecting information on the numerous variables of potential interest to a manager must carefully avoid excess precision. LQAS not only offers this attribute, but requires it.

The manager must choose the level of staff performance that defines adequate quality and the minimum level requiring a managerial response. For example, the manager may select 80% polio vaccination coverage as a standard of adequacy. He may choose 50% as the performance level at which managerial attention is a priority. This orientation is an intangible but important feature of LQAS.

LQAS's strength is also its limitation. With a small sample LQAS can be used to accurately detect the extremes of performance. In a health system with performance standards such as those described in the preceding paragraph, health workers who have reached or exceeded the upper performance threshold, 80%, are precisely identified so that resources are not unnecessarily invested in them. Conversely, health workers who reach or fall below the lower threshold, 50%, are identified so that attention can be given to these priority areas. However, this limitation is not particularly severe. This calibre of decision making is exactly what field managers require to maintain and improve their health systems. They need to know which communities are not at risk to health problems and which communities are at risk so that scarce resources can immediately be brought to ameliorate pernicious conditions in the latter without wasting them on the former.

The performance thresholds can be changed to suit local management needs. The following chapters use sample sizes ranging from 6 to 28 children and their mothers. They discuss how to choose a sample size and how to interpret the results. The mathematics of LQAS are also explained; I have taken precautions to eliminate technical language so that most readers can grasp the mechanics of LQAS despite having only an elementary understanding of statistics.

Most examples cited throughout this book concern the quality of care provided by paraprofessionals working at the community level. I selected this peripheral level of health care since it is the most difficult one to assess and provides the greatest logistical problems. Nevertheless, LQAS can be used to assess the quality of care provided by any health workers: physicians, nurses, hospital technicians, and the like. It can also be used to assess virtually any service including family planning and AIDS prevention interventions. However, before further technical discussion, the next section assesses the problems of managing public health programs in developing nations.

Defining Decentralized Service Delivery

National authorities of developing countries who are responsible for designing and implementing effective Primary Health Care programs typically subdivide the whole population into geographically defined communities. Whether they are large or small communities, every household in the country falls into the area of responsibility of at least one local health care unit. The exact type of health care unit may vary. A single hospital may serve several thousand people. A clinic or health center will generally serve an area with fewer people. Primary Care can be given to people who visit outpatient units where physicians, nurses, or technicians dispense a service, such as polio vaccination. Preventive services are often provided to people through outpatient units similar to hospitals. Moreover, health centers may sometimes be organized to reach out into the community to actively locate individuals at risk for health problems and to provide the preventive service.

In many developing countries, this latter active form of public health service delivery, is the foremost role of the most peripheral type of Primary Health Care unit, the Health Post or health area. The staff of that health unit, usually a community health worker (CHW) or auxiliary nurse, is responsible for identifying each household and its members within its defined area and for providing them with health care.

Table 1.1 Classification of Health Units by Active vs. Passive Health Care, Complex vs. Simple Services, and Specialized vs. General Health Problems

Health Unit	Active vs. Passive Health Care	Complex vs. Simple Services	Specialized vs. General Problems
Hospital	Completely passive to low level active	Very complex	General
Health Center	Low to moderately active	Moderately complex	Less general
Health Post	Moderately to highly active	Simple to moderately complex	Specialized

The various types of health units can be classified in three ways: active vs. passive; complex vs. simple, and specialized vs. general. The relationship of these dimensions with the types of health units is summarized in Table 1.1.

Hospital staff have very little direct active contact in their areas. This passive form of service is suited to a highly complex unit that provides tertiary, secondary, as well as primary care. The heath staff is presumably equipped to address a great many medical and public health problems.

A Health Center also tends to be passive in its service delivery, but often provides secondary and primary care only. Like a hospital, it is an organization whose health staff is trained to address a general set of medical and public health problems when clients present them. However, unlike hospitals, health centers refer clients with specific types of medical problems to other health units, namely, hospitals. Often they perform minor surgical procedures only, and no tertiary care. In some health systems the health center also has community outreach programs with a staff that contacts households in its catchment area.

A Health Post tends to be the most peripheral organizational unit of the health system. It generally is staffed by health workers trained to perform a very limited number of primary health care interventions and some highly focused treatment. These activities are associated with the leading causes of death and sickness. In many developing countries, a Health Post is highly active and, therefore, is responsible for reaching out into the community to identify high risk individuals and families, to deliver prevention service to them, and to treat specific diseases. On an occasional basis, this category of health worker also performs passive preventative and curative activities. Since a Health Post is highly specialized, it often serves as a referral facility to both health centers and hospitals.

These three categories of facilities, although broad, characterize many health systems in the developing world. A country may have additional levels of organization; however, for the purposes of this book, this simplified description of health systems will be sufficient.

The management principles discussed in this book are intended primarily for facilities responsible for providing universal primary health care in their community. These facilities will tend to be active rather than passive, simple rather than complex, and specialized rather than general. Throughout this volume, I will refer to this class of health facility as a local community health care unit or Health Post.

In order to reduce the rates of disease and death by inhibiting their specific causes or determinants, the staff of the local primary health care unit requires the following sets of information:

1. precise estimation of population sizes residing within each community served by the local public health facility and their stratification by sex, age, and marital status,

2. identification of the most serious, frequent, and preventable determinants of death and sickness prevalent in the client community,

3. definition of feasible procedures and specific plans to address these most serious, frequent, and preventable determinants, especially those among the individuals and families at highest risk of these conditions,

4. regular monitoring of services delivered within communities to ensure that interventions are implemented as planned and thus able to reduce health risks to communities,

5. diagnosis and amelioration of problems that reduce the efficacy of interventions,

6. impact assessment of interventions to determine whether they have achieved their intended effects and, therefore, should be replicated or adopted in other communities, provinces, or nations.

Although the health services research discussed in this volume is applicable to each of these activities, its main concern is to contribute to the fourth and fifth activities, namely, the monitoring and improvement of decentralized integrated health or Child Survival activities. Table 1.2 is a reference chart to help the reader determine how discussion in subsequent chapters can guide public health practitioners to the various aforementioned sets of information.

Primary health care programs are limited by the competence of the individuals planning and implementing them. Because these programs are administered within a health system, it is often difficult to determine whether or not individuals at each level of organization are performing their prescribed activities at an acceptable standard. Although problems reveal themselves within a health system either by poor outcomes or a low number and quality of services, the underlying causes of such problems are often a function of poor supervision, insufficient resources, improper education, and a high family/ health worker ratio. Hence, poor outcomes and inadequate service delivery within communities may often be a product of a series of other failures higher up in the health system that create a chain reaction which becomes evident locally in the actual service delivery. The relation between outcomes, outputs, and processes affecting the quality of services is discussed in detail in Chapter 2.

Table 1.2   A Reference Guide for this Volume

Information Sets	Primary Focus of this Volume	Secondary Focus	Not Considered in this Volume
1. Precise estimation of population sizes residing within defined communities ʹ served by public health facilities stratified by sex, age, and marital status.	Definition of community parameters (Chapter 5)	■ Principles of reliability and validity for data collection in LDC contexts (Chapter 3) ■ Procedures for developing a sampling frame (Chapter 5)	■ Stratification of populations by sex, age, and marital status
2. Analysis of the most serious, frequent, and preventable determinants of death and sickness prevalent in the client community.	Not applicable (Already determined by the epidemiologists of the National Primary Health Care Program for the cases considered in this book)	■ Procedures for developing Child Survival Programs (Chapter 2) ■ Principles of reliability and validity for data collection in LDC contexts (Chapter 3)	■ Identifying the biological and behavioral determinants of death and sicknesses ■ Performance of needs assessments within communities ■ Establishing and maintaining surveillance systems
3. Definition of feasible procedures and specific plans to address the most serious, frequent and preventable conditions.	Not applicable (Already determined by the Directors of the National Primary Health Care Program for the cases considered in this book)	■ Procedures for program development (Chapter 2) ■ Selection of appropriate approaches for program monitoring and evaluation (Chapter 2) ■ Principles for modeling programs (Chapter 3) ■ Principles of reliability and validity for data collection in LDC contexts (Chapter 3)	■ Performance of needs assessments within communities ■ Establishing and maintaining surveillance systems

Table 1.2   A Reference Guide for this Volume (continued)

Information Sets	Primary Focus of this Volume	Secondary Focus	Not Considered in this Volume
4. Regular monitoring of services delivered within communities to ensure that interventions are implemented as planned.	Chapters 2 through 9 in their entirety	Not applicable	Not applicable
5. Diagnosis and amelioration of problems reducing the efficacy of interventions.	Chapters 5 and 9 in their entirety	■ Conceptualization of potential approaches to diagnosis of implementation problems (Chapter 2) ■ Selection of appropriate approaches for program evaluation (Chapter 2) ■ Principles for modeling programs (Chapter 3) ■ Principles of reliability and validity for data collection in LDC contexts (Chapter 3)	Not applicable
6. Impact evaluation of interventions to determine whether they have achieved their intended effects and may be replicated in other locations.	Discussion of basic concepts and principles of program monitoring and evaluation (Chapters 2 and 3)	Not applicable	■ Program evaluation designs for evaluating health interventions

The failure or success of a health system is ultimately seen in the accuracy of the community diagnosis and in the coverage of local individuals and families with appropriate interventions by the staff of the health units directly responsible for specific communities. The health of people in communities is at risk when the performance of a health unit's staff is inadequate. Further, this risk is expected to persist regardless of the level of performance of any other health facility in the vicinity since the health care provided to people in one area is somewhat independent of the health care provided in any other one. Although the population of a community could use the health facilities in an area other than the one serving their own community, the chance of this happening is frequently small. People possess only partially the knowledge and understanding they need to judge the quality of the service they receive. Few are willing to bear the opportunity costs of traveling to other areas for health care.

The investigation of health services in communities by the staff of local health facilities is based on a simple assertion. When Child Survival interventions are provided at the community level, program managers must detect the communities in which implementation problems arise. Therefore, they need to assess the interventions at that level.

This assertion will become clearer through consideration of Figure 1.1, in which polio vaccination coverage in one block of 18 hypothetical health facilities is presented. If the average polio vaccination coverage among children under three years of age (80.3%) was assumed to be representative of service delivery throughout this hypothetical region, a program manager would conclude that coverage was acceptable, according to the arbitrary standard of 80% coverage. Nevertheless, as Figure 1.1 shows, coverage in three health unit areas fell below the 80% standard. Thus, the communities that lie within these three areas are at an unacceptable risk relative to the 80% standard due to the low vaccination coverage. The project administrator who can rapidly and accurately identify the substandard health units knows where to concentrate attention to improve coverage. Only by monitoring services at the lowest or

Figure 1.1 A Hypothetical Region with 18 Health Facilities of which Three Have Substandard Coverage*

90%	95%	35% Substandard	85%	95%	85%
85%	80%	90%	95%	30% Substandard	90%
80%	50% Substandard	85%	90%	90%	95%

*Average Coverage = 80.3%

most peripheral level of organization can the administrator know where to find the units with substandard coverage.

Coverage is more complicated than the above paragraphs suggest. As will be presented in Chapter 5, for some Child Survival interventions, "coverage" can be defined in a straightforward manner, while for others it is quite complex.

For example, coverage for an oral rehydration therapy program could be calculated as the proportion of mothers who adequately prepare the solution and administer it to their children when their symptoms so indicate.

However, the definition for measles vaccination coverage is not so obvious. Children should be vaccinated against measles, according to World Health Organization (WHO) norms, between nine and 11 months of age. Therefore, one measure of coverage could be the proportion of children vaccinated against measles in this age range. This proportion would inform a program manager whether CHWs were vaccinating children at the proper age. However, another appropriate measure of coverage is the proportion of children vaccinated regardless of their age. This measures children in a community currently susceptible to measles.

Various coverage measures will be discussed in Chapter 5 for several Child Survival interventions. Until that chapter, all references to coverage should be considered to use either of the definitions implied in the preceding paragraph.

Throughout this volume, I will refer to "Child Survival" and to "integrated health" interventions. The former term generally is used to refer to health programs with specialized health services delivered to communities, such as vaccinations and oral rehydration therapy. The latter term is used to refer to more comprehensive health service delivery consisting of the child survival interventions, plus a broad program of services, such as for older children and the elderly. I use the terms interchangeably because the methods and principles presented are intended for both types of programs.

Measurement Issues for Health Systems Managers

A national program director wants to know first whether or not services are being delivered adequately within each region to each regional population. Each regional director wants to know whether or not health services are being delivered adequately within each district. Each district director wants to know whether or not each primary health care unit is delivering services adequately to its client community.

The principles and methods investigated in this book will demonstrate how national, regional, and district program directors can acquire this knowledge rapidly at a cost that the society can afford.

Although it may seem logical to measure Primary Health Care coverage within local facilities, there are practical problems to overcome. One approach to measuring regional coverage is to estimate it from a single sample taken from households throughout the whole region. In Figure 1.1, a hypothetical region comprised 18 facilities. If the program director wished to measure coverage for each facility, then 18 samples would have to be taken, one from each facility. Hence, the cost of measuring coverage could increase potentially by 1800%, assuming no economy of scale in data collection. The work presented discusses Lot Quality Assurance Sampling (LQAS) as a rapid and potentially cost effective sampling method for determining whether the Primary Health Care coverage of community based health facilities is of adequate quality.

The mode of implementing community based primary health care units is recent, and often poorly understood. The earliest national health insurance scheme was instituted in Britain in 1911. This event provided the services of a general practitioner to every wage earner and self employed person in Britain earning less than £500 per year. By the 1940s, the idea of a national primary health care service was being explored in South Africa, Kenya, and India. Other nations developed their own versions that often attempted to provide simple curative and preventive services through a primary health center, often with outreach to subcenters. In the course of time, attempts have been made to incorporate various categorical programs into these primary health care systems. These include maternal and child health, nutrition, immunization, family planning, potable water supply, and sanitation. Some programs have been cross-sectoral, to interact with broader social and economic development issues, such as income generation.

In the early years of these programs, the program managers and their colleagues had more than enough to do to plan locations for health units, find and train staff, and to plan and supply the units to respond to the clinical problems brought into the health center by local patients. Finding trained staff to work in deprived rural and urban areas has always been, and still is, a major problem for program managers.

Neither program managers nor their staff were trained to identify each household or household member in the geographic area assigned to the health unit. But more recently some program directors, concerned to see that all households in their region or nation have been covered by health services, assert categorically that each health unit staff is to identify and reach every household and its members within their defined geographical jurisdiction. These households comprise the community for which the health unit undertakes responsibility. Primary health care practice when functioning in this mode can bear the description of being community based or community oriented.

The goal of an LQAS approach to program assessment, when applied to health units, is first and foremost to identify health units in which health service delivery is adequate and to distinguish them from units operating below a standard of coverage. The LQAS approach also makes it possible to identify coverage proportions within regions of whole nations with a precision not usually possible with conventional approaches.

The LQAS approach operates by determining the acceptability of coverage within the client community under the aegis of health care units. In the example given in Figure 1.1, the health service comprised 18 health units. The LQAS system provides the procedures for selecting a small random sample within each community selected for study and for interpreting the findings. It produces information that is applicable to the administrative needs of managers at all three levels of this health system: the nation, the region, and the community. Deciding what services to assess, what variables to measure, and what sampling procedures to use to collect the information is distinct from LQAS. However, deciding on each of the issues is essential for LQAS to be used. For issues of quality of care these measurement decisions are major issues that should not be confused with LQAS.

In conditions found in many developing countries, LQAS uses sample sizes no larger than 19 individuals for monitoring coverage of a community with a service; no more than six observations of a CHW are needed to control the quality of his service delivery technique. The data presented in this book are from the nation of Costa Rica. However, the techniques discussed in the following chapters are applicable in diverse nations throughout the developing world.

The findings from a comprehensive field test performed in Costa Rica are used to explain LQAS procedures. The project was developed from November 1985 to May 1986 through a collaborative effort of Harvard University, the Pan American Health Organization, and the Ministry of Health, and carried out from December 1987 through June 1990. Because the National Primary Health Care Program had already been in operation since 1972, the Directors of the Ministry of Health of Costa Rica decided that it was important to determine whether it was providing high quality services.

By describing the field test, this volume undertakes to explain six topics. Firstly, it discusses principles of management and measurement for managers of decentralized services. Secondly, it explains how LQAS may be used as a method to classify decentralized health facilities as either acceptable or below standard in their Primary Health Care coverage. Thirdly, it demonstrates how these same observations may be aggregated to produce statistics representing either a regional or a national level that are more precise than the current method in use by public health practitioners (Henderson and Sundaresan 1982). Fourthly, it presents a cost analysis for using LQAS in different country settings. Fifthly, it explains procedures for selecting optimal sample sizes for using LQAS. Sixthly, it proposes a framework to policy makers for national health system management that is feasible with regular use of LQAS.

Interventions Selected for Testing LQAS

As the field test of LQAS was organized in coordination with both the Director General of Health of the Ministry of Health of Costa Rica and the national representative of the Pan American Health Organization, the Primary Health Care interventions selected for assessment were identified jointly with them. The target population consisted of children designated by the Costa Rican Ministry of Health as the priority for Primary Health Care coverage, namely, children under three years of age and their mothers. The services studied included vaccination programs against polio, diphtheria/pertussis/tetanus (DPT), and measles; medical care of neonates and pregnant women; competency in the use of oral rehydration therapy (ORT); the recording in local health registries of vaccination dates, household composition, and of household visits by health workers; and growth monitoring.

Although the data concern Costa Rica, a main objective of this work is to explain how LQAS can be adapted to the conditions of other developing countries with more desperate conditions than those found in Costa Rica. This volume will try to advance this goal by investigating logistical, administrative, economic, and political requirements of LQAS to assess the quality of the services in the most peripheral units, or first level units, in the Primary Health Care system. In Costa Rica these are known as Health Areas. This health unit is identical to the Health Post. Although this latter term is used widely in the international public health community, the text refers to the peripheral health units in Costa Rica by their local organizational name, Health Area.

Many other nations throughout Latin America (e.g., Honduras, Bolivia, Ecuador, Guatemala, El Salvador, Peru, and Brazil) are now in the process of developing regular program monitoring and evaluation of their health care systems. Providing support for such initiatives requires us to learn from existing cases. The Costa Rican Primary Health Care system may be the best case from which to learn how to provide management support, and in which to field test LQAS.

Costa Rica has the longest enduring system of Health Areas and community registries in Latin America. Established in 1972 as part of the Rural Health Program, their 674 Health Areas contain recorded information about more than 330,000 families (Barrios, 1988). However, these data have yet to be analyzed either for programmatic or epidemiological implications. Moreover, the quality of their data has yet to be established. Due to its unique status of being the first to establish a community based health system, Costa Rica is a de facto "laboratory" for other nations. Thus, this book will synthesize certain aspects of the Costa Rican experience by identifying the characteristics of adequately functioning Health Areas which may then serve as a prototype for improving substandard Health Areas in Costa Rica, and for establishing norms for those planned by other nations throughout the world.

Since much of the later discussion requires a general understanding of how the Primary Health Care system is structured, a brief description is now presented. This discussion can also be read as the delineation of a system that is found throughout Latin America. Although some national Primary Health Care systems diverge substantially from it, the basic structure is found in many Latin American nations.

The Costa Rican Primary Health Care system, like many located throughout the world, is hierarchically organized. The Chief Executive Officer of the Ministry of Health is the Minister. However, his main function is as a health policy maker rather than as a manager of primary health care service delivery. The Minister is a political appointment whose tenure is limited to four years.

Day-to-day management of the health system is performed by the Director General of Health. The DG is an administrative appointee whose tenure extends beyond four years; in theory, this appointment is permanent. Although the DG is subordinate to the Minister, in practice, he is a very powerful actor in the Primary Health Care system since he and his colleagues determine the employment and the scope of work of workers at all levels of the Primary Health Care system.

Several departments within the Ministry support the Primary Health Care system such as the Departments of Nutrition, Maternal and Child Health, Immunizations, Malaria, and Water and Sanitation. These units perform two functions: firstly, they formulate a series of operational norms or standards by which the Primary Health Care system functions, and secondly, they ensure that required resources are available. Although these departments provide policy and logistical support, they are not responsible for the actual service delivery. This activity is performed by the Department of Primary Health Care through three subordinate levels of organization: regional offices, Health Centers, and Health Areas. Although these units perform functions other than Primary Health Care, the remaining discussion focuses on their functions only to the extent that they are related to the Primary Health Care system.

Five additional service delivery entities perform primary health care services in addition to Health Centers and Health Areas, although none of them are under the aegis of the Department of Primary Health Care. These include: 513 nutrition centers (Centro de Educación y Nutrición) that provide nutritional supplements; 45 other nutrition centers that also monitor growth and development, and provide programs to ensure motor skill development of children (Centro Infantil de Nutrición y Atención Integral); 49 mobile medical units in which a physician visits Health Areas twice a month for outpatient treatment; 55 mobile dental units that perform a similar function; and 60 mobile dental units that travel to schools for service delivery.

The second level of organization consists of regional offices. The nation is divided into six health regions: Central Sur, Central Norte, Huetar Atlántica, Huetar Norte, Brunca, and Chorotega. Each regional office is administered by a Regional Director who is a public health physician. Yet, as the Regional Director is responsible for numerous health affairs in his region in addition to ensuring that the Primary Health Care system is functioning, the subordinate post of Regional Supervisor, Primary Health Care, was established for day-to-day management of Primary Health Care. His role will be clarified momentarily after a brief description of the rest of the Primary Health Care system.

The third level of the organization consists of outpatient clinics called Health Centers. The principal actors in the Primary Health Care system at this level are chief nurses and local supervisors. The former are supposed to ensure that services are delivered by their subordinates (i.e., health assistants and auxiliary nurses) at a fourth level of organization according to ministerial norms. For example, a chief nurse should observe whether vaccinations are given to children within the prescribed age range and whether hygiene is adequate. A local supervisor monitors the technical quality of equipment and facilities necessary for Primary Health Care delivery. For example, they determine whether the cold chain is in operation and whether pharmaceuticals are amply supplied. Although the supervision is structured with supervisory responsibilities split between two actors, in practice, local supervisors perform both sets of tasks (Valadez et al. 1990).

The fourth level of the Primary Health Care system is the first level of client care. It consists of Health Areas in which auxiliary nurses and/or health assistants perform the actual Primary Health Care services of the health system. In many parts of Latin America, as well as the rest of the world, this level is referred to as the Health Post or Health Area. Until 1987, Health Posts were associated with Rural Health, and Health Areas were associated with Community Health. Although both Health Posts and Health Areas are now formally referred to as Health Areas, we will hold the earlier distinction for a moment to clarify the differences between them since these details are relevant to this study.

The Health Posts in rural areas usually stand alone in a single building generally consisting of a waiting room, an examination room, a small office with a desk and a file cabinet, a small pharmacy, storage space, and a toilet. Primary Health Care service delivery in Health Posts is the function of health assistants. One of these staff members is responsible for the work among about 500 families. If the number of families substantially exceeds 500, an auxiliary nurse is assigned to complement the work of the health assistant. In such cases the auxiliary has decision making authority.

Health assistants and auxiliary nurses are the main actors in the delivery of Primary Health Care at the first level of operations. The former receive approximately four and a half months of training and are not licensed; the latter receive nine months and are licensed. Health Posts with both an assistant and an auxiliary have a slightly different form of organization from those in which an assistant works alone. Health assistants normally visit households four days a week. Auxiliaries visit households three days a week. The remaining weekdays of both functionaries are spent at the Health Post in an outpatient clinic. Since auxiliaries spend more days in the Health Post, the families for which they are responsible are located closer to the Health Post than those of the assistant.

Health assistants and auxiliary nurses are responsible for visiting every household in their area once every three or four months in order to deliver a spectrum of Primary Health Care services including health education. Although they attend all homes, infants under one year of age are their priority. Indeed, they are supposed to ensure that infants complete their basic regimen of three polio vaccinations, three DPT vaccinations, and one measles vaccination within the first year of life. Since polio and DPT are prescribed by the Ministry of Health to be administered at two month intervals, health workers must return to the homes of these infants sooner than the normal visit of every three or four months to ensure that they are vaccinated on schedule.

Household members need not wait for the health worker's regular visit in order to obtain health care. They may visit the Health Post whenever they want; they also have the option of visiting the Health Center to request services.

Health workers also have management responsibility in the Health Post. They keep a running record of all services provided, maintain the vaccination cold chain, and order medical goods should the normal shipments provided by the supervisor be insufficient.

The staff of Health Areas in the urban Community Health Program are located in Health Centers and are also attended by health assistants and auxiliaries. Several Health Areas can be physically placed in the same Health Center although one health assistant or auxiliary is assigned to each Health Area. Although Health Areas in the urban community health program share one facility, each Health Area has responsibilities that are identical to those of its counterpart in the rural health program. Most important is the fact that each Health Area is responsible for a community that does not overlap the jurisdiction of any other Health Area.

Costa Rica has made great progress in improving its national health (Gonzalez-Vega 1985). Most of these achievements started with the implementation of the Rural Health Program in 1972, which initiated the extended program in primary care. In 1987, the program was thought to cover about 95% of the low income people. One finding of this study is that only 72% of the population is covered by the health system — nevertheless, an impressive achievement. From 1970 to 1983 the national infant mortality rate declined from more than 68.0 to less than 18.6 infant deaths per 1000 live births. Some of this reported reduction was due to reduced neonatal mortality, but a substantially greater proportion is accounted for by lower mortality among infants between one month and one year of age (Ferrero and Boada-Martinez 1985). During this same period, the incidence of many major infections declined and the marital fertility rate also declined (Sáenz 1985). At face value, health in Costa Rica appears to be continually improving. But such may not be the case for all subpopulations.

Costa Rica was the ideal nation in which to develop quality control methods for Primary Health Care and to formulate recommendations for other nations. The main reasons are that it has the greatest backlog of experience, a successful record in improving health, and a national and local political system supportive of improving Primary Health Care. At the same time, it has many of the characteristics of other developing nations: large periurban areas, poverty, dispersed rural populations, and difficult logistical conditions.

This book sets out to accomplish several specific objectives. Firstly, it will demonstrate the use of LQAS to assess the quality of Primary Health Care delivery in 60 randomly selected peripheral health units or Health Areas. An

LQA sample of 28 children and their mothers is used. Achieving this objective leads to the identification of training, logistical and information management procedures, and their costs. This set of information is expected to aid Costa Rica and other nations to decide whether LQAS is a feasible method for Primary Health Care quality control. Chapters 5-8 will inform the reader how to perform various assessments of integrated health services, such as classifying Health Areas as either adequate or inadequate for the following services: polio vaccination series, DPT vaccination series, measles vaccinations, visits by pregnant women to clinics, medical visits by neonates to clinics, competency of mothers and others undertaking child care in the use of oral rehydration therapy, visits to households by Health Area staff, and maintenance of the health information system. Chapter sections will identify problems in organizing a sampling frame for the LQA sample. Other sections present a critical review of training procedures for data collectors and for health care administrators interpreting and using LQAS results. Additional analyses concern problems encountered when collecting LQAS data within Health Areas and their communities. Such analyses may help other users anticipate and resolve problems when implementing the method.

A second objective is to identify in Chapters 4-7 optimal LQA sample sizes both for Costa Rica and for a hypothetical developing nation with a less developed primary health care system.

Thirdly, the book explains how to adapt LQAS for assessing the Primary Health Care technique of CHWs. Chapter 6 demonstrates how a regular supervision system was developed and implemented in the Costa Rican Primary Health Care system. Numerous methodological changes resulted when LQAS was adopted for supervision. One interesting finding was that the sample size was reduced from 28 to six observations.

A fourth objective is to demonstrate in Chapter 8 how the use of rapid program assessment methodologies facilitates management decision making at the local level and implies a more precise and specific bureaucratic role for the central office of the Ministry of Health.

The findings presented in the following chapters may lead the reader to judge LQAS as a method widely applicable to monitoring a variety of health care services.

This book is divided into two parts: I. Principles for Health Program Assessment, and II. Lot Quality Assurance Sampling for Monitoring International Health Programs.

Although the motivation for this book is to present the concepts, design, and field test results of applying LQAS in Costa Rica, it seemed necessary to place the discussion within the broader context of program monitoring and evaluation. The reasons for including Part I are as follows:

Firstly, the development of LQAS contributes to the formation of one small portion of a monitoring and evaluation algorithm. It is used to screen a Primary

Health Care facility using very small samples to determine whether it is providing adequate health services to the community for which it is responsible. However, program monitoring and evaluation involve more activities than screening health facilities for their adequacy. Part I indicates the broader spectrum of management issues that need to be considered when monitoring and evaluating international health programs. Part II shows how LQAS addresses some of those issues.

Secondly, although most of the concepts presented in Part I are not new, they have heretofore been discussed in United States and industrialized nation contexts only. Hence, issues concerning threats to valid inference have remained inaccessible to international public health researchers and practitioners. A strong motivation for including this section was to fill this literary void.

Thirdly, as already mentioned, the methodological concepts in Part I should indicate the types of precautions that need to be considered when collecting field data. Although not all of these precautions were pertinent to the LQAS data collection, as will become clear from a comparison of the two Parts, it would have been incorrect to discuss in Part I only those issues that were pertinent to LQAS data collection in Costa Rica. A field researcher or practitioner should consider the entire compendium of threats to validity since it is difficult to anticipate all those which will be encountered in any particular field situation.

Implementing international health programs can be likened to building a medieval castle, since the end product is not necessarily what was envisaged when construction began. The process of implementing a project uncovers problems and other considerations that determine the final product. Just like a castle that was built with two towers rather than the one that was originally planned, international programs can change substantially after they are implemented. For example, Chapter 5 discusses how 100 maps had to be updated by the project staff when we learned that the Costa Rican maps based on the 1984 census had not been fully updated by 1987, the time the work commenced. More than one month was required to update the maps in order to ensure an adequate sampling frame. This activity required employing a map maker who, with an assistant, reconnoitered all of the regions under study.

The result of including discussions of the methodological principles and LQAS theory and applications is a book that describes basic health program assessment principles (Part I) applicable to a broad range of field investigations, and a volume that explains a specific methodology, LQAS (Part II).

I should point out an important limitation of this book. Because it is confined to systems of monitoring and evaluation, it does not discuss in any depth the role of surveillance, needs assessment, or other information systems required in community public health. Such a discussion is beyond our scope, since surveillance and needs assessment systems can also operate outside the implementation of a top-down Primary Health Care system. For example, a public health practitioner could establish a surveillance system to identify the most serious, frequent, and preventable causes of death within a community. The plan for performing that investigation may involve establishing a scheme for routinely visiting all houses within a catchment area, systematically collecting health data, entering those data into a database, analyzing the local epidemiology, reporting the results to the community and to health administrators, and then planning appropriate prevention and treatment programs.

This book will not discuss those procedures except in those circumstances when such discussion does not distract from our main focus. Nevertheless, the principles presented in both Parts I and II could be applied to determine whether the surveillance system was operating correctly, and whether the information eventually collected was an accurate reflection of the conditions and operations within the community. ✧

Part I

Principles for Health Program Assessment

2

The Role of Program Assessment in Integrated Health Programs

This chapter discusses fundamental health program components and management activities, and demonstrates to health policy-makers and managers how LQAS can be used to collect information relevant to a few selected management principles. LQAS is presented as a monitoring tool to determine whether resources have been delivered to an adequate proportion of a client population with an appropriate level of quality.

For readers who are not interested in a review of management principles and of established approaches to monitoring and evaluation, please skip Part I completely. Continue with Chapter 4, which presents an in-depth discussion of LQAS statistical concepts written for a nonstatistician audience. Chapters 4 through 6 will also inform readers how to apply LQAS and interpret results.

Defining Monitoring and Evaluation Activities

The increased growth in size and complexity of international health programs has been accompanied by an increased demand for information on a program's performance. Typically this demand can be summarized under two broad headings: monitoring and evaluation. These headings may seem rather vague at first glance since both terms have been defined differently by many authors. I do not want to add to the confusion; the two concepts should be defined so that they are mutually exclusive and useful to health system managers. Historical reasons, usually program specific, may explain why such diverse concepts evolved.

Rather than critically overview each stream of thought, the most prominent approaches to monitoring and evaluation are synthesized under the two main headings. Later discussion presents in considerable detail distinctions between monitoring and evaluation. As introduction, monitoring determines whether a program has been implemented as planned, and evaluation measures its results.

In spite of their separate objectives these two activities are intimately related, both conceptually and operationally. LQAS is an approach to health system monitoring.

Although many international organizations like the World Bank, the World Health Organization, and the Agency for International Development (Casley and Lury 1982; Casley and Kumar 1987) have increased substantially the number of programs in which systematic monitoring and evaluation are required from their own staff or national counterparts, there continues to be a debate over what activities actually constitute monitoring or evaluation. One of the goals of this chapter is to try to define in precise terms the activities that should be performed and their basic principles. By so doing, Part II, concerning LQAS, will be understood as being pertinent to monitoring, rather than evaluation.

It is not coincidence that the value of monitoring and evaluation has been recognized during a period characterized by (a) increasing resource scarcity and high costs of health programs, (b) the realization by managers and policy makers that many health facilities either have not achieved their goals or have been unable to determine whether or not they have accomplished them, (c) increasing complexity of public health programs, (d) inability to assess the quality of programs or to determine whether they have been implemented as planned, (e) the need to know whether to replicate existing programs and generalize them to another context or to replace them with alternative programs, and (f) cost management.

The demand for program assessment came initially from national and international funding agencies requiring accountability. Now, others have promoted it too. Health specialists have long been interested in knowing the impacts of their programs on the reduction of morbidity or mortality on their client populations. Although in public health, epidemiologists have tended to embrace this role of health program manager, the principles presented in this book will not be found in traditional epidemiological texts (MacMahon and Pugh 1970).

Although monitoring and evaluation are valued by international public health administrators, there is not always agreement on what these activities actually mean. The following sections attempt to identify basic principles of public health program monitoring and evaluation. Although inevitably this list will be deficient and not address everyone's needs, the efforts will serve their purposes if enough material is provided for readers to apply to their own situations.

Although the concepts of monitoring and evaluation are often used interchangeably, each has different goals and requires a different data set. The purpose of *monitoring* is to determine whether health systems activities have been implemented as planned. In short, monitoring involves tracking whether resources are being mobilized as planned, and services are being delivered or products produced on schedule. The former we refer to as *input monitoring* and the latter as *output monitoring*.

Input monitoring of financial resources is very important in international public health programs since loans or grants that have been previously promised may be withdrawn or withheld due to unforeseen political decisions. Monitoring human and material resources is equally important since programs often require recruiting persons with certain specializations or procuring goods that are difficult to obtain. In some countries it is also assumed that money or labor will be obtained from the community, or that matching grants or loans will be obtained from other donors; these also need to be monitored. Thus, monitoring systems measure whether requisitioned resources are available for program activities, used in the expected quantities and at the expected intervals, and whether required activities are being performed as planned.

Output monitoring is important since continuation of funds is often contingent on having delivered a certain number of services (e.g., vaccinations, oral rehydration salt [ORS] envelopes, maternal education sessions) or produced a certain number of products (e.g., trained health workers, educational guides, latrines, water systems).

In more formal terms, *monitoring* is:

A management activity designed to provide ongoing feedback on the quality and progress of a health service delivery, and to identify the problems CHWs are facing during service delivery. Monitoring consists of operational and administrative activities that track resource acquisition and allocation, production or delivery of services, and costs.

Lot Quality Assurance Sampling is an instrument that can be used for input and output monitoring. In Chapter 6 the use of LQAS for input monitoring will be shown by assessing, for example, the availability of vaccines in Health Areas and the accuracy of CHWs' and their supervisors' knowledge of vaccination norms. Chapter 6 also demonstrates the use of LQAS for a particular type of output monitoring, namely, assessment of the quality of CHWs' technical skills in performing an intervention. Chapter 5 discusses LQAS's application for another type of output monitoring, namely, determining whether coverage in target communities of an integrated health program is adequate.

The purpose of *evaluation* is to measure the results of a health intervention, namely, whether the objectives have been achieved; whether it has produced other, additional impacts; the costs per program benefit or per program product; and diagnosis of problems that led either to inadequate implementation of interventions, or to the failure of achieving objectives. In formal terms *evaluation* is defined as:

An assessment of a health program's results, including the extent to which it is achieving or has achieved its objectives, whether associated costs are appropriate, and the underlying causes of problems detected through the monitoring.

Although evaluation analyses are directed toward judging the value of a specific intervention, the conclusions should also aid health system administrators to decide whether an intervention can be used in the design or selection of future programs most likely to reach certain objectives.

Evaluations can be summarized in three categories: impacts, costs, and processes. Only the first and third are considered here.

Impact evaluation, which is sometimes referred to as *summative* evaluation, is conducted to determine whether predicted objectives were achieved, and to identify what unexpected effects occurred.

For example, a primary health care program focusing on delivery of, say, immunizations to at least 80% of the population may expect to reduce the incidence of a targeted disease such as polio or measles. A perinatal maternal and child health program may expect to reduce both maternal and infant mortality rates. An impact assessment would measure whether each of these expectations was achieved.

Yet, unexpected effects could also occur. For example, other health indicators may improve, such as a reduction in the prevalence of third degree malnutrition. An impact evaluation would try to determine whether or not this outcome should be attributed to the primary health care intervention of interest.

Process evaluations assess trends of impacts, diagnose program problems, and identify other factors exogenous to the program that could have a bearing on either the program implementation or its impact. Impact measures can also be taken prior to the time when a program's objectives are not yet achieved. Process measures track the trend toward the expected impact while a program is still underway. Consider the example of a regional health director who expects that the infant mortality rate will decrease by 20% over a four year period as a function of a new decentralized health system. Although reaching this objective would not be expected prior to four years, the trend in improvement could be charted by measuring infant mortality at regular intervals during that four year period. By so doing, the regional director can detect whether milestones in IMR reduction are being reached at anticipated intervals. If milestones were not being reached, then health system managers could attempt to identify planning deficiencies or implementation problems that are impeding the program.

As implied above, in addition to tracking trends, process evaluations also identify and ameliorate unanticipated problems that could impede a program from reaching its objectives. This type of process evaluation is used when managers detect programmatic problems, such as when sufficient resources are not available or milestones are not reached. The main focus of such an investigation is diagnostic, namely, to identify the underlying causes of the problem. Such problems may be due to a breakdown in the provision of resources, or due to poor worker-employer relations which delay the implementation of the program.

A third category of program assessment, also referred to as process evaluation, is sometimes used interchangeably with the term *formative evaluation*. In the evaluation literature formative evaluation has been defined as a study that identifies existing needs within a community. Hence, a formative evaluation is synonymous with what some program planners call a needs assessment and some public health practitioners call an epidemiologic diagnosis. For example, social marketing experts may perform a survey to determine local preferences for a media campaign promoting the use of oral rehydration therapy or needs that they can then take into consideration to guide their design of the delivery of the public health services to identify and address the most serious, frequent, and preventable causes of death or morbidity.

In summary, six categories of monitoring and evaluation have been identified thus far: input monitoring of resources and material, output monitoring of the quantity and quality of service, impact evaluation of expected and unexpected results, process evaluation of expected trends, process evaluations that are primarily diagnostic, and process evaluations that are needs assessments. LQAS can be used for performing input monitoring and output monitoring.

Management Systems for Program Assessments

At the present time, many developing countries (with the encouragement of international agencies) emphasize monitoring activities. For example, managers of the Expanded Program in Immunization of the World Health Organization invest substantial resources into measuring immunizational coverage. Although public health officials would admit that they are ultimately interested in the subsequent impacts of immunization programs (i.e., the reduction of diseases and associated morbidity and mortality), many practitioners recognize that impact assessments are time consuming and complicated to perform since it is difficult to separate impacts attributable to immunization from those attributable to other health activities and regional development programs (e.g., housing, water, and sanitation).

Monitoring has been emphasized by donor institutions over evaluation. A contributing factor to this tendency is the general lack of trained personnel in developing countries for performing longitudinal studies, and to the incentive structure of international and national institutions for introducing priority national programs rather than assessing their long term impacts. Hence, planning, promotion, training, construction of facilities, and logistics have been the first orders of business. Although there is a certain logic underlying this orientation, serious implications arise as a result of giving substantially less attention to assessments of program impact. Without impact evaluation, scarce resources (including time and capital) may be invested in ineffective programs.

By contrast, the developed countries have invested in impact evaluation. This emphasis may be a function of their developed infrastructure that gives them the capability to note changes to the societal landscape. In developing nations the priority has been to generate programs addressing the perceived problems; planning and implementing them has absorbed the energies of almost all capable and sufficiently educated people.

In much of the evaluation literature, the distinction between monitoring and evaluation is either vague, nonexistent, or confused. The main purpose of the definitions of monitoring and evaluation used in this chapter is to convey clear meanings. Therefore, by being clear and precise, this book is intended to encourage and help practitioners organize their own monitoring and evaluation systems, and to communicate with each other effectively.

Monitoring and evaluation can be conducted at three levels. Firstly, at the community level, monitoring and evaluation are carried out by local managers directly responsible for ensuring service delivery by CHWs to individuals and families in small communities. Secondly, at the sectorial level (e.g., a region, a province), middle managers perform the assessments; their goals are to ensure uniform performance throughout the sector, to identify areas (e.g., districts) needing greater attention, and to determine overall impact (e.g., the impact on reducing a disease specific mortality) within the sector. Thirdly, at the national level, evaluations are concerned with the overall quality and impact of health facilities on the appropriate national indicators. Such assessments are particularly useful for refining national policies.

The following section presents main principles for program assessment and highlights some of the major issues in the selection and implementation of assessment strategies.

Program assessments should provide information needed by planners, implementors, and managers to determine whether or not a program has been implemented as planned, what problems need to be resolved, and what have been the expected or unexpected impacts on the communities affected by the intervention. For this reason, the best way to classify the different types of

Figure 2.1 A Simplified Program Development Cycle

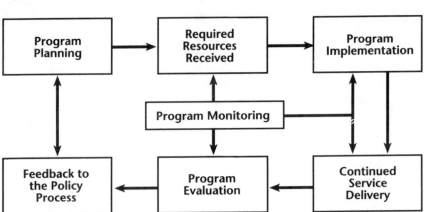

Table 2.1 An Elaborated Program Management Cycle

Program Stage	Monitoring Activity	Evaluation	Result
1. Program Planning	Determine whether all program subsystems have been formulated based on clear and explicit objectives and program interventions	Set program goals and objectives and have all interested parties review them	Develop comprehensive program and budget
2. Acquisition of Required Resources	Determine whether financing, personnel, office space, equipment, supplies, permissions, and contracts are available or will be available at appropriate intervals	Identify and resolve underlying problems impeding resource acquisition	Invest capital, sign contracts, commit to commence, terminate or continue the program
3. Program Implementation	Determine the following: ■ all program subsystems have begun as planned ■ all scheduled interactions of personnel are occurring ■ all interventions between CHWs and the target population or support institutions are occurring ■ all outputs are delivered in expected quantities and with expected quality ■ required resources continue to arrive at planned intervals and in adequate amounts	Identify and diagnose underlying problems in implementation	■ Redesign program ■ improve management ■ negotiate with problematic participants ■ change program personnel ■ alter the funding schedule ■ continue program service delivery as planned
4. Continued Service Delivery	Determine the following: ■ all program subsystems are functioning properly ■ (bullets 2 through 5 above)	Diagnose underlying problems in service delivery	(Bullets 1 through 6 above)

Table 2.1 An Elaborated Program Management Cycle (continued)

Program Stage	Monitoring Activity	Evaluation	Result
5. Program Evaluation	Ensure that data necessary for assessing all program indicators are being or have been collected	■ Determine whether impacts reach specified objectives ■ explain failures to achieve objectives ■ identify unexpected impacts ■ assess sustainability of program and of impacts ■ determine accountability	■ Redesign program for continued operation ■ continue program unaltered ■ halt program activities ■ write program report
6. Feedback to the Policy Process	■ Ensure that all appropriate institutions receive expected results ■ solicit comments from appropriate institutions	Assess comments from participating institutions at all levels of organization from national and international to local, for information leading to improved understanding of program deficiencies and unexpected impacts	■ Continue self sustained program ■ identify new objectives ■ replicate program ■ abandon program

evaluation methodologies is to relate them to typical information needs at different stages in the program management cycle.

Once the policy makers have accepted a health program in principle, it generally proceeds through six distinct stages: planning; obtaining required inputs (e.g., financial, technical, materials, and other resources); implementation; continued delivery of the planned intervention; evaluation of the impact on the target population and its environment; and feedback of these results into the policy process. Following this sixth stage the cycle can begin again if the program is to be continued, replicated, or altered according to criteria based on the assessment results (see Figure 2.1).

The management cycle is much more complex than this simple graphic. There are interactions among each of the stages of the cycle resulting from, among other things, the monitoring and evaluation that take place at each stage. Refer to Table 2.1 for a more comprehensive treatment of the program design cycle.

Each stage in the development cycle requires the collection of specialized planning, monitoring, and/or evaluation data. Studies typical of what is required at each of these stages are now discussed.

At the **planning stage** four activities are performed. Firstly, the practitioner collects information to define the boundary and characteristics of individuals who will form the target community; this task defines the denominator in calculations of rates and proportions. Secondly, the condition the health service is intended to resolve or diminish is identified; this task constitutes the goal. Thirdly, the program's objectives are formulated; these are explicit quantitative endpoints to reach. And fourthly, additional information is collected for formulating the program design that is supposed to produce the desired change in the target community. Any program, whether explicitly stated or not, embraces assumptions about the ways in which the target community will respond to it, the relative efficacy of different implementation methods, and the ways in which the health system is likely to affect and be affected by the social, economic, and political environment within which it operates. These assumptions can be based on theories, hunches, and previous experiences about how problems developed and can either be eliminated or prevented (Kaplan 1963).

The essential planning concepts include the *model, goals,* and *objectives*. A *model* is a planned intervention based on explicit theories of the determinants of specific health problems and how to ameliorate them. A model of a health program should make explicit what activities need to be carried out, their duration, and specific time intervals in which impacts should occur and what resources to invest. Therefore, a program model incorporates a testable hypothesis that when implemented can be either refuted or vindicated.

Goals are broadly stated changes to which a program is expected to contribute. For example, a goal of the Pan American Health Organization has been to eradicate polio from the Western Hemisphere by 1991. *Objectives* are the magnitude of an impact expected from a program expressed in quantitative terms. In the above example, a PAHO objective would be to vaccinate with 3 doses of polio 80% of all children in Haiti during their first year of life. Monitoring activities at this stage ensure that objectives are explicitly formulated and that all key program subsystems and their associated budgets have been formulated.

The second stage of the management process involves *obtaining resources* to support program activities. In this context another basic term is introduced:

Inputs: The resources required to implement a program as planned.

Although this definition is simple, it is not trivial. Managers are responsible for ensuring that all financial resources, personnel, and material are available at required quantities to place into operation the model that has been planned. In order for managers to perform this task, all inputs must be explicitly stated irrespective of whether they are individuals, vehicles, money, office space, energy, printed material, or resources.

The program input monitoring system should determine whether personnel and material are either available as planned or are due to arrive according to schedule.

Input Monitoring System: A set of procedures that checks whether the necessary resources are available or on schedule, thus making program implementation possible.

The third step of the management cycle involves program **implementation**. Once the required resources are available, interventions can commence. Typically, health workers are trained to perform a set of activities or to furnish a set of products; together they comprise the *outputs*.

Outputs: The services or products that a health worker delivers to a target community that are intended to produce the expected impact.

Perhaps the best way to understand the concept of output is through examples. In an integrated health program the following are outputs. Vaccinations of children under three years against polio are outputs of the Expanded Programme on Immunization (EPI). Mothers correctly preparing and administering ORT are outputs of the Control of Diarrheal Disease (CDD) program. Trained CHWs reliably collecting and recording epidemiological and health service information are outputs of the program information system component. Educational sessions for women about perinatal care are outputs of the Maternal and Child Health (MCH) of the program. Health workers plotting the growth and development of children in the community also are outputs of the MCH component.

Monitoring implementation includes five activities (see Table 2.1). Firstly, it ensures that all program subsystems have commenced (e.g., training, procurement, logistical systems, and service delivery are in operation).

Secondly, it determines whether interaction between personnel or subsystems is occurring. For example, planning groups should often include participation of personnel from different locations in the health system. In an integrated health program such interactions may involve experts in maternal and child health, the EPI, diarrheal disease control, health worker training, distance education, social marketing, epidemiology, and information systems.

Thirdly, programs often require interaction with the target community they are intended to benefit. In the case of planning an integrated health program, participants could include political leaders, teachers, local health care producers, women's and men's groups representatives, church leaders, and elected neighborhood representatives (Valadez 1985b). Hence, local leaders need to be contacted and community meetings organized. In some cases leaflets or posters should precede meetings that briefly explain the program goals and the community's role in achieving them.

Fourthly, monitoring detects whether the outputs are actually being delivered to the targeted individuals in the community and at an adequate quality. In the example of an immunization program, monitoring determines whether an expected proportion of children is being vaccinated on time. This monitoring activity was one motivation for developing LQAS.

Fifthly, although all interventions are operating, they may come to an abrupt halt if resources fail to be supplemented as scheduled. Monitoring should ensure that managers are looking forward to subsequent stages of the program management cycle and that preparations have been made to obtain resources as they become needed.

Assessment activities at this stage are primarily diagnostic. Should the monitoring system detect problems in any of the preceding five areas, managers investigate for their underlying causes and provide suggestions for their resolution. In terms of the concepts used throughout this book, this form of assessment is a *process evaluation*.

The fourth step in the management cycle is *operation and maintenance*. Once health interventions are in operation, the monitoring system ensures that necessary resources arrive as scheduled and that planned activities are performed, as discussed under "program implementation." Special emphasis is given to determining whether outputs are being produced at expected quantities, such as through comparing the number of outputs with predetermined quotas. In other words, the monitoring system must comparatively assess the quantity and quality of services and products relative to the expectations previously defined in the program plan. Such monitoring identifies the volume and speed of delivery and production.

Managers continue with problem diagnosis as in the preceding section. In addition, they perform a second type of process evaluation, namely, measurement of the trends of impacts. Although health programs will not reach their objectives early in the implementation process, they are generally expected to have an early impact on a target population, even if it is slight.

Both types of process evaluation (i.e., diagnosis of outputs and trend analysis of outcomes) are mutually supportive. Diagnosis of, say, low production of outputs may eventually focus on activities critical to a program's performance although they may not be explicit in the implementation plan. For example, worker relations and worker-manager relations are, in part, a function of the styles and personalities of the people involved. Low production of outputs or impacts may be due to labor relation problems.

Both monitoring and evaluation involve assessing processes. Hence, both perspectives are included in the following definition.

Process: A measure indicating (1) whether the number of services delivered and the products provided are at expected levels, e.g., predetermined production quotas are reached, or (2) problematic components of the health system that lead to inadequate outputs or impacts.

The fifth component of the management cycle is *assessing results*. Such evaluations can take place at micro and macro levels. Chapter 8 discusses LQAS information for use at both levels. This fifth component involves micro level evaluations.

Once program interventions are being implemented, the quota of inputs has been used, and the outputs have been delivered, their results can be evaluated. These include the actual costs associated with service delivery or production, and impacts on the client or target group.

Impacts are sometimes referred to as *outcomes*. I try to use the term "impacts" only, since some audiences confuse "outputs" with "outcomes." The distinction between output and impact should be clearly understood. Programs are planned to deliver services or produce products, with the expectation that doing so will produce changes in the population. These expectations are based on the theories and assumptions upon which the original program model is based. For example, a maternal immunization program vaccinates pregnant women to prevent tetanus in their newborns as well as themselves. The output is vaccination of pregnant women; the outcome or impact is a reduced neonatal and maternal mortality attributable to tetanus.

In assessing impact the manager determines whether or not program objectives have been reached, and if they were not, the reasons for such failure. This activity involves not only measuring whether or not expected changes occurred in the target population but also determining whether such changes should be attributed to the interventions or to other extraneous factors.

Impact or Outcome: The expected effect of a program on a target population.

The distinction between monitoring and evaluation should now be clear. Monitoring assesses whether inputs, outputs, and processes are in place as planned so that the observer can conclude whether or not the interventions have been implemented as planned. Subsequently, it is possible to measure whether the program has achieved the expected impact. This second measure is obtained as part of an evaluation. These processes are charted in Figure 2.2.

Impact Evaluation: Assessing whether expected program impacts have occurred and can justifiably be attributed to the interventions or to extraneous factors.

In strict terms, evaluation cannot really take place until the monitoring is completed. One must know whether interventions have been adequately implemented before their impacts can be assessed. Managers should not assume that the program was executed as planned. Activities, resources, personnel and goals may have been consciously or unconsciously added or deleted.

I emphasize this point for a practical reason. Often an evaluation is performed to determine whether or not to recommend a program as a prototype for other locations or to terminate it. In each case, managers must be sure to identify the program model and its goals.

A microeconomic analysis can also be performed at this stage of a program, for example, charting the progress of a program in relation to the disbursement

Figure 2.2 Relation of Inputs, Outputs and Results

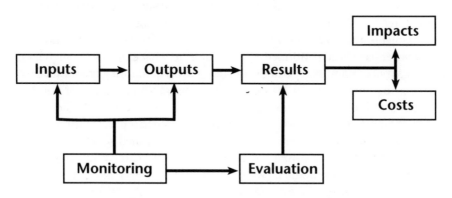

of funds so as to determine whether the program will be able to provide all planned services within the approved budget. This is an obvious but frequently overlooked point, since financial analysis and the above types of monitoring are often conducted independently of each other.

Other forms of assessment at this stage of the management cycle involve determining the efficiency with which inputs and outputs are being delivered. Efficiency could be defined in terms of:

1. costs per unit of output (i.e., cost-effectiveness),

2. speed of delivery of inputs and outputs,

3. quality of the program's services and products,

4. duration of interventions,

5. the accessibility of interventions to the target population, and

6. the types of problems which arise and proposed solutions.

The sixth and final step in the program management cycle consists of *evaluating impacts at a macro level.* Policy makers also need to understand the overall impacts of health services on the target population and their communities, but in different terms from those of local managers. For example, they may need to assess the impact of a single intervention on diminishing a national problem. In many cases, the potential impacts at the macro level (i.e., on families of all income levels) will be less than those observed in specific communities.

In macro analyses a manager may also want to assess questions of scale. For example, if a program was implemented in an area several times larger than in a prototype, the impact might be proportionately less since it may not be possible to hire a sufficient number of workers who are as competent or as motivated as in the prototype. Hence, a policy maker may need to anticipate whether resource expenditures should vary across target sites and, indeed, whether candidate sites should exhibit special population or environmental characteristics.

It is also important to understand how a program is affected by, and affects, the social, economic, and political environment within which it is implemented. Conclusions and recommendations produced during evaluations should be structured to take into account social, economic, and political conditions. Assessments must present feasible recommendations; otherwise they might as well never have been performed. For example, to what extent is the high level of grass roots community participation in a growth monitoring program due to the existing local tradition for community action? What amount of political support or hindrance could program managers expect from local officials? In other locations how much local support do they need to replicate the program?

In summary, macro evaluations should be performed to identify policy implications from the existing program. For example, should the program be replicated? If so, how should it be replicated? What changes should be made in the objectives, the scale, the organizational structure, or program components that comprise the model? As one might expect, evaluations do not mark the end of a program; they are only a phase of a continuing cycle of administrative activity.

A Brief Review of Monitoring and Evaluation Methods

When monitoring program inputs and outputs, it is usually necessary to develop an information system that can collect and process information on a basic list of necessary resources to determine whether capital is flowing into the program at central and local levels at expected quantities and according to a set schedule. Similar information is needed on whether personnel are being hired and trained as planned, facilities are being constructed or rented, and material is in place at the correct time. The level of complexity of this monitoring will vary according to the complexity of the program and the resources available for the monitoring.

Information for monitoring, such as what is collected with LQAS approaches, should be collected at regular intervals and forwarded to managers and administrators. A monitoring system can also be expanded into a comprehensive control system by designing the flow of information to provide key administrators and policy makers with information they require. In a decentralized organization, the local manager is provided with monitoring information. It should also be possible to provide regional and national administrators with summarized reports of the program monitoring so that they may be advised regularly as to the progress being made toward achieving regional or national objectives.

The monitoring system can also be expanded into an information system which reports indicators of program efficiency and recommendations to management on the type of corrective measures which should be taken.

Monitoring information about inputs should include the timeliness of their arrival, their ultimate cost, and their quality at the time of arrival. Such information could help managers anticipate a potential problem in health service delivery and, therefore, whether delays may be expected prior to producing or delivering outputs. Similarly, outputs can be ranked in terms of their accessibility to the target community, such as whether services are being delivered at expected frequencies. Throughout the country health facilities could be rank ordered by the adequacy of their inputs and outputs. Managers could assume that this information indicates the relative progress of the health units in each community. If analyses were desired to explain the relative program performance in each city, these indices of inputs and outputs could be investigated relative to various socioeconomic characteristics of the target communities and environmental characteristics of the cities (in addition to analyses of the processes involved in creating the inputs and outputs).

Statistical analyses of a CHW's performance relative to the social and physical environmental characteristics of local communities would be possible if sample surveys were designed, administered, and analyzed in conjunction with administrative records.

Although emphasis has been placed on numerical measures thus far, non-numerical focus groups and participant observation methods should also be performed. These techniques are particularly worthwhile for managers who need or want to describe organizational procedures being followed by CHWs. They also give policy makers anecdotal reactions of the staff and participants.

In assessments of impacts on a target group, variants of experimental or quasi-experimental designs are sometimes used (Campbell and Stanley 1966, Cook and Campbell 1979, Valadez 1985a). With these approaches, measurements are taken from a community before and after it is exposed to the health services. These measures are compared with a comparison or control community similar to the former community apart from the intervention. The assessment is intended to indicate what would have happened without the health services. Differences between the intervention and control groups after services have been delivered are used to infer the impact.

Most of the standard monitoring and evaluation methodologies rely upon a single or a very small number of techniques with very little attempt made to evaluate the validity or reliability of either the techniques or the conclusions derived from the data collected with them. This limitation of traditional approaches indicates the importance of using a multimethod, multitrait approach in which both a variety of measurement techniques and a number of independent indicators of the same impact measure are obtained. The triangulation of the results from more than one analysis indicates whether the estimates of a program's performance are consistent. In circumstances in which the triangulated results lead to similar conclusions, a manager can be more confident in the findings.

Another seldom analyzed issue involves understanding interactions between the program and its environment. Such investigations assess whether an intervention's impact or lack of one is associated with the special characteristics of the population or the environment in which it has been organized and, therefore, is not transferable to other locations. For example, the health system in Chapter 1 may not be transferable to Ecuador from Costa Rica due to the different geographical, political, and economic conditions that exist in both locations. In later chapters I will try to indicate how to adapt LQAS procedures to different national settings.

Many of the key concepts used in this and the following chapters have been developed for investigations outside of the health sector (see Campbell and Stanley 1966, Cook and Campbell 1979, Valadez 1985a). Although these principles are applied most frequently to quantitative research, they can also be applied to qualitative evaluations. Nevertheless, regardless of the investigative tools, fundamental issues must be taken into consideration to guide the use of various instruments to produce reliable and credible results. The following concepts are used in one or more of the following chapters:

Intervention Group: An intervention group consists of individuals or communities exposed to the program's outputs (i.e., interventions, services, or products).

Comparison or Control Group: A control group includes individuals or communities who are as similar as possible to the intervention group but who are not exposed to the program's outputs.

Randomization: Random assignment involves using appropriate randomizing procedures to select individuals or groups for intervention and control groups. The use of randomization ensures that the average characteristics of all the individuals in the study are represented in both the intervention and control groups. Random assignment is always desirable although not always possible.

Matching: Whenever random assignment is not possible, the manager must assume that the intervention and control groups differ in many ways other than the fact that one is exposed to the intervention and the other is not. In this event, both groups can be matched by as many of their characteristics as possible to ensure that the two groups are as similar as possible. That is, members of the intervention and control groups are selected on the basis of their shared traits. The characteristics on which the participants should be matched should include those which could possibly explain a difference in outcome between the intervention and control group other than the intervention. For example, a growth-monitoring intervention in which the intervention community consists of individuals who have been trained to regularly measure and plot children's growth, and to take action should they falter, may not perform substantially better than a control community of residents who may have learned growth monitoring when they participated in a perinatal care program that also instructed mothers how to monitor their children's growth.

Pretest I: Information about both groups is collected before the intervention begins for those variables which are expected to be affected by the program. At the same time information is also gathered about the socioeconomic and other characteristics of the target population in both the intervention and control groups, to assess whether these differences might affect the outcome variables.

For example, differing maternal education and income could explain the trends in the infant mortality rate in either group regardless of the intervention.

Pretest II: The term "pretest" is also used in instrument development. In this context it refers to the stage of an investigation in which an instrument (e.g., a questionnaire) has been developed, but needs to be field tested to determine both whether it measures what it is intended to measure (validity) and whether it can reproduce measures on subsequent applications in the same population (reliability). Testing the questionnaire's validity requires the manager to perform a pilot study in field conditions to determine whether respondents understand the questions being asked. Redrafting ambiguous and unclear questions is usually sufficient to resolve such problems. The second type of study is more difficult. Testing the questionnaire's reliability involves performing a survey of a small pilot sample twice, with the second interview occurring a short time after the first. The purpose is to determine how much the responses differ from those obtained in the first round. Instruments which produce repeatedly the same measures of the same variable are considered to be reliable measures.

Post-Test: Following implementation of the program and the delivery of outputs, information is collected about both the intervention and control groups and compared to pretest data to assess the impact. These data should be collected at that point in time when an impact could be expected. For example, a maternal vaccination program aimed at reducing neonatal tetanus deaths through vaccination in the second trimester of pregnancy should have a perceivable impact in the first one or two weeks after delivery since newborns are immunized transplacentally by their mothers. Therefore, a lowered disease specific infant mortality rate should be expected.

Also, the socioeconomic and other population characteristics of the target community should be measured to determine whether or not the intervention and control groups continue to share commensurate characteristics at both the pretest and post test. This latter point is important since either group can be replaced during the time interval between which the program began and the post-test data were collected. Therefore, a change in infant mortality could be associated with middle class families replacing low income families.

One limitation of many assessments is that the managers do not consider how the interventions alter the composition of the intervention or control groups. Although the purpose of the control group is to eliminate some of the external effects, it is difficult to determine all the characteristics to monitor so as to account for differences that occur later. For example, if the control group area should become flooded or if a new factory offering more employment opportunities opens near an intervention group, how should the manager take into account the impact that these events may have, not only on the number and types of individuals in the intervention and control groups, but also on their life style?

How should these influences be taken into account in the analysis? Although such contamination of an assessment's design is common, it is frequently impossible to separate unintended effects from the intervention's effects. Managers should always report unanticipated findings and events so that policy makers, planners, and other users of the results can judge how to interpret them — and take precautions when interpreting a manager's conclusions.

Another limitation with many assessments is that they rely exclusively on one method of data collection, generally sample surveys. Any one data collection method has its limitations. Information about income or fecal disposal, for example, may be difficult to obtain through a questionnaire. Collecting information from multiple sources, using multiple instruments, is preferable. The assumption is that if multiple sources of information indicate similar results, then one can be more confident in the conclusions of an assessment. Despite the fact that dangers of using unimethod approaches are widely known and accepted, analysts seldom use systematic consistency checks of their data.

A third weakness of many assessments is that they frequently do not analyze the effects of local influences on the programmed work. Although information may be obtained on the type of contact the participant had with the program (e.g., did he attend meetings, how did he obtain needed information to perform his task), it is unusual for analyses to investigate ways in which the organizational processes may have affected the impact. For example, health systems using a strategy for decentralized primary health care service delivery involve training community health promoters who organize the community census, educate mothers about hygiene, encourage participation in the EPI, refer pregnant women and neonates to health professionals, and the like. Their work requires skills in community organizing and in soliciting the participation of families. In practice, the overall participation of families in communities may differ substantially. Such variation may be due to the characteristics of the community promoter, the characteristics of the community members, the reactions of local political groups, and other related social institutions. Some community families may participate as individual units. In others, families may prefer group settings. In instances in which latrines need to be built, the participants may organize the work as a family activity. Others may hire workers. These variations (which may range from systematic sabotage of the program by local political leaders in one area to very active support and the provision of additional resources in another) are seldom enumerated (see Valadez 1984) and the suspected influences go unreported. Such explanations would be assisted if a program journal were maintained by the program manager in which all such variations were recorded. National counterparts, such as the director general of the Ministry of Health or regional directors of health, find such qualitative information important for interpreting quantitative reports. ✧

3

Models, Control and Validity

An inability to think abstractly about a program may blind a health program manager from measuring pertinent variables explaining performance. The very substance of theory consists of deducing essential causal agents, their interaction, their relative temporal order, and a hypothesis about what the health intervention is expected to produce. The theory upon which a health program is based determines the variables to be measured and how they interact. Potentially, it can suggest the measurement methods and the subsequent analyses.

In this chapter, health programs are described as *models*. This chapter also explains the practical applications of modeling principles. The first section discusses modeling as a step in program development in which five aspects of a program are identified: program components, their interaction, the required resources, the outputs they should produce, and the impacts expected.

Also, principles are presented that may lead to the elaboration of program plans. These concepts are intended to help managers anticipate and resolve measurement problems early in the development cycle. Later in the chapter, discussion turns to field conditions and to errors in the design of program assessments which should be avoided in order not to invalidate an evaluation.

Readers familiar with the quasi-experimental literature will notice that many of the concepts applied were developed originally by quasiexperimenters. However, that literature has been presented for audiences interested in reforms and interventions formulated for developed countries rather than for developing countries. The latter group of nations has environmental conditions that are substantially different from those found in the developed West. Therefore, one goal of this chapter is to translate basic methodological precepts into a form that is applicable to circumstances that international public health practitioners encounter when carrying out applied scientific research.

Modeling Health Systems

Programs planned to improve health conditions are based on theoretical models of health processes. Even though the underlying theory is often not stated, the decisions made about the amount and type of inputs, implementation procedures, and even the size and characteristics of target or client groups are based upon a set of assumptions about influences that affect a program's results. A program model makes explicit the community and its population or environmental conditions that a program is intended to affect (e.g., infants under three years of age), the direction of the effect (e.g., reducing infant mortality, increasing the proportion of children under three years with measles vaccination, increasing the availability of clean water), and the variables that lead to these effects (e.g., community-based public health programs, infant immunizations, and construction of a water purification facility). In traditional terms, the variables measuring the expected effect are dependent variables; those leading to the change are independent variables.

For example, let us assume that a nation has high infant mortality attributable to tetanus neonatorum. Maternal vaccination programs for tetanus toxoid are known to be an effective method for reducing infant mortality from this cause. Implicitly, an organization needs to be formulated to obtain the vaccinations in sufficient quantity, to administer funds, to train and manage personnel, to publicize the vaccination program to attract mothers, and to plan logistics for vaccinating the target population. The model in this instance is the entire vaccination program and its client communities. Its expected impact is based on medical knowledge about the etiology of infectious diseases and their control; on logistics that maximize the potential for adequate coverage with vaccines of the mothers within the populations of the target communities; and on the provision of adequate monetary, human, and material resources for implementing the plan. In this example the logistics could consist of activities such as estimating the amount of vaccine required for a target population, preparing a cold chain, a host of organizational issues dealing with the delivery of the vaccine to the target population, and the vaccinating of the communities themselves.

Five tasks are needed to construct a program model. The first one involves developing an explicit statement of program goals — the ultimate achievements a program is expected to produce. The second task consists of stating program objectives — the quantifiable bench marks used for judging a program's success. The third activity is an enumeration of program inputs for each intervention — all the necessary program resources (e.g., money, material, personnel, infrastructure). They comprise the independent variables of the program. As seen in the above example, inputs generally are derived from interdisciplinary sources (e.g., medical, administrative, logistical).

In the fourth task, the phasing through time of each input is explicitly stated. In other words, a time chart or a flow chart should be constructed that indicates the quantity of input required, the point in time it is required, the length of time it takes to receive the input, and the dependency of any input on preceding inputs. This fourth task specifies the quantity and the order in which inputs should be introduced. The variation among the inputs can be quite substantial since some inputs will continue (e.g., program management and operating capital) at a constant quantity while others will be present at one time (e.g., computer programmer) or intermittently at different phases and in variable quantities (e.g., technical advisors on epidemiology).

In the fifth and final task, the impacts expected from the intervention program are defined. The effects comprise the dependent variables. Impacts, as explained in the preceding chapter, consist of both expected and unexpected results. During the planning of a program model expected impacts are identified. Subsequent analyses of results may aid in replanning the program by making explicit the impacts that were not anticipated. Conversely, when objectives are not achieved, the model needs editing to eliminate the anticipated impact and the program components that were supposed to produce it, or to modify the model by adding additional support components that could increase the possibility of achieving an objective.

In summary, a model explicitly identifies inputs, outputs, processes, and impacts; how they are related; and the crucial role of each component in the program plan. Probably the most distinctive feature of a model is its explicit description of how the variables that compose it interact to produce impacts. These implicit components and interactions that compose the intervention ought to be the focus of quality control. Later chapters show how LQAS can be used for this purpose. Presenting interventions as models expedites quality control by making clearer the targets of the assessments.

On the Importance of Controls When Assessing Integrated Health Programs

This section discusses a basic monitoring and evaluation principle, namely, *control*, that will be useful for health professionals using LQAS or many other program assessment approaches. Because health programs are often planned either to deliver a certain quantity of outputs or to produce certain impacts, health system managers need to understand the processes that lead to them and be capable of exercising control over the program components that produce them. The term *control* has several different meanings in scientific investigations. Although many principles of control presented in the following section were originally discussed by managers performing quasi-experimental research, they also have a broader application to health system managers.

A first meaning of control involves identifying both the populations that are exposed to the program and those that are not, and the duration and intensity of the intervention. One purpose of such control is to identify or choose individuals to receive the services of a health program and to select others for a control group that will not. For later evaluation it is often advisable to use selection criteria that result in both groups having similar characteristics. Such control helps to separate the effects that are due to the program intervention from those due to exogenous effects. For example, when assessing an integrated health program, the manager has to define clearly the individuals that comprise the community for which a given health facility is responsible. Sometimes these individuals live together in a barrio or neighborhood; at other times they live in dispersed rural settings. A manager exercises control by distinguishing people or villages with access to health services from those who do not. If such distinctions are not clearly recognized, data concerning individuals using a health facility could be mixed with data concerning people from a non-user group. A spurious conclusion would result showing no or low effectiveness of a health facility's program in maintaining or improving the health status of the community.

The second usage of control refers to shielding the intervention environment from extraneous influences. In a traditional laboratory a barrier can be constructed to prevent contamination of an experiment. For example, a shield can be erected to prevent penetration by outside influences. The purpose of such control is to measure the effects of an intervention that is not confused with outside influences. In an integrated health program, this form of control can be exercised by coordinating the responsibilities of different health managers and their staffs to ensure that the communities for which they are responsible do not overlap. If such were the case, it would be difficult to determine whether any one health facility was delivering services adequately to its community since more than one facility was providing services. This very issue had to be considered when identifying the catchment areas of the health areas assessed with LQAS and reported in Chapter 5.

In another example, assume that a health education program is implemented in the same set of communities in which a waste management program has also been established. Both programs are intended to reduce the absolute number of annual diarrhea episodes. Since both programs are implemented in the same environment, it is not possible to separate out the effects due to one or the other.

The third type of control involves eliminating those factors which can confuse interpretation of cause and effect. These alternative explanations call into question the cogency of a health program for the following reasons: (1) its inability to realistically accomplish its objectives, (2) its inability to demonstrate that an impact is attributable to its interventions, (3) its use of inappropriate statistical analyses to assess whether an impact occurred and can be attributed to the program, and (4) its results not being generalizable to other program sites since the characteristics of the health facility site are associated with production of its impacts. These four validity problems illustrate, respectively: construct validity, internal validity, statistical conclusion validity, and external validity. Of these four categories, internal validity threats are perhaps the most important to prevent since they render data useless. Each of these categories of validity is now briefly discussed.

Construct Validity

In health program assessments, construct validity involves determining whether a particular program is capable of receiving inputs, producing or delivering proposed outputs, or effecting impacts. Program planners need to justify the expectation that a program model should lead to the delivery of certain services, the production of specified products, or the achieving of desired impacts. Programs with unfeasible expectations lack construct validity.

Construct validity problems that undermine the credibility of programs can either be logistical or structural. Logistical threats to construct validity include inappropriate delivery or maintenance systems, inadequate number or qualifications of personnel, and other problems that impede the implementation of interventions. In other words, a logistical threat results from faulty planning so that inputs and outputs are inadequate in either their quantity or quality to produce the program's impacts.

For example, a primary health care program that is transferred from a mountainous area to a tropical region may lose construct validity by not including additional vehicles and personnel to ensure delivery of vaccines and other drugs in tropical terrain. The program model may also lack construct validity by not including additional drugs to prevent or treat infections associated with a tropical climate, or by including other inputs required for mountainous areas which are useless in the tropics. In this example, the mode of transportation for delivering services (in this instance, vaccinations) to the target population may be inadequate.

Structural threats to construct validity occur if a program plan contradicts already established principles, say, the relationships between a program's outputs and the impact it is supposed to produce. The construct validity problem is that the program's model is intended to produce an impact that practice suggests is not probable.

For example, an oral rehydration therapy program that emphasizes distributing oral rehydration salts (ORS) envelopes, but that does not educate mothers to prepare the solution, will probably be ineffective in reducing the diarrhea mortality rate.

Construct validity is the sine qua non for achieving a program's objectives and should be attained prior to its implementation. Although construct validity may not be possible to assess at the outset of a program, the monitoring system should be aimed to detect both theoretical and logistical weaknesses at any time during the implementation. For example, a monitoring program should detect whether inputs are at sufficient levels to produce a necessary output. Subsequent improvements, if introduced expeditiously, could render an otherwise futile intervention successful. In the example presented earlier, the manager of the tropical primary health care program could augment the program's facilities with four-wheel-drive jeeps for transportation during the rainy season, and additional antibiotics and other medicines to treat endemic infections.

Internal Validity

As discussed earlier, the purposes of program evaluation include assessing whether or not expected or unexpected results have occurred and, in cases where objectives were not achieved, what were the reasons. These purposes can only be achieved if alternative explanations of observed consequences are made explicit and investigated.

Problems due to internal validity arise from measurement errors. In broad strokes, a measurement error occurs whenever a change in an impact measure can be attributed to a factor that is exogenous to the program. Such influences are measurement errors because they obscure whether or not a result is associated with a program's model or with some other irrelevant, but plausible, factors. Influences that impede program assessments are referred to as *internal validity problems*. They are threats precisely because they prevent appraising the validity of the model. A discussion of several threats, all of which are summarized in Table 3.1, follows.

Table 3.1   Summary of Modeling, Control and Validity Principles and Problems

Principles	Category	Measurement Problem
Goal	Expected health status change	Inability to plan or discriminate among policy options
Objective	Measurable program bench mark	Inability to evaluate
Construct Validity	Ensuring logistical and structural capability to justify expectations	Program unfeasible due to inappropriate quantity of resources introduced and products produced
Internal Validity	History	Results attributable to national trends
	Local history	Local social, economic, political events within either the intervention or control group that explain differences in impact measures
	Maturation	Results attributable to internally motivated changes in participants
	Testing: preferred response	Response due to perception of testing instrument
	Testing: test wisdom	Response due to low retest reliability

Table 3.1 Summary of Modeling, Control and Validity Principles and Problems (continued)

Principles	Category	Measurement Problem
Internal Validity (continued)	Instrumentation	Results attributable to change in the measuring instrument through interviewer improvement, instrument modification, or instrument deterioration
	Selection: control vs. group variation	Results attributable to the diverging characteristics of the study populations rather than to the program
	Selection: inadequate predictor variable variation	Inability to determine whether or not a variable explains program impact
	Selection bias in epidemiology	Group assignment procedure associated with the impact
	Regression to the mean	Extreme values of the pre-implementation group gravitate toward the population mean
	Attrition or mortality	Results attributable to change in the composition of program participants
	Diffusion	Results due to contamination of control group by program intervention
	Rivalry	Results attributable to the control group improving its own condition instigated by competitive rivalry with the intervention group
	Compensatory equalization	Intervention introduced into the control group thus eliminating potential for comparison with intervention group.
	Resentful demoralization	Conditions worsening among control group participants demoralized from knowing they were not permitted to receive the intervention
	Political indifference	Managers impeding or not implementing a program because it is perceived as irrelevant to their own priorities
	Political interference	Actions of political actors impeding program implementation and thereby changing the program model in ways that managers cannot control

Table 3.1   Summary of Modeling, Control and Validity Principles and
Problems (continued)

Principles	Category	Measurement Problem
Internal Validity (continued)	Seasonal cycles	Results attributable to seasonal variation rather then the intervention
	Interactions: selection-maturation	Results attributable to increasingly acute differences between the intervention and control groups
	Interactions: selection-history	Initial differences between participants are obscured due to entry of program participants at different points in time
Statistical Conclusion Validity	Ensuring correct selection of statistics to investigate essential evaluation questions	Improper interpretation of statistics leading to incorrect conclusions
External Validity	Interaction between interventions	Program impacts influenced by the sequence in which activities are implemented
	Interaction of setting	Program impacts and treatments influenced by variations in environmental, administrative, and demographic conditions of the site
	Interaction of selection and interventions	Program impacts associated with the characteristics of local populations
	Interactions of history and interventions	Program impacts associated with the historical conditions in the site area

History

The first internal validity problems concern historical influences. Two categories of validity issues include macro or national history, and local history or local tradition. For the first type of historical issues, consider the change in a health indicator, such as a reduction in infant mortality. It could be due to the overall trend in development within a nation rather than to a specific health program. Although a change may be construed as a program's impact, it could also be due to extraneous factors influencing the nation as a whole. For example, assume that the success of a program of child health care was measured by the number of infants examined at ambulatory clinics. Also, assume that during the life of the program the nation had undergone reductions in the birth rate, the infant mortality rate, and the growth rate. The internal validity problem arises since the frequency of outpatient care can be affected by these demographic changes. A declining population growth rate from a lower birth rate will result in a smaller percentage of children in the population. Since there are fewer children, one could expect a reduction in the frequency of outpatient care given to young children, compared to the earlier time period. A decrease in the absolute number of visits by the target population could be attributed erroneously to their disaffection for the health care program since each year fewer visits were recorded. A more appropriate measure would be a change in the age distribution of the facility's client population. This change would be exhibited by a differential increased use by adolescents, adults, and the elderly.

The second category of validity problems, local history or local tradition, exhibits itself in quite different ways from national history problems. Local history involves events within the community that either augment or depress impact measures in it. The basic principle of this local history problem is that new or enduring conditions in the communities could explain variation in the impact measure. Consider the following three examples.

Improved transportation (comfort or speed) may explain local attendance at health centers, rather than improved service delivery. Development of a new road may promote diffusion of information to a control population that previously had been insulated from the intervention, thereby diminishing the relative magnitude of the impact of a health communication intervention in a target community. Introduction of radio or television into a target population may create additional reinforcement for the local population to reach program goals that were not originally structured into its outreach component. For example, local public health education programs promoting the use of oral rehydration therapy (ORT) may be augmented by national media reinforcing the messages of health workers. Or a local population striving to be socially mobile and receiving messages from popular culture may be more inclined to participate in child survival interventions than those living according to traditional local norms.

Maturation

Results that are due to internally motivated changes in the participants (e.g., their growing older, wiser, fatigued, or bored) and are not attributable to the interventions are maturation effects. Although maturation may either augment or mitigate the perceived effectiveness of a model, it is detrimental to program assessments since it obscures the true conditions.

For example, consider a decentralized health program implemented in a series of pilot areas of a nation. Program administrators should be sure to choose areas that are not overrepresented with residents who have previous successful participation in health programs. Residents' involvement in health education events, vaccination sessions, and community finance schemes may be explained by either of two maturation effects. Firstly, participants' previous experiences in community participation may explain the program's success rather than the education and management components of the program alone. Secondly, previous community participation experience of local managers may explain the program's success rather than the training and management modules of the intervention design. In order to throw light on whether maturation explains the results, the manager in this example should investigate the histories of participating communities to identify whether their experiences and those of the program administrators potentially explain the successful completion of the intervention.

In another example, the success of a decentralized health care program may be associated with the high parity of participating mothers (i.e., the number of children to whom a mother has given birth). Program impacts may not have been uniform across mothers of varied parity. If "success" is measured in terms of reduced infant mortality, then a lower infant mortality rate of participating families might be due to the variation in their experiences. The maturation effect in this case is that the mothers using the program who have had more children may be more capable of coping with the complications associated with childhood disease, and knowing when and how to solicit local medical aid, than less experienced mothers who are not participants. More experienced mothers may be either more or less receptive to alternative practices than the less experienced mothers.

Maturation issues were considered when designing the test application of LQAS, discussed in the next chapters of this book. Potential maturation problems were eliminated by randomly selecting Health Areas from throughout Costa Rica as test sites. Therefore, the distribution of variation of Health Areas that exist in Costa Rica was included in the assessment.

Testing

Two categories of testing issues are discussed in this section: the preferred response and test wisdom. Although the first type of measurement error is more pertinent to the use of LQAS, both categories are presented in order to be comprehensive.

Any measure requiring an informant's response may be affected by his perception of the testing instrument. Regardless of whether observations are made before or after an intervention is implemented, the validity of a measure is threatened when an informant's response is slanted by his reaction to the measurement process. Such reactions are called *testing threats*.

The testing problem of preferred response can occur in a number of ways in health programs. Whenever some residents in a community are selected through interviews for participation in an intervention, such as a food supplementation program, other potential candidates may make fallacious links between the earlier responses of their associates and their selection into the program. Such links may lead them to suspect that a specific response will either include or exclude them from an intervention group. Therefore, later candidates tailor their responses based on their assumptions. This informant reaction is called a *preferred response*.

For example, a colleague working in West Africa told me he had noticed that the pre-intervention measures of the population exhibited little variation (e.g., families were said to be uniformly of the same size, age distribution, income, and the like). In subsequent interviews after the program commenced, participants responded more accurately since the selection process had finished. Variation in the population increased. Impacts of the intervention could not be analyzed since the staff could not determine whether the difference in pre-intervention and post-intervention measures was due to the program or to the preferred response bias. Such a threat commonly exists when selection to receive a benefit is based on family size, marital status, age, income, diet, or medical history.

In another example, participants in a food supplementation program in Bogota, Colombia (Herrera et al. 19ᵕᴗab, 1983; Mora et al. 1974, 1978ab, 1979) during the 1970s were chosen on the basis of their medical history, family size (i.e., families had to have more than one child), and current calorie intake. If the squatter settlers who were chosen later in the program had suspected that the criterion for selection was low caloric intake or low food consumption, they could have given erroneous responses to interviewers to increase their potential for inclusion in the intervention, and thus receive food supplements. Respondents could, therefore, have matched their responses to those of neighbors who were selected. By speculating about the criterion, candidates may have given inaccurate responses to ensure their receiving the food supplements.

This case also illustrates another preferred response incident. Following implementation of the program, Mora and his associates (1978a) found that the caloric intake in the intervention group had increased only slightly. The investigators concluded that the supplements intended for children were treated as economic resources rather than as food, namely, they were either given away, shared with other family members or with neighbors, or sold. Another interpretation is that informants continued to report low caloric intake because they thought their participation was due to their continued reporting of low caloric intake. This interpretation was investigated and rejected through comparing data from 24 hour recalls by participants of their diet and dietary surveys (Mora et al. 1978a).

Another category of testing threat is *test wisdom*. Although it is probably more familiar to investigators working in educational or training programs in which retention of skills or knowledge is tested, test wisdom is also applicable to health programs. There are two types of test wisdom relevant for assessing Child Survival programs. The first one occurs when individuals learn from the assessment process itself. Sometimes when a community participates in a series of interviews or surveys, residents learn how to respond to the questions asked of them. Therefore, over a series of questionnaires, they may respond more accurately to the latter instruments than to the former ones. Such a testing problem is more severe in Child Survival programs that assess the knowledge and practices of individuals. An improvement in knowledge or the competency of program participants could be due to improved skill in responding to formal questions over the course of the program.

The second category of test wisdom affects assessments of information quality. For example, the study of LQAS reported in Chapter 5 assesses the quality of the information recorded in community health facilities by CHWs about the Child Survival interventions or about the people receiving them by asking mothers to verify the information. Some responses concerned the number of annual visits of health workers to the household, the number of individuals living in the household, and the years of the mother's education. However, variations in the responses among households for those types of data are not necessarily due to real differences. Frequently, they are due to the lack of precision of a respondent. I have had the experience of a mother citing fewer children than she really had even though all were present with her during the interview. The reliability of responses, therefore, needs to be verified, as it was in the LQAS field test.

Reliability is generally measured by asking a sample of the respondents to answer the same set of questions on two occasions. Test wisdom threatens these investigations when participants answer by recalling their previous responses rather than reacting independently of them. In the test of LQAS, 10% of the 1680 households were resampled by a management team assigned to maintain the quality of the data collection process in each of the 60 Health Areas sampled. In order to control for potential influences of test wisdom, areas were resampled between one and three weeks after the original interview. Any Health Area that did not exhibit 90% or greater reliability suggested inadequate data collection, thereby requiring the full sample of households in the area to be visited again.

Instrumentation

Although a manager may hope that interviewers will improve their skills over the course of the data collection, if such changes were to occur, the data could be hopelessly biased. Whenever an instrument changes during the data collection period, a measurement error occurs. An instrumentation problem occurs whenever variation in a variable may be due to changes in the measurement instrument rather than either to existing variation in the environment or results of an intervention.

Three categories of instrumentation problems are *interviewer improvement*, *instrument modification*, and *instrument deterioration*.

Interviewer improvement is a problem for assessing programs in which interviewers received the bulk of their training in the field or are allowed to innovate in order to find the interview style they prefer. If either of these conditions are suspected, an instrumentation problem may exist. Information collection at later points in time would be performed by an interviewer with different standards as compared to the earlier period of data collection.

Another type of instrumentation problem arises when a manager, after taking several measures with one instrument, decides to change it either by replacing it, by altering certain features of it (e.g., modifying the questions in an interview schedule or questionnaire), or by including additional questions so as to study variables not initially included in the data set. Such alterations may lead to spurious differences between pre- and post-implementation observations, thereby obscuring differences that are attributable to an intervention.

Although changing an instrument may reduce the comparability of two data sets, it need not do so. The order of questions and their content can affect the responses to those that follow. Some methodologists suggest that questions appear in a random order; others recommend that sensitive or personal questions appear at the end, thus permitting the informant to become accustomed to replying before intruding on his privacy with intimate questions (e.g., income, sexual practices, occupation, household budget). Since the order and content of questionnaires can influence responses, changing either the order or content by adding or deleting questions may alter subsequent responses.

To minimize these dangers, as many questions as possible should remain in successive questionnaires or interviews, and in the same order. New or rephrased questions should appear at the end of the instrument, if feasible. Thus, the data acquired in both pre- and post-implementation observations would thereby remain the same while also obtaining additional information.

A final category of instrumentation validity threat involves changes to an instrument due to its deterioration. For example, tape measures can shrink or stretch due to climatic change; gauges can produce uncertain readings when their units become difficult to read due to dirt, scratches, chipping, and cracking of their measurement scales; or spring or battery driven instruments may slow down with extended use.

Selection

Both health service researchers and epidemiologists recognize selection bias as a threat to the validity of an investigation, yet they define it differently. Since integrated health programs bring both groups together, each group should be aware of the other's usage. Despite their differences, both health service researchers and epidemiologists agree that selection bias occurs when an outcome can be attributed to the composition of intervention and control populations rather than to the treatment.

For the former group, selection bias exhibits itself in two ways. Firstly, the diverging characteristics of intervention and control groups rather than a program output could explain an impact. For example, the lower infant mortality rate in a town with a new primary health care program compared with a control town using a traditional program may be due to the difference in educational attainment of the town's people rather than to the intervention. Had the program been introduced into towns with similar levels of education, perhaps less reduction in the infant mortality rate would have resulted. Therefore, change in the dependent measure may be attributable to the characteristics of the individuals being studied rather than to the program. In this example, a between group difference in educational experience is a potential threat to validity since it, in interaction with the intervention, may explain variation between intervention and control town mortality rather than the intervention alone.

A second selection bias exists when the target population has small variation in social characteristics so that it is not possible to assess whether an effect is due to an intervention or due to these social characteristics. The basic principle is that a manager can determine whether a social variable is responsible for an effect only if that variable exists in sufficient variety to measure whether the program impact varies with it.

An assessment could control for this selection threat by including participants with a range of personal characteristics. Subsequently, it would then be possible to analyze whether or not the outcome variable was associated with a particular population characteristic.

In an example similar to what Clignet and Long (1975:11) experienced in Senegal, consider a primary health care program in which the District Medical Officer concludes that mothers with few children tend to bring newborns to the local health post for examination within 30 days of their birth. Such an observation could lead to an unjustified conclusion that mothers who have many children are too burdened by household responsibilities to visit health posts. In other words, the manager believes that the behavior of families may not be due to the incentives introduced by the program, but to the families' characteristics. Another explanation, however, is that the health post visits are associated with programmatic factors that inconvenience mothers with large families. In my own experience, I have found that mothers are sometimes annoyed by the Health Area environment rather than burdened by their household responsibilities. Health facilities that do not permit older children to accompany their mothers may diminish the number of larger families using the facility. The two competing interpretations cannot be assessed unless the program first analyzes a distribution of family sizes to assess systematically whether or not a negative correlation exists between family size and program use.

The third type of selection bias is relevant to epidemiological research. For many epidemiologists, selection bias refers to procedures that assign individuals to the study populations in such a way that the point estimate of risk does not measure true risk of mortality or morbidity of individuals who have been exposed to specific agents. For example, consider an epidemiological study of the hypothesis of a negative relationship between heart attack and exercise that compares an active population of Argentinean gauchos (or steel workers, or longshoremen) with a sedentary population of workers in the service sector of Buenos Aires. Assume that the relative risk for the service sector workers is 2.0 (a level of risk which is twice that of the active population) with a 95% chance that the true level of risk lies within the range of 1.6 to 2.2. Although these results support the test hypothesis, a selection bias offers an equally probable explanation. The lower risk of heart attack in the active population may not be due to life style factors, but may be due to the adaptive pressures of their professions that make them less likely to retain anyone at risk to heart attack. Gauchos have an invigorating life style. Such a life style would select against men without a fit heart. Hence, the study examines a group of people who exercise, but who also live in a habitat with selective pressures favoring people a priori with a low likelihood of heart disease versus one with a wider distribution of medical histories. Such selection bias prevents making any rational conclusion, since individuals potentially prone to heart disease are eliminated from the group by the group itself. There is no method for rectifying this problem after it has occurred. Therefore, it is essential to consider the potential for selection biases during the planning of a study.

A selection bias occurs when the criterion with which individuals are assigned to a study or control group is also related to the dependent variable (e.g., heart attack). In this instance the group assignment criterion (i.e., occupation) is negatively related to the outcome variable. Therefore, the assessment is biased. In the above example, the gaucho population was designated as the study group, yet membership in that group was possible because they had strong hearts. A proper selection criterion would tend neither to include nor to exclude individuals on the basis of their health. Therefore, their selection would be unrelated to the dependent variable.

Although this category of selection bias has been developed for epidemiological research, it has broader application. In another example, assume that one impact measure for a housing program is the improvement of health conditions within the community. The working hypothesis of the program model is that low density housing that includes basic infrastructure (i.e., clean water and sewerage) is negatively associated with the incidence of diarrhea and respiratory disease. Before the program is introduced, the program managers study two existing communities in the city: one which already has improved housing and another for which the housing will eventually be intended. The focus of the study is to determine whether the former community has significantly lower incidence of the two diseases. The problem with the selection of these communities is that the former one may already have better hygiene, be better educated and nourished, and exhibit better mothering practices. Their incidence of both diarrhea and respiratory disease is low for many reasons associated with the fact that they live in higher quality housing. The selection bias is that the group with better housing may consist of individuals who are motivated not only to improve their housing conditions, but also to improve more broadly their quality of life. Thus, they may already have characteristics that explain superior health levels rather than their housing alone.

In summary, three categories of selection biases have been discussed. In the first one, differences in the traits of control and intervention groups are alternative explanations to a programmatic effect. In the second category, insufficient variation of a community trait exists in the intervention and control groups, making it impossible to determine whether it is an alternative explanation. In the last one, the trait used for choosing individuals for the control and treatment populations is related to the expected effect rather than the exposure to a risk factor.

Regression to the Mean

Choosing a group of individuals to participate in a program intervention on the basis of their extreme characteristics (e.g., diet, income, disease, housing condition) may ultimately reduce internal validity. *Regression to the mean* is a phenomenon in which exceptionally high or low performance gravitates toward average performance over time. The closer a study group is to either tail of a distribution of performances, the greater the likelihood that subsequent scores will be closer to the average characteristics of the overall community from which it was chosen, regardless of the intervention that is introduced. A person could perform exceptionally above or below his or her capability. A mother may demonstrate, through response to a single interview, excellent comprehension of principles of hygiene or child care, or conversely, she may score very low. However, if her knowledge is tested on multiple occasions, her score may fall in the middle range of her capability. This same phenomenon can occur for almost any activity. Therefore, if a person is selected to receive a program intervention on the basis of a single extreme score, it is feasible that their performance will change subsequently, regardless of the intervention to which they have been exposed.

Individuals or groups may under- or overperform at any point in time. Such extraordinary performance is not their typical behavior. The basic principle is that a target group chosen on the basis of extreme characteristics will include individuals whose behavior is nontypical for them. On subsequent observations these individuals will exhibit their average behavior. In addition, the performance of a group of individuals with extreme scores will regress to the mean of the community from which they were drawn. For this reason, measurements taken after program implementation could lead the manager to erroneously conclude that the altered performance of the intervention group is an effect of the program. However, regression to the mean is an equally plausible explanation.

Integrated health programs may be particularly susceptible to regression effects when they focus on people with the most marginal housing, health, economic, and educational conditions. Procedures to select candidates below a certain income level, or who have a particular health risk, may increase the potential for regression effects by including extreme cases and excluding those that are typical for a local community.

Attrition or Mortality

Differences either within or between intervention and control communities can produce erroneous conclusions when individuals who move into or out of the program are not considered in the analysis. For example, improvements to the primary health care system may be related to subsequent reductions in infant mortality and increased life expectancy at birth. Yet, improved health services may also attract wealthier people with a different set of personal characteristics who buy out lower income residents and thereby replace them. Therefore, the population change rather than the intervention may explain the improved community health.

Failure to analyze attrition of participants or program mortality is to ignore the fundamental question of how people adapt to a program. Attrition may allude to either alternative preferences or to dissatisfaction with the services offered. Several reasons could explain why the target population leaves the community. For example, they may simply prefer the money offered to them to sell their housing rather than the program's benefits. Or the program's improvements to the community may have led to increased expenditures that forced the relocation of the initial population. The former reason signals an alternative preference while the latter one indicates dissatisfaction with the program.

Attrition or mortality could have been examined in this example had residents been restrained from selling their housing for a period of time (e.g., 5 years). Doing so would eliminate the first explanation: an alternative preference. The latter one would be exhibited by an increase in the abandonment of housing. This reaction occurred in 1978 in a housing project built in the northern Argentinean town of Federación. The population abandoned their housing en masse (cf. La Nación 1978, Valadez 1985a) due to the culturally inappropriate architectural design.

These threats are particularly applicable to public health programs. Integrated health programs could appear to perform well due to unreported deaths of children, or due to underreporting of migrant laborers' children. Such a potential reinforces the importance for maintaining up-to-date and well-supervised community based information systems.

Diffusion

Urban programs are not necessarily confined to the urban areas they are intended to serve. Their influence can extend beyond the specific neighborhoods for which they were planned or even beyond the city's limits. Therefore, it may be possible for a control community to be affected by the intervention intended for another community. Unintended program influences on other communities are a threat to internal validity when this effect reduces the difference between the intervention and control areas, thereby making the intervention appear less effective.

This problem, although difficult to avoid, emphasizes the need for choosing control communities in which the chances of contamination are negligible. Such controls require ensuring that a barrier prevents or reduces the flow of information between the intervention and control communities. In practical terms this principle is difficult to put into operation. Unless natural barriers already exist it can be very difficult to block information flow. However, precautions can be taken. Comparison groups should have no commercial links, so that trade is minimal. No airports, waterways, accessible roads or trails should connect them. They should not share infrastructure that encourages representatives of either community to exchange news or to establish cooperative agreements. Infrastructure includes the following systems: energy, sewerage, water.

Diffusion is similar to another internal validity threat already presented, namely, history. The difference between them is that historical threats to validity involve contamination of the program context by exogenous events. These effects can depress (or augment) the difference between the comparison groups. Diffusion involves contamination of the control group by endogenous events (i.e., the program intervention) to the intervention group. These effects, as mentioned, tend to depress rather than augment differences between the comparison groups. Thus, in many ways diffusion and history are based on similar principles of control, namely, to establish barriers that prevent contamination flowing from the intervention to the control setting.

Rivalry and Compensatory Equalization

These two threats to internal validity problems share the characteristic that an intervention is introduced into the control group after initially being deprived of it. Because the control group is also affected by the intervention, it becomes difficult to judge the outcome of the program. Since each of these validity problems has different derivatives, the manners in which they can be prevented differ. Therefore, they are discussed separately.

Rivalry between intervention and nonintervention groups can be a threat to the internal validity of a program assessment when individuals in a control community become aware that an intervention has been introduced into another community group and, through their own initiative, improve their own living conditions. The result produced by this self-initiative is to diminish the difference in the impact between the intervention and control communities.

Compensatory equalization occurs in either of two ways. Firstly, when local political leaders in the control communities are pressured either by their own constituents or by other competing political leaders to improve local conditions, they may insist that the program also be implemented in the control area.

Secondly, program administrators themselves may perceive in the course of their work that it is unethical to deprive the control group of intervention. The Berggrens and their associates experienced just such a problem in Haiti as they attempted to reduce infant mortality due to tetanus (Berggren et al. 1981). They eventually vaccinated their "control" population, and hence treated it as another intervention group. They controlled for the potential validity problem of treating the control group by examining both groups in a time series design. As they had observations at several pre-intervention time points, they were able to argue for the success of their program using a time series analysis (Cook and Campbell 1979:207-232). The potentially confounding influence of history was not an issue since no events occurred during the program that could otherwise explain the reduced mortality attributable to immunization against tetanus.

The basic difference between rivalry and compensatory equalization is that for rivalry the initiative for improvement of the control group comes from within that group. Compensatory equalization occurs when policymakers and program decisionmakers are responsible for contamination of the control group.

Resentful Demoralization

The control community learning about the program introduced into an intervention community does not always result in rivalry or compensation equalization. The control community's conditions can worsen due to demoralization. Such an effect can lead to spurious statistical analysis by fallaciously making it appear as though the intervention community has improved due to the program when it could actually have remained unchanged. The control group's condition deteriorates, thereby magnifying the difference between the post-test observations of the control and intervention groups, thus leading to an erroneous conclusion that the health status of the intervention group has improved.

Political Indifference or Interference

Local managers or political actors can affect health program assessments when their attitudes or other agendas subtract or add activities that alter the program model. Two categories of these problems include political indifference and political interference.

Political indifference is a problem when managers consciously refuse to implement an intervention because it is perceived as either too risky, inconsequential to their own goals, or disruptive to their life style. An intervention can be seen as risky if it has not been field tested, or if the manager has no assurance of his superiors' political support. Therefore, the manager believes he may have political costs to pay should the intervention prove ineffective or not have political support. An intervention can be judged inconsequential if program planners have not sufficiently explained the benefits that can be derived from proper implementation. Therefore, the manager develops no incentive for proper implementation. An intervention is disruptive when the manager is either passive, already overburdened by work, or not supportive of institutional reform. Therefore, the intervention is seen as more work which he prefers not to perform.

Political interference can be explained by an experience from the LQAS field test. A small group of Health Areas in the north of Costa Rica near the Rio San Juan at the Nicaraguan border was excluded from the sampling frame. During 1987 these areas were technically a war zone. A health worker had been killed a few months before the field test began. These Health Areas were eliminated since the goal of the field test was to assess implementation problems of the primary health care program rather than the effect of the war on the health system. The former problem was an endogenous problem that managers could address. The latter one was exogenous to the health system and could not be ameliorated by them.

This category of validity problems is similar to local history as discussed earlier. The difference is that local history refers to influences affecting the local population and the culture as a whole. Political interference refers to the actions of specific political actors that affect community health workers and their managers.

Seasonal Cycles

Seasonal variations can also produce confusing results since cyclical increases or decreases, if not detected, could be erroneously interpreted as a program impact. For example, the infant mortality rate fluctuates throughout the year. In some nations it is higher during the summer dry season and lower during the wetter winter, the former season having stagnant water and the latter one having more abundant clean water. If pretest data are collected during the summer and the post-test data during the autumn, the analysis could erroneously attribute the reduced mortality to the program rather than to the seasonal cycle. In this example, "seasonal cycles" are a threat to internal validity because one cannot determine whether the fluctuation is a result of the program or of a natural process.

Another example is taken from the Yacyreta Hydroelectric Program. This binational program involved the construction of a 72km wide dam across the Rio Paraná, an international boundary between Argentina and Paraguay. The flood waters were expected to affect substantially the economies and design of cities located along the river shore. Hence, the program required comprehensive planning in addition to designing the dam alone. Failure to consider the potential elimination of income by the program could have had severe consequences for health. Industries using the river bank, such as brickmaking, were known by local people to be an important source of income that would be especially affected (Valadez, 1985a). However, empirical validation of this local knowledge was possible only if data were not collected during the rainy season when brick making ceased. If program planners had not made their assessments during the rainy season, they potentially would have overlooked the traumatic effect due to the elimination of the local economy.

Interactions

In addition to the individual internal validity problems discussed in the preceding sections, threats may be produced through interaction of these threats with each other. Two of them are now discussed.

The interaction of *selection* and *maturation* threatens an evaluation when initial differences between intervention and control populations increase over time. This makes it increasingly difficult to decide whether any impacts have occurred, and whether they are attributable to an intervention. The basic characteristic of this category of internal validity problems is that although initial differences between intervention and control communities are not associated with variation in an outcome variable, over time they become increasingly associated with it.

For example, assume that a program includes two communities in which integrated health programs have been initiated. However, in one of them a social communication and mass media program has been introduced to reinforce the messages of local health promoters. Further, assume that the control community has a history of community organization and participation (e.g., a self-help housing program, an active health committee), while the latter community does not. The management question is whether the social communication and mass media program augmented the integrated health interventions and promoted a more rapid reduction of infant mortality.

Although the different histories of either community in self-help activities may have no immediate effect on the program, over time both communities may exhibit similar trends in mortality, but for different reasons. The outcome of the intervention community may be due to the social communication program. However, the outcome in the control community is due to its past experiences. The latter group of residents grew more capable of supporting the integrated health program over time because the existing community organizations learned how to apply their past self-help experiences to support the child survival interventions. Therefore, this selection-maturation characteristic may explain the lack of difference in the outcomes of the two communities rather than that the social communication intervention was ineffective.

Selection and *history* can threaten internal validity when an intervention is implemented in phases. The principal problem is that the initial differences between participants are obscured since they receive the intervention at different times. The problem is that one can not determine whether selection, history, or both explain variations in the outcomes of the different phases of the intervention.

Let us examine a hypothetical housing program that is expected to improve the local health status of children. Two portions of the same population are matched and compared at the same point in time. Yet, the first subpopulation receives the intervention in phase one, and the second receives it a year later in phase two. Subsequent data analysis shows that income and the health status of children have increased in each group, but with the following provisos: children in the second group have a substantially higher average birth weight and a significantly higher weight for height. In short, the second group is apparently out-performing the first one although it received the intervention later. Two possible interrelated interpretations for these results are:

Firstly, local conditions in the second group may have improved since the initial participant selection during phase one, thus explaining their higher values. Such an improvement could have occurred if benefits intended for group one diffused to group two prior to the formal implementation of the interventions resulting in locally initiated activities. These activities, in tandem with the program, may have given group two the momentum to catapult it ahead of group one once it received external support, despite the fact that it began at a later point in time. Conversely, conditions in the first group may have deteriorated resulting in differing demographic compositions.

Secondly, the characteristics of the participating population may have changed so that the second phase individuals no longer conform to the selection criteria. For example, individuals with higher incomes could have replaced the more marginal population immediately following the intervention.

With the available information, a manager cannot determine whether or not the outcome measures arise from initial differences among populations (i.e., community organization), or from historical events that occurred in the second group subsequent to the pre-implementation observations, or from better implementation of the intervention in phase one versus phase two. Indeed, the pretest data may or may not be pertinent to the evaluation since the characteristics of group two may have changed in the interim.

An implication of the above validity problem is that following careful selection of participants, subsequent checks are necessary to ascertain whether the participant populations are still suitable.

The above interaction of validity problems are examples. Other complex threats remain that can either diminish or enhance the perceived effects of development programs. As the reader may have already concluded, each intervention may have its own specific internal validity problems. Hopefully, the categories of internal validity threats presented here will be sufficient for a manager to detect potential threats to valid inference. Managers should inter-nalize the basic principles presented. By so doing, with time they may develop a capacity for creatively adapting them to detect other interactions and threats that may be specific to a particular program.

Statistical Conclusion Validity

Only a brief discussion of this category is presented. Statistical conclusion validity refers to making improper inferences from statistical results and, therefore, reaching erroneous conclusions. It also refers to the improper use of statistical tests for assessing program outcomes.

Managers may unknowingly violate statistical conclusion validity (or any other type of validity). This might occur, for example, when they find it necessary to perform statistical tests while in the field although they may not be sufficiently experienced in such matters. For this reason, they should include in their own field notes, in memos, and in written reports the exact procedures used and their assumptions. Anything less can render a report useless, for not only can the evaluation not be replicated by others, but also readers cannot assess for themselves whether the correct statistical tests were used.

External Validity

Although any assessment has satisfied all of the above considerations of validity, and the child survival interventions have reached their objectives, administrators should not assume that the same results will occur when the interventions are implemented in other locations. The external validity of a program refers to the extent to which findings can be generalized to other settings, people, and times. Four external validity threats are now discussed.

Child Survival programs typically consist of several categories of activities. For example, they may include outreach activities concentrating on health education, immunizations, diarrheal disease and control, prenatal and postnatal care, growth monitoring, and the like. All of these distinct activities have their own influences on participants. Together they may also have cumulative effects. The overall effects of the program could change with the order in which the different interventions are phased into the program area. In other words, the "interactions between interventions" may affect the generalizability of a program's result. A program could control for this external validity problem by standardizing the phasing of the interventions.

If the ordering of interventions is not considered, subsequent replications of the program may not achieve previously observed impacts, thus leading the manager to suspect that the program model is invalid.

The effectiveness of a program may also vary with communities as well as with the nations in which it is implemented. Another external validity problem concerns the *interaction of the setting and the intervention*. For example, LQAS methodology has now been taught in Ministries of Health in countries of Latin America and Africa. But should we expect the procedures to be implemented with managers experiencing similar difficulties? Procedural problems may differ throughout the world due to variations in population size, administrative structure, competency level of health personnel, ecology, and physical layout of the cities. In a workshop in Bolivia during 1989, I found that greater investment in the development of a supervision system on the Altiplano would probably be necessary since none was apparently functioning on a regular basis. Similarly, I found that the supervision systems in both Guatemala and Costa Rica needed improvement. I suspect that LQAS used in Bolivia would reveal logistical and transport problems previously unknown to the work team, and that these problems are different from those encountered in Costa Rica, as discussed in Chapters 5 and 6.

Numerous additional factors may affect the generalizability of a program from one location to another. For example: do nations with Western histories vary in their reactions to a program relative to those with Islamic histories? Similar queries could be raised for nations varying by agricultural, industrial, or mercantile traditions; family system; and educational systems. All of these aspects must be considered when assessing the external validity of programs.

A difficult to resolve external validity problem is found in programs having to select participants systematically and to eliminate candidates with particular characteristics from their sample. Thus, the intervention's participants have characteristics that are not comparable to the distribution of characteristics of other people in the whole population, or to other populations where the program might be replicated. The section on internal validity concerning selection bias discussed the importance of choosing participants that exhibit a wide variety of characteristics, rather than restricting the selection criteria to a narrow range. Such variation is also needed for assessing external validity. Income, medical histories, social economic status and rural-urban experience must be sufficiently varied to assess the relative effects of these factors on the outcome measures. In this way, it may be possible to develop a rational basis for discussing the external validity of a program and anticipating the settings in which it may or may not be expected to succeed due to characteristics of the target population. This third external validity problem can be summarized as an interaction of selection procedures and program interventions.

When programs are replicated in different locations, they are affected by the history and culture of that local community. The final external validity problem concerns an *interaction of history and the program.* Energy crises, political climate, inflationary trends, and other international programs may all have an influence on the program's outcome. For example, the LQAS field test, presented in Part II of this book, was developed during a time in which health professionals in the central and regional offices of the Ministry of Health had reached a consensus that an overall assessment of the integrated health system was needed to aid administrators to further develop and improve child survival services. Therefore, the field test began in a political climate that was very supportive, and middle managers were not threatened by the implementation of assessment procedures. Although it is difficult to conclude what impact the favorable political climate had on results reported in Chapter 5, public health practitioners using LQAS or any assessment method should take precautions to ensure that methods are implemented faithfully and at the same time to cultivate an atmosphere in which program assessments are viewed as an attempt to enhance child survival rather than penalize health workers.

In short, a clear and definitive statement of one's conclusions and one's doubts due to particular historical events always strengthens an evaluation. This information may help policy makers decide whether a model should be replicated, and if so, whether or not modifications to the program would be advisable.

The basic principles of modeling, control, and validity presented in this chapter are summarized in Table 3.1. A purpose of this section was to identify validity problems. Solutions were not systematically presented as they vary from program to program.

Since program planning, monitoring, and evaluation are all practical activities, they are often constrained by resource availability, by the timing of analyses required by policy makers, and by the prejudices of administrators against specific approaches to program assessments. Although it may not always be possible to implement an optimal assessment design, a manager should be capable of identifying the limitations of any assessment. Such caveats are essential for both administrators and policy makers who may be faced, as they often are, with making decisions with inadequate information. ✧

Part II

Lot Quality Assurance Sampling for Monitoring International Health Programs

LQAS Principles

Lot Quality Assurance Sampling (LQAS) was initially used in industry beginning in the 1920s. When applied to assessments of integrated health programs, it can help local managers and national health policy makers in four types of judgments: (1) assessing whether services have been delivered to children and women in communities on schedule, namely, at the time in their life when services are most needed to reduce health risks; (2) deciding whether a sufficient proportion of the client population has received services; (3) determining whether services were delivered properly; and (4) analyzing whether they could result in their intended effect. With these types of information, both local and national managers can determine whether the Child Survival Program is functioning adequately.

Regardless of the level of the health system which is being assessed, the primary sources of data should be at the periphery. As discussed earlier, quality control of health care service delivery ought to occur locally because communities are at risk to health problems when their health workers perform inadequately.

The first unit of operation of the primary health care (PHC) system in Costa Rica is known as a Health Area. In other countries of Latin America this peripheral unit is referred to as the Health Post. In some African countries it is called a Health Hut. The following discussion refers to Health Areas only. However, it is applicable to all peripheral health units. The health workers being assessed in Costa Rica are community health workers and auxiliary nurses; however, any category of health worker could have been monitored, including physicians and nurses.

Any inspection procedure in which a population is sampled, rather than totally studied, has inevitable errors and risks. These risks include provider and consumer risks. The provider is at risk when a Health Area is identified as inadequately covering the people for which it is responsible with specified PHC interventions (e.g., vaccinations) when in actuality it is performing adequately.

In this case, the Health Area staff suffers the reputation of being substandard, and health administrators spend scarce resources on "improving" a Health Area that does not need it. The consumer or community is at risk when assessments conclude that a population is adequately covered when, in fact, it is under-covered (Dodge and Romig 1959:1, Miller and Knapp 1979, Stroh undated). Therefore, the population remains vulnerable to a disease or health related problem from which its members think they are protected. Although a good sampling plan should reduce these risks to a minimum, there are other important considerations when selecting a methodology for monitoring and evaluation: measurement and analysis of costs, ease of training and use of instruments, time requirements to complete the task, and defining practical thresholds for provider and consumer risks.

In the following sections, LQAS is presented as a method for controlling the quality of PHC at first level facilities directly responsible for service delivery. This section was written for public health practitioners who need to understand the statistical principles upon which LQAS is based. For that reason, very little mathematical notation is used. For a more formal mathematical discussion of LQAS see Duncan (1965), Dodge and Romig (1959), or Lemeshow and Stroh (1989).

In order to demonstrate the need that LQAS may be satisfying, we first discuss the Expanded Programme on Immunization (EPI) cluster sampling design, as recommended and used by the World Health Organization (WHO) (Henderson and Sundaresan, 1982) to measure the level of immunization coverage in large populations. It may also be applied to relevant parameters of almost any PHC program.

This discussion of the merits of these two methods of assessing the level of vaccination coverage is conducted on the basis of two assumptions: (1)the staff of each Health Area undertakes responsibility for protecting (or covering) every child of appropriate age in the Health Area's jurisdiction with the specified immunization procedures which this project has undertaken to monitor, and (2)the Health Area staff achieve a uniform level of coverage throughout their whole area of jurisdiction. This second assumption will be changed after the basic features of LQAS are presented.

Using EPI Cluster Sampling

The EPI method requires a random selection of 30 clusters within what is usually a large geographical area that is often served by several Health Areas. Within each of the 30 clusters or sites, the first of seven individuals of a predetermined target group (e.g., child under five years of age) is randomly selected. The other children are then systematically selected on the basis of their proximity to the first child (WHO undated) within each of the 30 clusters or sites. A sample of 210 individuals is normally required. This method has been used more than 60 times in 25 countries and has been judged to produce reliable results (Henderson and Sundaresan 1982, Lemeshow et al. 1985).

The results produced by EPI cluster sampling methodology are useful for ascertaining the extent of coverage in a large area with a relatively small sample of households. The low costs and speed of the measurements make it a more attractive instrument than simple random sampling. Stroh (undated) recently argued that EPI cluster sampling is still too costly; it also has other limitations. In the event of low coverage, it does not identify the administrative units (Health Areas) delivering PHC interventions adequately. Hence, in the event the EPI method detects low coverage, a second stage investigation is needed to identify problematic health units. For example, accountability analyses are sometimes performed of every health facility to detect those either under-supplied or lax in service delivery. Or the substandard region may be the target for a national immunization day (PAHO 1988). Regrettably, this second stage of activities has not yet been considered in discussions of the cost of EPI cluster sampling.

For nations with a community based PHC system, such as Costa Rica, the Health Area is the key administrative unit to evaluate (Commission on Information for Costa Rica 1988). Although EPI cluster sampling could determine the extent a geographical region was under-covered, it would not identify the Health Areas responsible for the under-coverage. Further, it would also be possible for a geographical region to exhibit adequate coverage, while leaving undetected several inadequately performing Health Areas. The reason for this possibility is intuitively clear. With the exception of the first child, none of the seven observations is selected randomly. Therefore, they are not representative of the coverage in the catchment area of any of the 30 clusters. Also, seven observations are too few to estimate coverage within any cluster with precision.

Another reason explaining why Health Areas would remain undetected is that the 30 clusters sampled, using the EPI approach, are often not selected with reference to the area of jurisdiction of particular Health Areas. The samples could include individuals from a few poor quality Health Areas and other individuals from a great number of higher quality Health Areas. In such a case, the sample will tend to be evaluated as being adequately covered for that intervention, since most individuals were from Health Areas performing at higher quality. Therefore, it is feasible for the 30 clusters to be evaluated as adequate although a number of Health Areas are performing poorly.

All sampling techniques have error, including LQAS. For EPI cluster sampling, errors of provider and consumer risks can be defined in terms of their precision at $\pm 10\%$, and the confidence level at 95% (Lemeshow et al. 1985: 479, WHO undated:3, Henderson and Sundaresan 1982). Therefore, if a cluster sample found a large region to have 70% coverage, it is 95% probable that actual coverage is within the range of 60% to 80%. Assuming that acceptable coverage was 80%, the provider could be at risk if he were to invest in improving PHC in the area which he found was 70%. He would be at risk because the region may already have 80% coverage since it is within the confidence interval of 60% to 80%. Alternatively, the consumer could be at risk were the region's PHC system not improved, since actual coverage could be as low as 60%.

LQAS has the same set of risks as EPI cluster sampling. Further, these risks depend on the same variables. The difference lies in the definition of the population being sampled and the inferences applicable to that population.

Limitations of EPI cluster sampling have been documented recently. For example, it is not particularly useful for identifying smaller administrative units where success or failure has occurred. Also, it is usually too large an undertaking for a local manager or supervisor to entertain (Lemeshow and Stroh 1989:72, Stroh, undated:3).

LQAS methodology resolves these particular problems since it can be applied either to small or large populations using a small sample size; further, minimal training is necessary. LQAS has been applied in industry by inspectors who have little skill and education (Dodge and Romig 1959). In the following chapters I will demonstrate that it can be used in developing countries by local supervisors of health workers. Prior to the field test reported in this book, that was an open question (Lemeshow and Stroh 1986).

Using LQAS

Three uses of LQAS will be discussed in this volume. All three of them involve assessing the quality of repeatedly performed activities by health workers.

The first application is used for assessing whether a health worker in a Health Area is adequately implementing child survival interventions planned by the Ministry of Health, such as whether children are receiving their first dose of polio vaccination at two months of age. This measure of susceptibility to health problems I call *service adequacy*.

The second application determines whether a targeted group in the community has been sufficiently covered with an intervention irrespective of when the individuals received it, such as the polio vaccination coverage of children under three years of age. This I refer to as *coverage*.

The third application assesses the quality of a health worker's technique in the performance of his work, such as whether he measures and plots the growth of children properly. These are only two examples of specific activities that LQAS can appraise in monitoring the growth and development of children in the community. This use of LQAS is practical for regular supervision of health workers.

LQAS sampling uses the binomial formula. The rest of this chapter explains statistical principles underlying it, and how to modify it for different applications. All of this presentation will concern LQAS as used for measuring *coverage* only. However, the principles are the same for assessing service adequacy and technique although sample sizes may change.

Assume that coverage for a Health Area is defined as "p". In a Health Area with an infinitely large population the probability "P_a" of selecting a number "a" of vaccinated individuals in a sample of size "n" is calculated as:

$$P_a = \frac{n!}{a!\,(n-a)!}\ p^a \times q^{n-a}$$

where:

p = the proportion of actual coverage in the Health Area
q = $(1-p)$
n = the sample size
a = the number of individuals in the sample who received the service
n–a = the number of individuals in the sample without the service (in LQAS this expression is often referred to as "d").

LQAS aids the investigator in choosing the sample size and the permissible value of n–a and interpreting the results. In order to use LQAS, five initial decisions must be made. Firstly, the health system manager must select the intervention to assess and, secondly, the health unit responsible for its implementation. In some decentralized health systems the unit is the Health Area. However, in some cases a regional or national unit is responsible for implementing an intervention, such as in the case of a health worker training program.

Thirdly, he must identify the target community to receive the intervention being delivered by the health unit under assessment. The community includes individuals residing in the catchment area assigned to the health unit. A Health Area often includes more than one village plus the dispersed rural population living around it.

Fourthly, the manager must define a triage system for classifying facilities whose communities are at the highest risk because they are receiving low quality services, or are at moderate risk, or are at the lowest risk because they are receiving adequate services. These different levels of the triage system can be defined in focus groups by Ministry of Health policy makers using practical criteria. A high risk community is one in which a Health Area is judged to be substandard and a priority area for improvement. This threshold has varied in the different countries where I have discussed applications of LQAS. In Costa Rica, high risk communities were those in which coverage with an intervention was 50% or less of the targeted individuals. In Bolivia, a 20% threshold was proposed by a work group. Thresholds for identifying the lowest risk communities also varied from 80% coverage in the case of Costa Rica to 50% coverage for Bolivian health units.

Fifthly, the manager must define levels of acceptable provider and consumer risk, as discussed earlier in this chapter. In the case of Costa Rica both risks were under 10%.

Following these five decisions, a series of *Operating Characteristic Curves* (OC Curves), or their corresponding probability tables, can be constructed with the binomial formula. The use of binomials, OC curves, and probability tables will be explained in this chapter. From this information the manager can select the sample size (i.e., n) and the number of uncovered individuals (e.g., without polio immunization) allowed in the LQAS sample before deciding that a Health Area has substandard coverage (i.e., d). In the following example the use of these decisions will become clear.

Assume that the Ministry of Health is assessing health facilities by the coverage of their catchment areas with specific health services. The selected health service in this case is polio vaccination. The target population defined by the Ministry of Health consists of children under three years of age. The Ministry of Health defines the upper and lower levels of the triage system as 80% and 50%. Communities with the lowest risk are those in which coverage is $\geq$80%; those with highest risk have coverage of $\leq$50%. The Ministry of Health defines acceptable provider and consumer risks as <10%.

Having made these decisions, LQAS theory will inform the manager as to the proper sample size and the decision rule for judging each catchment area as adequate or inadequate. LQAS decision rules are always used in the same manner. In any sample a certain number of observations are permitted in which a child received inadequate services. If that number is exceeded, the Health Area is classified as inadequate; otherwise it is considered to be adequate.

For example, the assessments discussed in Chapter 5 use the following LQAS design. In a sample of 28 children from the catchment area of a Health Area, if nine or fewer have not received the target service, then classify the Health Area's coverage as adequate. Using this rule, managers will identify correctly areas with $\geq$80% coverage more than 95% of the time. Conversely, they will also identify areas with $\leq$50% coverage more than 95% of the time when they judge as inadequate Health Areas in which more than 9 of the 28 children lack the service.

The binomial formula calculates probabilities of accepting Health Areas whose communities have differing levels of coverage according to the LQAS decision rule. For example, these probabilities indicate the proportion of Health Areas with different levels of coverage, ranging from 100% through 0%, that will be either correctly or incorrectly classified as having adequate coverage. The classification errors (the provider and consumer risks) are derived from these probabilities. The probability of accepting a Health Area with coverage at the lower level of the triage system, in this case 50% coverage, is the maximum amount of consumer risk. On the other hand, one minus the probability of accepting a community with coverage at the upper threshold of the triage system, in this case 80% coverage, is the provider risk.

As an example, assume a sample of 14 children and a decision rule in which three or fewer unvaccinated infants (d = 3) are permitted. Using the probabilities found in Table 4.1, one can see that a Health Area in which the community is 80% covered will be classified as adequate 70% of the time. The provider risk is 30% = 100%–70%. The consumer risk is, at most, 3% since 97% of the Health Areas with inadequate community coverage (50%) will be accurately identified.

If the decision rule is changed to permit four unvaccinated individuals in the sample, the provider risk decreases to 13%, since 87% of the Health Areas with 80% coverage will be correctly identified. However, consumer risk increases to 9% since 91% of the Health Areas with 50% coverage will be accurately classified.

When comparing the two decision rules for a sample of 14 children, the alternative of permitting, at most, four unvaccinated children is preferable since it conforms to the guidelines presented earlier. Both provider and consumer risks are approximately 10%. Another reason for choosing a decision rule of 14:4, instead of 14:3, is evident from column five of Table 4.1. The total risk is

Table 4.1 Example of the Application of the LQAS Statistics to Detect the Probability of 80% or 50% Coverage of Health Area Residents with Respect to a PHC Vaccination Program According to Sample Sizes of Health Area Residents Ranging from 8 to 28, and Numbers of Cases Not Receiving a Hypothetical Intervention Ranging from 0 to 10

Sample Size of Appropriate Residents	Number in the Sample Not Receiving the Intervention	Probability of Detecting Health Areas with 80% Coverage (a)	Probability of Detecting Health Areas with 50% Coverage (b)	Total Classification Error $(1-a)+(1-b)$
8	0	0.17	1	0.83
	1	0.50	0.96	0.54
	2	0.79	0.83	0.38 *
	3	0.94	0.64	0.42
12	0	0.07	1	0.93
	1	0.28	1	0.73
	2	0.56	0.98	0.46
	3	0.80	0.93	0.28
	4	0.93	0.81	0.27 *
	5	0.98	0.61	0.41
14	0	0.04	1	0.96
	1	0.20	1	0.80
	2	0.45	0.99	0.56
	3	0.70	0.97	0.33
	4	0.87	0.91	0.22 *
	5	0.96	0.79	0.25
19	0	0.01	1	0.99
	1	0.08	1	0.92
	2	0.24	1	0.76
	3	0.46	1	0.55
	4	0.67	0.99	0.34
	5	0.84	0.97	0.20
	6	0.93	0.92	0.15 *
	7	0.98	0.82	0.20
28	5	0.50	1	0.50
	6	0.68	1	0.32
	7	0.81	0.99	0.20
	8	0.91	0.98	0.11
	9	0.96	0.96	0.08 *
	10	0.99	0.90	0.11

All probabilities have been rounded.
Asterisks indicate the optimal decision rule for a sample size.

represented as provider risk plus consumer risk. The lowest total risk for 14:4 is .22. Both 14:3 and 14:5 exhibit higher total risks of .33 and .25, respectively.

Both the provider and consumer risk categories can be modified by altering the sample size (i.e., n), and/or the number of defectives permitted (i.e., d). For example, referring to Table 4.1 once again, if n = 12 and d = 3, 79.5% of the acceptable Health Areas and 93% of the defective ones would be accurately identified. When comparing the provider and consumer risks for samples of 12 and 14 with the same value of d, the risks change from 20.5% and 7% to 30% and 3%, respectively. All probabilities in Table 4.1 are found in the Appendix.

Provider and consumer risks should be chosen by the health policy makers who are responsible for managing the national health system. In my experience, the director general of health and the managers of ministry departments responsible for service delivery can make the most informed decisions about these risks by forming a consensus in a focus group.

If resources are scarce and the efficiency of the health area system is unknown, the management priority may be to improve only the most substandard Health Areas, and thereby ensure that scarce resources are not being directed erroneously to adequate Health Areas misclassified as inadequate. In this instance selecting a small sample size and a large d that produces a corresponding low provider risk could be an appropriate selection. For example, with n = 8, d = 3, 94% of the adequate Health Areas sampled will be detected, but at a cost of identifying only 64% of the inadequate ones.

From a public health policy standpoint it could be inappropriate to give priority to maintaining low provider risk without also considering consumer risk. Depending on the resources that are available, an argument could be made for detecting as many inadequate Health Areas as possible despite the increased risk of misclassifying adequate ones. However, health system managers pressured by shrinking budgets are often interested in keeping provider risk as low as consumer risk. For example, with n = 28, d = 5, about 100% of the inadequate Health Areas with 50% coverage would be identified, but at an unacceptable cost of misclassifying 50% of the Health Areas with 80% coverage.

The binomial formula was used to calculate the probabilities in Table 4.1 for samples ranging from 8 to 28. In each case the upper and lower thresholds of the triage system are the same (i.e., 80% or 50%).

In the above example the LQAS design is n = 12, d = 3, which results in a provider risk for Health Areas with 80% coverage of 20.5%. Therefore, 79.5% of these adequate Health Areas would be accurately identified. The calculations for obtaining these risks are explained in detail in the following sections. The probability of selecting in a Health Area zero individuals without a target service in a sample of 12 individuals in a community with 80% coverage of the population is:

$$P_a = \frac{n!}{a! \, (n-a)!} \; p^a \times q^{n-a}$$

$$P_a = \frac{12!}{12! \, (12-12)!} \; p^{12} \, q^{12-12} = (1) \; .80^{12} \times .20^0 = .0687$$

The statistical notation will be explained in the next section. The probability of selecting in this Health Area 1 person without a PHC service in the sample is:

$$P_a = \frac{12!}{11! \, (12-11)!} \; .80^{11} \times .20^{12-11}$$

$$= (12) \; .80^{11} \times .20^1 = .2062$$

The probability of selecting in this Health Area 2 persons without the intervention in the sample is:

$$P_a = (66) \; p^{10} q^{12-10} = (66) \; .80^{10} \times .20^2 = .2835$$

And, the probability of selecting in this Health Area 3 persons without the service in the sample is:

$$P_a = (220) \; p^9 \, q^{12-9} = (220) \; .80^9 \times .20^3 = .2362$$

Therefore, the probability of selecting, in a Health Area with 80% coverage, *3 or fewer persons* lacking the service in the sample is the sum of the above results:

$$(.0687 + .2062 + .2835 + .2362) = .7946 = 79.5\%$$

Similarly, the probability of selecting 2 or fewer persons without the service in the sample is:

$$(.0687 + .2062 + .2835) = .5584 = 56\%$$

These probabilities, .795 and .56, are found in Table 4.1.

The binomial formula was also applied to calculate the probability of finding 3 or fewer children without the target service in the sample of 12 taken from a Health Area with a true coverage of 50%. This calculation is:

$$(.0002 + .0029 + .0161 + .0537) = .0729 = 7\%$$

Only 7% of the time will 3 or fewer children without the intervention be found in a sample of 12. Hence, a Health Area with 50% coverage would not be classified as adequate 93% of the time (or 100% – 7%).

From these two calculations it becomes clear why adequate (80% coverage) and highly inadequate (50% coverage) Health Areas can be sorted. Because in a sample of 12 children, 3 or fewer of them will be found without the service

79.5% of the time in Health Areas with 80% coverage, when more than 3 children in the sample have not received the service, the Health Area is more likely to have substantially less than 80% coverage. Therefore, a manager can be confident in judging it as inadequately covered.

In summary, LQAS is a statistical procedure that uses cumulative probabilities calculated with the binomial formula with which a health system manager can select a sample size and a decision rule to reliably identify health providers who adequately cover their client population and those who inadequately do so. To use LQAS, the health manager must define: (1) the intervention to assess, (2) the health unit to assess, (3) the client population, (4) a three level triage system defining adequate, inadequate, and very inadequate coverage, and (5) acceptable provider and consumer risks. Item 5 is information obtained through LQAS calculations using the binomial formula. Item 4 is an essential policy decision that precedes the calculation. Items 1-3 are decisions that do not affect the LQAS application; however, they are fundamental to determining the information collected and interpreted with LQAS.

This section has only discussed communities with 80% and 50% vaccination coverage. The next section considers communities with 0% to 100% coverage.

Using Binomials in LQAS

Health system managers like other producers should be interested in estimating whether their products are consistently at or above a certain acceptable standard of quality. Although they may not expect every health service like every product to have the same high quality, they want a large proportion of them to meet their production standard. Should low quality services or goods be produced sufficiently often, the consumer could lose confidence in the manufacturer, and the product would be perceived as unreliable by both the producer and the consumer.

The producer, which in our case is the health system manager, also must accurately identify high quality production units. These are the units that do not need additional investment for maintenance. Resources directed to them are wasted since they are already functioning adequately.

Therefore, the manufacturer needs a method for determining whether a production unit is meeting production standards. A basic question is, how many items should be inspected to provide adequate monitoring of the production system? To inspect every item would be too expensive and impractical. How many items would be too few?

The binomial formula helps answer this question. Assume that a health worker is supposed to produce vaccinated children. Every so often he misses a child and produces an unvaccinated one. The local supervisor accepts the fact that the health worker is imperfect; nevertheless, he expects that at least 80% of any lot or community of children will be vaccinated. Production below that level would indicate a problem sufficiently severe to justify investigating and improving the health worker.

Assume further that a particular community is infinitely large and has exactly 80% vaccinated children, but the supervisor does not know it. This last assumption is realistic since a public health official would not know exactly how many children in his catchment area are vaccinated against polio unless each vaccination status is confirmed.

The supervisor will sample the children and determine whether the lot meets the production standard of at least 80% vaccinated coverage. In a random sample of children from this community, one would not be surprised to find unvaccinated children mixed in with vaccinated ones, since the health worker sometimes misses children. But how many unvaccinated children ought to be permitted in the sample before the supervisor decides that too many are present and that the health worker's performance should be judged as inadequate?

The binomial formula calculates the probability of selecting a certain number of unvaccinated children from a community that is composed of, say, 80% vaccinated children.

Once again, the binomial formula is:

$$P_a = \frac{n!}{a!\,(n-a)!}\ p^a \times q^{n-a}$$

where in the current example:

P_a = the probability of selecting "a" vaccinated children in a sample of "n" children

p = the production standard for vaccinated children, which in this example is 80% (i.e., the proportion of acceptable items)

q = the expected proportion of unvaccinated children ($q = 1 - p$)

n = the sample size

a = the number of vaccinated children in the sample (i.e., the acceptable performance)

$n-a$ = the number of unvaccinated children in the sample (i.e., the unacceptable performance; in LQAS this expression is referred to as "d").

One portion of the binomial formula deserves a brief discussion, namely, the expression:

$$\frac{n!}{a!\,(n-a)!}.$$

This expression is the number of permutations or possible combinations in which "a" (vaccinated children) can appear in the sample "n". For the uninitiated, factorials may be difficult to understand. Let's assume $n = 3$; therefore $n! = 3! = 3 \times 2 \times 1$.

If $n = 5$ then $n! = 5 \times 4 \times 3 \times 2 \times 1$.

If a sample of 14 children from an infinitely large community contained 14 vaccinated children, the supervisor might ask himself, what is the likelihood that the community had exactly 80% coverage? By convention when $a = n$, the expression is equal to 1. The assumption is that there is only one way in which all elements sampled can be "a". Using the binomial formula he calculates the following probability:

$$\frac{14!}{14!\,(14-14)!} \times .80^{14} \times .20^{14-14} =$$

$$.80^{14} \times .20^{14-14} = .044 \times 1 = .04.$$

Hence, a sample of 14 in which all children are vaccinated has a .04 chance of being taken from a community in which exactly 80% of the children were vaccinated.

If the sample of 14 children contained 13 vaccinated individuals, the supervisor would know that the probability of taking this sample from a community with exactly 80% vaccination coverage is:

$$\frac{14!}{13!\,(14-13)!} \times .80^{13} \times .20^{14-13} = (14)\,.055 \times .2 = .154$$

Figure 4.1 Binomial Distribution for n = 14 for Communities Ranging from 0.8 to 0.5 Vaccination Coverage

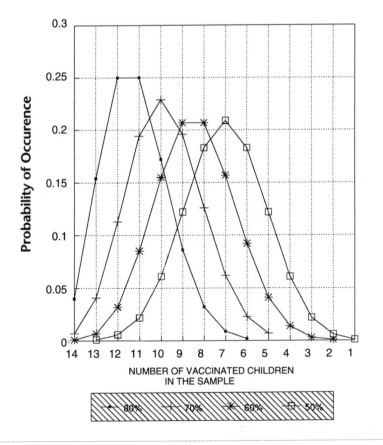

The probability of this distribution occurring in a sample from a community with 80% coverage is larger than in the preceding example, but is still quite small.

This probability is a result of the following properties of a binomial distribution: if we sample 14 children from the community with 80% coverage an infinite number of times, the mixture of vaccinated and unvaccinated children in the collection of samples will form a binomial distribution. In Figure 4.1 and Table 4.2 binomial distributions are exhibited for four communities in which the coverages are 0.8, 0.7, 0.6, and 0.5.

Table 4.2 Probabilities for Selecting Vaccinated Children in Samples of 28 and 14 from Communities Ranging from 0.8 to 0.5 Vaccination Coverage

Samples:	n=28	n=28	n=28	n=28	n=14	n=14	n=14	n=14
Proportion Vaccinated	0.8	0.7	0.6	0.5	0.8	0.7	0.6	0.5
28	0.002							
27	0.014	0.001						
26	0.046	0.003						
25	0.099	0.012	0.001					
24	0.155	0.032	0.002					
23	0.186	0.065	0.008					
22	0.178	0.107	0.020	0.002				
21	0.140	0.145	0.043	0.004				
20	0.092	0.163	0.074	0.012				
19	0.051	0.155	0.110	0.026				
18	0.024	0.126	0.140	0.048				
17	0.010	0.088	0.152	0.080				
16	0.004	0.054	0.144	0.114				
15	0.001	0.028	0.118	0.139				
14		0.013	0.084	0.150	0.044	0.007	0.001	
13		0.005	0.053	0.139	0.154	0.041	0.007	0.001
12		0.002	0.028	0.114	0.250	0.113	0.032	0.006
11		0.001	0.013	0.080	0.250	0.194	0.085	0.022
10			0.005	0.048	0.172	0.229	0.155	0.061
9			0.002	0.026	0.086	0.196	0.207	0.122
8			0.001	0.012	0.032	0.126	0.207	0.183
7				0.004	0.009	0.062	0.157	0.209
6				0.002	0.002	0.023	0.092	0.183
5						0.007	0.041	0.122
4							0.014	0.061
3							0.003	0.022
2							0.001	0.006
Totals	1.002	1.000	0.998	1.000	0.995	0.998	1.002	0.999

(Totals do not add exactly to 100% due to rounding.)

In the lot with 0.8 coverage, the most frequent selection in a sample of 14 consists of either exactly 12 or 11 vaccinated children. Any other combination occurs with progressively less frequency. Combinations of 12 or 11 vaccinated children each occur 25% of the time. Thus, the supervisor could not be sure that the children came from a community with 80% coverage since the probability of making that selection is only .25.

Many other communities with low coverage proportions also produce selections of exactly 12 or 11 vaccinated children. For example, communities with 81% or 79% coverage will also have a probability of about .25 of exhibiting either 12 or 11 vaccinated children in a sample of 14. In Figure 4.1 one can also infer that the binomial distributions for communities with 0.7, 0.6, and 0.5 coverage also include selections of 12 vaccinated children in a sample of 14, albeit the probability of such occurring is small (.113, .032, and .006, respectively). The probability of selecting 11 vaccinated children from these communities is also small (.194, .085, and .022, respectively). Although the likelihood of selecting such a combination of children from each of these communities is smaller than in the 80% lot, that combination occurs sufficiently frequently to prevent the supervisor from deciding confidently whether the community from which the 12 or 11 vaccinated children were selected had exactly 80% coverage.

This same property holds for other portions of the distribution. For example, a selection of 9 vaccinated children and 7 unvaccinated children from a lot with 80% coverage has a .086 chance of occurring. Communities with other coverage proportions, such as 70%, 60%, or 50%, have a slightly higher likelihood of producing such a combination of children, namely, .196, .207, and .122, respectively (see Figure 4.1 and Table 4.2).

Thus far, the supervisor has a small chance of deciding correctly whether or not the community from which he selected 12 vaccinated children had exactly 80% coverage. Too many other combinations could occur in a sample of 14 from a community with 80% coverage. Also, communities with other coverage proportions have a similar likelihood of having 12 vaccinated children selected from them.

How does increasing sample size affect this probability? Assume that the supervisor doubles the sample to 28 children. Figure 4.2 displays four binomial distributions for communities with 80%, 70%, 60% and 50% coverage. The probabilities used to construct these distributions are found in Table 4.3. The supervisor has the greatest likelihood of correctly identifying the community with 80% coverage should he choose exactly 23 vaccinated and 5 unvaccinated children. Although the probability is .186 that such a combination will be selected from an 80% lot, there is zero probability that the lot had only 50% coverage. It is also not very likely that the sample was taken from a community with 60% coverage (P_a = .008).

The conclusion is that although the larger sample size produces observations that distinguish 80% lots from 50% lots, the supervisor cannot be sure of his conclusions, since the probability of selecting any combination of vaccinated and unvaccinated children is very small (e.g., n = 28, vaccinated children = 23, P_a = .186).

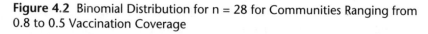

Figure 4.2 Binomial Distribution for n = 28 for Communities Ranging from 0.8 to 0.5 Vaccination Coverage

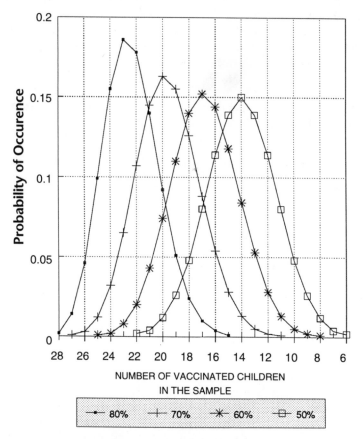

The solution to the supervisor's problem of identifying inadequate health workers is advanced by noticing that the probabilities of selecting various combinations of vaccinated and unvaccinated children from a community that has a specific coverage proportion (e.g., 80%) is binomially distributed. All the probabilities add to 1. A single probability indicates the proportion of samples from a community of a given coverage that will have a specific number of vaccinated children. LQAS does not use single probabilities, but cumulative probabilities.

Cumulative Probabilities

Table 4.3 exhibits the cumulative probabilities for the single probabilities recorded in Table 4.2. A cumulative probability is the probability that at least one of a set of events occurs in a sample.

For example, from Table 4.3, we know that the probability of 28 vaccinated children and zero unvaccinated ones being selected in a sample of 28 from a community with 80% coverage is .002. The probability of selecting 27 vaccinated children is .014. Therefore, the probability of selecting either 28 or 27 vaccinated children is .002 + .014 = .016. Since the probability of selecting 26 vaccinated children is .046, the cumulative probability of selecting 28, 27 or 26 is .002 + .014 + .046 = .062. The cumulative probability increases with the range of selection options. The cumulative probability of selecting 20 or more vaccinated children from the 80% lot is .912.

Table 4.3 Cumulative Probabilities of Selecting Indicated Numbers of Vaccinated Children for a Sample of 28

Number of Vaccinated in Sample	Coverage 80%	Cumulative Probability	Coverage 70%	Cumulative Probability	Coverage 60%	Cumulative Probability	Coverage 50%	Cumulative Probability
28	0.002	0.002						
27	0.014	0.016	0.001	0.001				
26	0.046	0.062	0.003	0.004				
25	0.099	0.161	0.012	0.016	0.001	0.001		
24	0.155	0.316	0.032	0.048	0.002	0.003		
23	0.186	0.502	0.065	0.113	0.008	0.011		
22	0.178	0.680	0.107	0.220	0.020	0.031	0.002	0.002
21	0.140	0.820	0.145	0.365	0.043	0.074	0.004	0.006
20	0.092	0.912	0.163	0.528	0.074	0.148	0.012	0.018
19	0.051	0.963	0.155	0.683	0.110	0.258	0.026	0.044
18	0.024	0.987	0.126	0.809	0.140	0.398	0.048	0.092
17	0.010	0.997	0.088	0.897	0.152	0.550	0.080	0.172
16	0.004	1.000	0.054	0.951	0.144	0.694	0.114	0.286
15	0.001		0.028	0.979	0.118	0.812	0.139	0.425
14			0.013	0.992	0.084	0.896	0.150	0.575
13			0.005	0.997	0.053	0.949	0.139	0.714
12			0.002	0.999	0.028	0.977	0.114	0.828
11			0.001	1.000	0.013	0.990	0.080	0.908
10					0.005	0.995	0.048	0.956
9					0.002	0.997	0.026	0.982
8					0.001	0.998	0.012	0.994
7							0.004	0.998
6							0.002	1.000

The cumulative probabilities for the four communities with different coverage proportions are represented in graphic form in Figure 4.3. The most distinct feature of this figure is the relative cumulative probabilities in the four distributions. For example, although a supervisor with a sample of 28 has more than a 90% chance of selecting 20 or more vaccinated children from a community with 80% coverage, he has only 1.8% chance of selecting this combination from a 50% community. Therefore, the supervisor can be confi-

Figure 4.3 Distribution of Cumulative Probabilities for n = 28

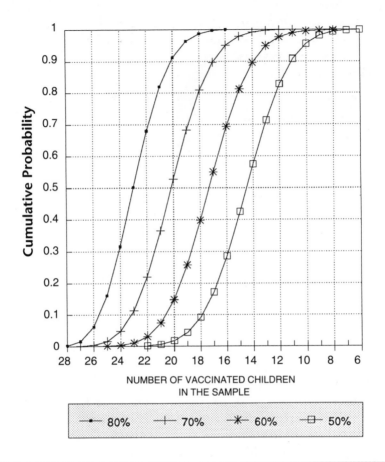

dent that the community under inspection is highly unlikely to be a 50% lot and that it is much more likely to be an 80% lot.

Discussions have thus far shown the differences between the probability of making a specific observation and the cumulative probability of making any one of a set of observations from a sample of a community with a specific coverage. From the point of view of a supervisor determining whether or not a community is of an acceptable standard, neither of these probabilities alone is sufficient. Although the supervisor would know the probability of selecting, say, at least 21 vaccinated children in a sample of 28 from an 80% vaccinated community, in fact he would not know the proportion of vaccinated children in the community; nor would he know the probability of making the same selection from a community with any other coverage level unless he inspected their vaccination distributions. The question still remains: what instrument can a supervisor use to determine efficiently whether or not the community under inspection either meets or exceeds a service delivery standard, with the only available information being the sample size and the number of inadequate products in the sample?

Operating Characteristic Curves (OC curves) provide such a method. An OC curve depicts classification errors. In order to use an OC curve an inspector must first make the following decisions:

1. What is the health service being assessed?

2. What is the production unit and the catchment area?

3. What is the production standard the production unit must reach?

4. What is the production standard below which it should not fall?

5. What is an acceptable level of classification error (or provider and consumer risks)?

Once these five decisions have been made, the supervisor then examines various OC curves for different sample sizes and for different values of "d" (the number of defective elements permitted in the sample before judging the lot as unacceptable). One would like to think that there may be a straightforward, mathematically elegant manner of selecting the sample size and "d", but such is not the case. There are always trade-offs that will have to be considered between these two factors, as well as provider and consumer risks. An exercise will be presented for selecting a sample size and a value for "d" later in this chapter.

Varying the Number of Permissible Inadequate Observations

Figure 4.4 contains a set of five OC curves. Each curve was constructed for a sample size of 28 and for a particular number of inadequately covered children permitted in the sample for the Health Area to be accepted.

The x-axis is the proportion of the target community that has not received a service. A community with 80% coverage is 20% not covered. A 40% community is 60% inadequate and so forth. The y-axis is the probability of accepting a lot as adequate for a particular sample size for a particular number of target individuals without the service. For example, the five curves in Figure 4.4 refer to different numbers of uncovered clients permitted in a sample of 28 (i.e., 0, 3, 6, 9, and 12 uncovered). Returning to the example of vaccination coverage, assume that management has decided that an adequately covered community contains not more than 20% unvaccinated children. Also, use the curve with 9 unvaccinated children permitted. In order for the supervisor to accept the lot, 9 or fewer unvaccinated children will have to be found in a sample of 28. This pattern will occur about 95% of the time in a community with 80% coverage. A 10% unvaccinated community will be classified as acceptable about 100% of the time with this rule since 9 or fewer children are almost always found in a sample of 28. From Figure 4.4 we observe that a 30% unvaccinated community lot will be classified as acceptable 68% of the time; a 50% unvaccinated community will be classified as acceptable about 5% of the time when the supervisor uses a 28:9 decision rule.

An OC curve depicts classification errors in a graphic form for communities with all different coverage proportions. If the reader were to draw an imaginary line from any point on the curve (for all lots greater than 20% inadequate coverage) down to the x-axis, the length of that line indicates the probability of misclassifying an inadequately served community as acceptable. If you draw an imaginary line from any point on the curve (for all lots with 20% or less inadequate products) upward to the horizontal line parallel to the x-axis that originates at 1.0 on the y-axis, the length of that line is the probability of misclassifying an acceptable lot as inadequate.

For example, a grid is superimposed over Figure 4.4. For an LQA sample of 28:9, six points encompassed by a square are intersected by a vertical line,

Figure 4.4 Operating Characteristic Curves for 5 Communities with Different Decision Rules for n = 28

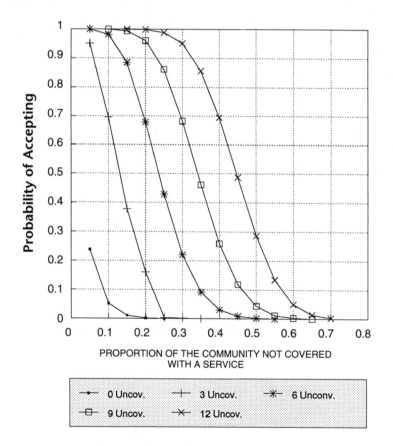

namely, proportions .1 through .6. For proportion .2, the length of the vertical line below the square is about .95; the length above the square is about .05. The former value is the probability of accepting as adequate the community with 20% of its residents uncovered by a service. The latter value is the probability of rejecting the community as being inadequately covered.

These two forms of classification errors were referred to earlier in this chapter as provider and consumer risks (i.e., the classification of acceptable lots as inadequate, and the classification of substandard lots as acceptable). These same classification errors are also referred to in some contexts as alpha and beta errors, or specificity and sensitivity, or type I and type II errors.

The magnitude of classification errors varies both with the sample size and the maximum number of individuals without the service permitted in the sample. In Figure 4.4 the sample size is held constant at 28. Using 20% not covered as the minimum acceptable quality level one can see that consumer and provider risks vary substantially with the number not covered permitted in the sample. For example, with zero defects permitted, the consumer risk is very low; all communities with more than 20% of the client population without the target service are accurately classified as unacceptable. However, the corresponding provider risk is very high; no communities with 20% of the individuals without the service (i.e., uncovered) are accurately classified as acceptable. Less than 5% of communities with 10% inadequate coverage are accurately classified as acceptable. Although the consumer is well protected, the provider risk is too high.

As the number of individuals without the service permitted in the sample increases, consumer risk increases and the provider risk decreases. To use a quality control procedure, policy makers must select:

1. the upper threshold of the triage system, which is the maximum proportion of a community that a health worker is permitted to leave uncovered with a health service (e.g., 20%, which is equivalent to 80% coverage), and an acceptable provider risk for classifying it (e.g., 10%); and

2. the lower threshold of the triage system, which is the proportion of uncovered individuals in the community that marks the point of severe health service deficiency (e.g., 50%) and an acceptable consumer risk for classifying it (i.e., 10%).

The practical reason for these decisions is that policy makers need to:

1. forego investment into improving health worker performance in areas where coverage is acceptable, and

2. invest resources into improving health service delivery where it is most deficient.

In the above example, health managers established a triage system in which the worst ($\geq$ 50% uncovered) and the best health workers (< 20% uncovered which is equivalent to coverage of $\geq$ 80%) were identified so they could either be the focus of remediation or left alone, so as not to invest capital in needless improvements.

The range of communities between 20% uncovered and 50% uncovered comprise the non-priority health workers. Figure 4.4 indicates how these middle quality systems are classified. The closer that the health worker's performance is to 80% coverage of the community (20% uncovered), the greater the probability he will be classified correctly as adequate. The closer he is to 50%, the greater the likelihood he will be classified as inadequate.

With LQAS there is no middle ground. A health worker is classified either as adequate or inadequate. Once standards are created to define the two ends of the triage system, the communities lying in the grey area in between are also judged. In whatever way these lots are classified, one can assume that the classification is appropriate. For example, Figure 4.4 exhibits an OC curve for a sample of 28 individuals and a decision rule permitting 9 individuals without the service under assessment. An 80%:50% triage system is displayed, thereby leaving the range between these two thresholds as the grey area. A 30% uncovered community will contain 9 individuals or fewer without the service about 68% of the time, and the health worker will, therefore, be judged as acceptable that frequently. This classification would not be inappropriate despite the fact that the community has less than 80% coverage, and is below the upper threshold that permits no more than 20% of the target population to not have the service. However, the community is not a priority to improve since it did not fall below 50% coverage. The same quality health worker will be classified as inadequate 32% (100%–68%) of the time. That classification also would not be inappropriate. Although the health worker is not a priority for improvement, he certainly does not meet the standard of 80% coverage. The system producing this quality lot eventually would have to be improved — either now or later. The bottom line is that the health workers of grey area lots may be classified as either acceptable or not, without much consequence. Either classification of these health workers could be argued as appropriate, since addressing their problems is not a priority.

Varying Sample Size while Holding Consumer Risk Approximately Constant

The previous section demonstrated the influences on OC curves of altering the number of individuals without the service under assessment permitted in a sample of a given size before classifying the health worker's performance as inadequate. Both alpha and beta errors (provider and consumer risks) were affected. Discussion implied that the supervisor had to find a balance between provider and consumer risks through altering the number of individuals left uncovered that he is willing to permit in a sample. That balance was obtained by selecting a "d" (number of "defectives" in the same sample), which placed both types of errors (or risks) closest to the selected standards (e.g., 5% consumer risk and 5% provider risk).

Another method of altering the shape of an OC curve is by changing the sample size and "d" simultaneously. In Figure 4.5, the four OC curves were constructed in the following manner. A desirable consumer risk for a community with 50% lacking the service was defined as 5%. Then for four different sample sizes (7, 14, 28, and 50) the number of individuals without the service permitted was selected to maintain a consumer risk of 5%. The provider risk continuously decreased with the increasing sample size. Referring to the x-axis in Figure 4.5, if 20% of the sample is inadequate, note the difference between each succeeding OC curve. At n = 7, d = 1, the provider risk is 42.3%; at n = 14, d = 4, the risk reduces to 13%. The risk is .293 less with the larger sample. At n = 28, d = 9, the provider risk is 3.9% — a reduction of about .09. The provider risk at n = 50, d = 19, is .1% — a further reduction of .03.

The decision of which of these curves is acceptable to decision makers is a function of policy concerning the desirable levels of provider risk and consumer risk and the investment into sampling that the nation wants to make. This issue will be discussed in Chapter 7 in a cost analysis of LQAS. Figure 4.5 demonstrates that the reduction of provider risk through increasing sample size is not

---

Figure 4.5   OC Curves with Consumer Risk Held Constant at about 5% to Determine Effect of Sample Size on Provider Risk

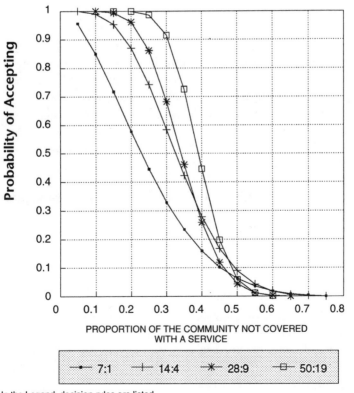

PROPORTION OF THE COMMUNITY NOT COVERED
WITH A SERVICE

| ● 7:1 | + 14:4 | ✳ 28:9 | ◻ 50:19 |

In the Legend, decision rules are listed
as "sample size : defects permitted"

linear. Doubling the sample size from 7 to 14 reduced provider risk by a factor that was three times greater than when the sample was doubled again to n = 28.

The process of selecting a sample size for LQAS and "d" is a process that involves many trade-offs between classification error and cost, between provider and consumer risks. Once the decisions are made about how large a sample to take and the size of "d", the individuals taking the sample and using the data only need to know "n" and "d". They do not need to know the details of how "n" and "d" were chosen.

Defining Provider and Consumer Risks

The supervisor for primary health care services needs a mechanism for selecting "n" and "d" that produces an optimal balance between provider and consumer risks. In order to facilitate this decision I have calculated a set of tables to create OC curves for sample sizes ranging from n = 5 to n = 50 (Appendix). These probability tables can also be used to calculate provider and consumer risks ranging from 5% through 95%. With these variations in sample size and provider/consumer risks the reader can select an optimal sample size for a given set of risks and the corresponding number of unvaccinated children or inadequate products permitted in the sample before the production system is classified as inadequate. Table 4.4 contains an abbreviated version of one set of outputs for a sample size of 28; values of "p" range from .40 to .95, instead of .05 through .95.

When the acceptable production proportion is 80%, and 9 defects are permitted in the sample of 28, the provider risk is .039 = 1 − .961; when inadequate coverage is defined as 50% the consumer risk is .044. The total risk is .083 = .039 + .044.

In my experience, the best means of identifying provider and consumer risk is to work with policy makers to identify the upper and lower ends of the triage system by selecting the minimal coverage proportion in a community they consider adequate, and the threshold of under-coverage that identifies communities at high risk due to very low coverage. Assume that the upper and lower triage thresholds are 80% and 50% coverage, respectively. Policy makers then select various sample sizes and determine which option results in the smallest total risk, misclassifies the fewest health workers, and is rapid and cost effective. As discussed earlier, they also need to identify optimal consumer and provider risks. For this example, assume two scenarios. In the first one, each maximum risk is < .05; with the second, each one is <.10.

The choices for "n" and "d" are exhibited in Table 4.5. The five columns display various sample sizes and values of "d" as well as their corresponding provider, consumer, and combined risks. For the first scenario, in which maximum provider and consumer risks are <.05 each, n = 28, d = 9 is the optimal choice. Within this sample size both risks for d = 9 are <.05, and the combined or total risk is smaller than 28:8 and 28:10. For n = 27 no value of "d" results in both risks being < .05; so it is not a viable option. When n = 29, d = 9 also pro-

Table 4.4 LQAS Table of Probabilities for Forming OC Curves and for Calculating Provider and Consumer Risks n = 28

d	Cumulative Probabilities for Values of p with d Defects										
	.40	.50	.55	.60	.65	.70	.75	.80	.85	.90	.95
0	.000	.000	.000	.000	.000	.000	.000	.002	.011	.052	.238
1	.000	.000	.000	.000	.000	.001	.003	.015	.063	.215	.588
2	.000	.000	.000	.000	.001	.004	.017	.061	.187	.459	.837
3	.000	.000	.000	.001	.004	.016	.055	.160	.377	.695	.951
4	.000	.000	.001	.003	.014	.047	.135	.315	.587	.858	.988
5	.000	.000	.003	.011	.039	.113	.264	.501	.765	.945	.998
6	.000	.002	.009	.031	.092	.220	.428	.678	.885	.982	1.000
7	.000	.006	.024	.074	.182	.365	.600	.818	.951	.995	1.000
8	.001	.018	.058	.148	.309	.528	.750	.910	.982	.999	1.000
9	.003	.044	.119	.259	.461	.682	.862	.961	.994	1.000	1.000
10.	.008	.092	.213	.399	.616	.809	.932	.985	.998	1.000	1.000
11	.022	.172	.340	.551	.753	.897	.971	.995	1.000	1.000	1.000
12	.050	.286	.487	.695	.857	.951	.989	.999	1.000	1.000	1.000
13	.102	.425	.636	.813	.926	.979	.996	1.000	1.000	1.000	1.000
14	.187	.575	.765	.898	.966	.992	.999	1.000	1.000	1.000	1.000
15	.305	.714	.865	.950	.986	.997	1.000	1.000	1.000	1.000	1.000
16	.449	.828	.930	.978	.995	.999	1.000	1.000	1.000	1.000	1.000
17	.601	.908	.969	.992	.998	1.000	1.000	1.000	1.000	1.000	1.000
18	.741	.956	.988	.997	1.000	1.000	1.000	1.000	1.000	1.000	1.000
19	.852	.982	.996	.999	1.000	1.000	1.000	1.000	1.000	1.000	1.000
20	.926	.994	.999	1.000	1.000	1.000	1.000	1.000	1.000	1.000	1.000
21	.969	.998	1.000	1.000	1.000	1.000	1.000	1.000	1.000	1.000	1.000
22	.989	1.000	1.000	1.000	1.000	1.000	1.000	1.000	1.000	1.000	1.000
23	.997	1.000	1.000	1.000	1.000	1.000	1.000	1.000	1.000	1.000	1.000
24	.999	1.000	1.000	1.000	1.000	1.000	1.000	1.000	1.000	1.000	1.000
25	1.000	1.000	1.000	1.000	1.000	1.000	1.000	1.000	1.000	1.000	1.000

duces risks of <.05 and a combined risk that is .003 less than in the 28:9 option. However, since 28:9 satisfies all policy criteria, there is no meaningful advantage to increasing the sample size to 29 and incurring additional related costs.

The provider and consumer risks in Table 4.5 were calculated from the probabilities presented in Table 4.4 and in the Appendix. For example, for n = 28, all values of risk can be derived from Table 4.4. To find consumer risks for 28:8 go to the column in which the value of coverage is .50 — the lower threshold of the triage system in this example. Locate the row for which the value of "d" is 8. The corresponding cell has a value of .018. This is the consumer risk, since in 1.8 assessments out of a 100 a supervisor will find 8 or fewer individuals without the service in a community with 50% coverage.

Provider risk is determined in the same way using the probability tables; however, with one slight modification. Firstly, locate the value of "p" corresponding to the upper threshold; in this example p = .80. In this instance, identify the cell in Table 4.4 corresponding to 28:8. The resulting value, .910, indicates that in 91 samples out of 100, 8 or fewer individuals without the service will be found in a sample of 28 taken from communities with 80% coverage. Therefore, the probability of misclassifying these adequately covered communities is 1 − .91 = .09. Nine times in 100 the provider will classify adequately covered communities as underserviced. The costs resulting from this classification error belong to the producer.

For the second scenario, in which maximum desirable producer and consumer risks are <.01, 19:6 is the optimal solution. Within n = 19, d = 6 has less combined risk than 19:5 and 19:7, and both individual risks are <.10. Also, for n = 18 no value of "d" results in risk <.10. Although 20:6 does satisfy this criterion, no meaningful advantage results by increasing costs and the sample size to 20.

Although policy makers and program managers have understood the concept of risk, they have had difficulty deciding upon their own risk levels. They almost always select provider and consumer risks in a vacuum by juggling financial and political considerations. Policymakers, and others, have been forced to formulate decisions using foreign and abstract statistical concepts with which they had no previous experience. Further, their decisions were based on probabilities without a sense of the economic and human costs associated with them. It may be very important for applications of LQAS to present policy makers with the economic costs of data collection and of provider risks relative to consumer risks that are based on empirical rather than theoretical grounds.

Another method for selecting among different LQAS designs uses the practical criterion of estimating the maximum number of misclassified health workers that result from each one. For example, assume that of 60 health workers under assessment, 30 cover 80% of their communities, and 30 cover 50%. The expected number to be misclassified is displayed in Table 4.5 as a result of the producer and consumer risks. These estimates were calculated in

Table 4.5 Examples of 18 Provider, Consumer, and Combined Risks for Six Sample Sizes and the Resulting Number of Health Workers Misclassified from the 60 Assessed: Assumption is that 30 Have Achieved 80% Coverage and 30 Have Achieved 50% Coverage

n	d	(a) Provider Risk	Misclassified Health Workers	(b) Consumer Risk	Misclassified Health Workers	a+b	Total Misclass- ified Health Workers
27	8	.074		.026		.100	
	9*	.030	1	.061	2	.091	3
	10	.011		.124		.135	
28	8	.090		.082		.172	
	9*	.039	1	.044	1	.083	2
	10	.015		.092		.107	
29	8	.012		.108		.120	
	9*	.031	1	.049	2	.080	3
	10	.068		.020		.088	
18	5	.133		.048		.181	
	6*	.051	2	.119	4	.170	6
	7	.016		.240		.256	
19	5	.163		.032		.195	
	6*	.068	2	.084	3	.152	5
	7	.023		.180		.203	
20	5	.021		.196		.217	
	6*	.058	2	.087	3	.145	5
	7	.132		.032		.164	

*Optimal value of d for a given sample size.

the following manner: For n = 28, d = 9 the producer risk is .039 and the consumer risk is .044. The expected number of misclassified health workers is: (30 x .039) + (30 x .044) = 1.17 + 1.32 = 1 + 1 = 2. Calculations of misclassified health workers are rounded to whole numbers since health workers are not divisible into fractions.

Table 4.5 further justifies selecting n = 28 since it misclassifies fewer health workers than n = 27 and misclassifies the same number as the larger sample of n = 29. For the same reasons n = 19 is preferable to n = 18 and n = 20.

The more difficult decision consists of selecting between the n = 28 and n = 19 LQAS designs. Health system managers would have to decide whether the costs of sampling 9 additional individuals in each of 60 health areas is justified by misclassifying 3 fewer health workers. These trade-offs are discussed again in Chapters 5 and 7.

Calculating Coverage Proportions and Confidence Intervals with LQAS Data

This section demonstrates procedures for calculating coverage proportions using LQAS data. Because the number of children varies from one Health Area to another, the formula requires that the results from any one Health Area be weighted by the number of children in the community of that Health Area. As an example, consider calculating the proportion of children vaccinated against polio. In Table 4.6, coverage in five hypothetical Health Areas has been assessed using a sample size of 19. Each one has already been judged using a LQAS decision rule of 19:6.

Table 4.6 An Example of Calculating a Weighted Coverage Proportion

Key: n = LQAS Sample Size
      d = Number of Unvaccinated Children Found in the Sample
      N = Number of Children in the Community

Health Area	n	d	$\frac{n-d}{n}$	N	wt.	wt. $\frac{n-d}{n}$
1	19	4	.79	150	150/660	.18
2	19	5	.74	176	176/660	.20
3	19	9	.53	123	123/660	.10
4	19	2	.89	111	111/660	.15
5	19	10	.47	100	100/660	.07
	95	30		660		.70

Coverage across several Health Areas is measured by taking the coverage in each Health Area, multiplying it by the fraction of the total population found in the Health Area, and adding this product across all Health Areas. It is not appropriate to publish or make decisions on the basis of coverage in a single Health Area (i.e., $\frac{n-d}{n}$) because in each case the proportion is not precise since it is based on a sample of only 19. The confidence interval for any Health Area is so wide as to render the proportion meaningless.

The greater precision of the coverage is due to the larger number of observations that results from combining the small LQA samples from several Health Areas. However, I should emphasize that the utility of LQAS is its ability to identify rapidly deficient health facilities within a larger area. The fact that coverage can also be precisely calculated for the whole area of several health facilities is a secondary benefit.

The calculations in Table 4.6 estimate coverage in the catchment area of these five Health Areas as 70%. The 95% confidence interval for this result would be calculated as follows:

$$CI = \pm 1.96 \times \sqrt{\sum \frac{wt._i^2 \times p_i q_i}{n_i}}$$

where:

1.96	=	z score for the 95% confidence interval
CI	=	confidence interval for a coverage proportion for a region with multiple Health Areas
wt_i	=	the weight for the ith Health Area described in Table 4.4 in which the numerator is the number of children in the Health Area and the denominator is the number of children in all of the Health Areas studied
p_i	=	the coverage proportion for the ith Health Area: $(n-d)/n$
q_i	=	$1 - p_i$
n_i	=	the sample size from the ith Health Area.

In this example the 95% confidence interval for the 70% coverage proportion is $\pm 8.9\%$. Using the preceding formula, the calculation is:

$$\pm 1.96 \sqrt{[\frac{(\frac{150}{660})^2(.79 \times .21)}{19}] + [\frac{(\frac{176}{660})^2(.74 \times .26)}{19}] + [\frac{(\frac{123}{660})^2(.53 \times .47)}{19}] + [\frac{(\frac{111}{660})^2(.89 \times .11)}{19}] + [\frac{(\frac{100}{660})^2(.47 \times .53)}{19}]}$$

$$\pm 1.96 \sqrt{.0005 + .0007 + .0005 + .0001 + .0003} = \pm 1.96 \times .046 = \pm .089.$$

This same formula can be used for calculating the confidence interval for any Health Area. The proportion for any Health Area need not be weighted since the calculations do not include any other Health Area. Using the data in Table 4.6., the confidence interval for the third Health Area is $\pm 22.4\%$, which is calculated as follows:

$$\pm 1.96 \sqrt{\frac{.53 \times (1 - .53)}{19}} = \pm 1.96 \times .115 = \pm .224$$

Since the coverage proportion is 53% within the third Health Area, true coverage with 95% level of confidence may be assumed to range from 30.6% to 75% coverage. This wide interval renders useless the proportion calculated for any single Health Area. LQAS was never intended for calculating such proportions. It uses binomials for estimating whether a coverage threshold has been reached by a single health worker.

This characteristic is both LQAS's strength and weakness. However, the argument of this volume is that the strength is impressive and the weakness unimportant. The management decisions that should be made at the local level concern determining whether a health worker's performance is adequate. Coverage proportions, in my experience, are more relevant to managers at more centralized levels of the health system. As demonstrated in this section, a single collection of LQAS information provides data that are suitable for judging a health worker's performance and for calculating coverage proportions across the catchment areas of several health workers.

The next chapter is an in-depth analysis of one thorough nation-wide application of LQAS that should help managers apply it when assessing child survival programs in any less developed nation.

The selected sample size of 28 is larger than would be used regularly in the field. For the same application a sample of 19 would be as useful. This sample size of 28, with d = 9, was selected since it was the first one that permitted both provider and consumer risks that conformed to the statistical convention of being less than 5%. The classification of health worker performance as acceptable or inadequate using this sample, therefore, forms a reference standard. The risks can be set higher than 5% in other applications of LQAS. Decision makers will have to perform the difficult task of identifying risks they can tolerate with sample sizes smaller than 28. Although all data collection procedures have risks, LQAS forces decision makers to be specific about both the risks they will undertake as providers and the risks they ask the people living in the communities served by the health system to shoulder.

In closing this chapter, I would like to summarize basic LQAS principles. One management goal of a PHC system is to monitor the care that local health units provide. For this purpose, individuals should be sampled in such a way as to make inferences possible at the level of the health care unit. LQAS can be used to judge the quality of service provided by health workers within an administrative unit, such as a Health Area. By taking the judgments of all units within a large area into consideration, it is also possible to estimate the coverage of the entire area. LQAS can be used to monitor administrative units either individually or collectively. This is an important feature. In practical terms, the PHC quality in a single Health Area's population can be measured, and the quality in several Health Areas responsible for several communities in a region can also be assessed. ✧

5

LQAS Field Methods for Assessing Child Survival Program Coverage

Costa Rica was the selected site for a comprehensive field test of LQAS. This Central American country was chosen for several practical, policy, and methodological reasons. Although the decline in infant mortality from 1972 to 1989 (72/1000 to 14/1000) is well known, no systematic assessment of the quality of the services offered to the country had been undertaken, nor had there been an examination of how well these services had been delivered. For that reason, the Minister of Health invited the Harvard School of Public Health to collaborate with the Ministry of Health to jointly carry out an assessment of the national primary health care program. From a methodology perspective, Costa Rica was an appropriate choice since it has field conditions typically found in many developing nations. Dense, wet tropical areas can be found in the East, cool mountainous areas in the Center, and dry lowlands to the West. Its decentralized health system is probably the best functioning system in the developing world. Any problems we encountered in applying LQAS in Costa Rica could occur in other countries. The following demonstration of the use of LQAS could provide a standard for applications in other developing nations.

All assessments commenced with the Health Areas, the most decentralized level of the Primary Health Care program. LQAS was used to screen Health Areas by the quality of the performance of community health workers. When used in other countries, health posts, health huts, health centers, district hospitals, or almost any other level, could be assessed. In Costa Rica, Health Areas composed the relevant level of organization. Similarly, health promoters, midwives, auxiliaries, nurses, nutritionists, technicians, or physicians could be the focus of the screening. However, in Costa Rica these health workers were not pertinent. Standards from the Ministry of Health and the World Health Organization (WHO) were used to judge the Health Areas. After these units were classified according to their adequacy, the same LQAS data were used to calculate precise coverage proportions of several interventions at both the national and regional levels.

This chapter demonstrates how to use LQAS for two of the three types of quality control presented in Chapter 1, namely, service adequacy and coverage. The distinction between these assessments is discussed in a later section of this chapter concerning vaccination programs. Due to the different operational research designs used for assessing the third category, the adequacy of Community Health Worker (CHW) technique, this latter type is presented in Chapter 6.

Quality Control of Child Survival Interventions

Budgetary limitations indicated that 60 of the 674 Health Areas could be visited. The quality of primary health care of children under three years of age and their mothers was assessed for the following services: delivery of the complete series of polio, DPT, and measles vaccinations; competent use of oral rehydration therapy; referrals of pregnant women and newborns to doctors; and, prescribed home visits by CHWs in each of the Health Areas selected. A work team led by the Director General of Health and composed of officials from the Departments of Maternal and Child Health and Primary Health Care (PHC), and the Commission on Information, defined adequate coverage as a standard of 80% or better. The lower threshold used to define priority Health Areas with inadequate service delivery was 50%. Using these upper and lower limits, and consumer and provider risks of $\leq 5\%$, a sample size of 28 children with a maximum of nine uncovered children permitted in the sample was selected as an optimal LQAS design. The upper and lower limits of the triage system (80% and 50%) were developed during a focus group discussion with a Ministry work team, and were agreed upon through a consensus.

Figure 5.1 exhibits the corresponding operating characteristic curve. I should emphasize that the sample size of 28 was chosen for this first comprehensive use of LQAS to maintain conventional alpha and beta errors of <.05 (i.e., .039 and .044, respectively). However, I would not recommend this sample size again. The 28 households in the catchment area of each Health Area required about 8.2 person days of interviewing. A sample size of 19 individuals permitting six uncovered individuals saves about 2.7 person days of work with a small increase in alpha and beta errors (.07 and .08, respectively). Assuming that exactly half of the 60 Health Areas studied have 80% and 50% coverage, a 28:9 rule will misclassify $(30 \times .039) + (30 \times .044)$ Health Areas or $1.17 + 1.32$ Health Areas; with rounding these fractions of Health Areas to integers, the misclassification is $1 + 1$ Health Areas. With a 19:6 rule, the misclassification would be $2.04 + 2.52$ Health Areas (or $2 + 3$ Health Areas with rounding). The cost of reducing the sample size 32% is a misclassification of three more Health Areas. Within Costa Rica, or presumably many developing countries, the resulting increased provider and consumer costs would be negligible, therefore, making the 19:6 rule the preferable LQAS design for a 80%:50% triage system.

Figure 5.1 Four OC Curves for Samples of 6, 19 and 28, and "d" varies from 1 to 12

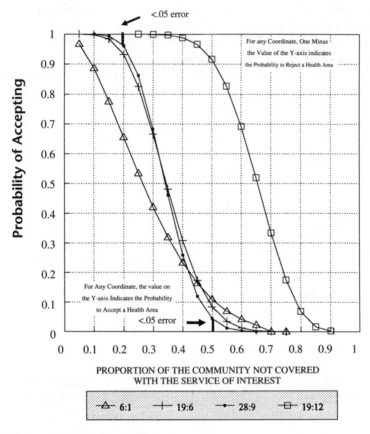

In the Legend, decision rules are listed
as "sample size : defects permitted"

During the last few years, I have worked with work groups in other Latin American countries to define triage systems with acceptable consumer and provider risks. In Bolivia, the work team, through a consensus forming meeting, selected an upper threshold of 50% coverage and a lower threshold of 20%. A sample size of 19 with 12 uncovered individuals was an appropriate LQAS design. For comparative purposes, Figure 5.1 exhibits both the 19:6 and the 19:12 LQAS designs in addition to the 28:9 design. All four of the OC curves displayed were developed using the Appendix of this book. The 6:1 design is included for comparative purposes although it will not be applied un–til Chapter 6. As explained in Chapter 4, the y-axis values for all communities consist of the probabilities in the tables found in the Appendix.

Although samples smaller than 28 are probably appropriate for most applications, the 28:9 LQAS design selected for this first comprehensive application of LQAS provided an optimal opportunity for identifying operational problems. The main reason is that it is the largest sample size that would be used regularly. Therefore, it had the greatest likelihood of exhibiting logistical and other problems. We took every opportunity to choose an LQAS design that would manifest the limitations of the method.

The following sections present field methods used and examples of results obtained from data analyses. Discussion will be detailed to permit the reader to replicate the procedures. Since the data are relatively easy to analyze once they are obtained, discussion emphasizes the problems encountered in obtaining the data in field conditions and in reporting results to health system managers. The resulting precision of the estimates of national and regional communities is presented in later sections of this chapter.

Choosing a Sample and Data Collection

A two-stage sampling design was used since all 674 Health Areas could not be included in the study. The first stage consisted of selecting 60 Health Areas from the universe of Health Areas. The second stage consisted of selecting 28 households with children under three years of age within each of the selected Health Areas. During the time of this study, the Rural Health Program and the Urban Health Programs were administered by different offices in the Ministry of Health. We therefore stratified the Health Areas accordingly. Since 48% of the Health Areas were urban and 52% were rural, we selected a sample of 29 urban Health Areas and 31 rural Health Areas.

A detailed discussion of the organization of the Costa Rican health system was presented in Chapter 1. On average, one Health Center administers nine Health Areas with a range of three to about 15 Health Areas. In general, urban Health Centers manage many more Health Areas than do rural ones. The variation in number of Health Areas under any one Health Center produced a problem.

A simple random sample of Health Areas would tend to overrepresent the largest Health Centers. Most of the sample would have been Health Centers near the largest metropolitan centers, San José and Puntarenas. They would have been overrepresented in both the rural and urban health strata since both the Rural and Community Health programs had Health Areas in both metropolitan areas. The team stratified the Health Areas to ensure that the variety of Costa Rican environmental conditions were represented in the sample drawn from each of the six health regions. Although further discussion of this stratification would not be of general interest, future users of LQAS should be aware of this problem and a general strategy for resolving it.

Some Health Areas had two CHWs rather than one. As discussed in Chapter 1, this combination most often consisted of a health assistant and an auxiliary nurse. In further discussion both assistants and auxiliaries are referred to as CHWs. The problem was as follows. The production unit is the health worker; he or she is ultimately responsible for PHC coverage; therefore, the unit of analysis had to be the CHW. However, not every CHW should have an equal probability of being included in the sample since CHWs from the same Health Area are likely to share too many characteristics. It is quite possible that PHC coverage is associated with the location of the Health Area. Those that are more remote or that have poor roads will have fewer supplies and have a more difficult time in covering their population than their counterparts living in more developed areas. Hence, the coverage of any two CHWs sharing the same Health Area could interrelate; therefore, they should not appear in the same sample. Only one CHW per Health Area should be permitted to appear in the sample.

In the end, the sample included 60 Health Areas from throughout Costa Rica, in both urban and rural conditions. In any selected Health Area with more than one CHW, a random selection determined the individual to be included in the sample.

A requirement of LQAS is that the sample, in this instance 28 children under three years and their mothers, be representative of the population of the community whose coverage is being assessed. A sampling frame therefore had to be constructed from which each child had an equal chance of being selected. A sampling frame consists of a list of the sampling elements from which the 28 children will be selected.

Since we found no satisfactory existing sampling frame in which all or most children under three years of age were already listed, one had to be constructed. Since it was not practical to develop an actual list of all Costa Rican children under three years of age, a proxy list was formed listing the houses in each catchment area. The main assumption was that the density of the children is the same as the density of housing. This assumption is reasonable for low income populations found in developing nations and covered by Primary Health Care Programs. It was also a reasonable assumption for Costa Rica. Nevertheless, this assumption should be assessed for other contexts in which LQAS will be used. The theory was that a house could be selected from the sampling frame, and if no child of the appropriate age lived there, then a systematic search would be performed to find the child who lived nearest to it. This will be discussed in more detail in the section concerning sample selection.

Existing sampling frames were inspected to determine whether they could be adapted to serve the project. These included maps from the malaria campaign, existing maps within Health Areas prepared by the CHW to identify the client population he served, maps of governmental organizations such as town planning organizations, and the maps from the 1984 census.

We rejected each as insufficient in its current state. We did not use most of the maps of the malaria campaign since they were out of date (malaria was no longer a national problem by 1987). In other countries, maps developed by the malaria campaigns could be used as sampling frames.

Handmade Health Area maps were also not used. The majority of the hand-drawn maps were out of date, and, therefore, it was highly probable that many families in target Health Areas would not be listed in them. Furthermore, the sampling frame had to be independent of the health system since the Ministry of Health intended to assess the health information system and to determine the proportion of families identified by each health worker.

Maps from local governmental organizations were not used since they had little credibility. The 1984 census maps were rejected since they were incomplete. Firstly, not all of the new housing identified by census workers had yet been transferred to the official national maps. Secondly, housing was constantly being built and, therefore, did not yet appear on the maps. Nevertheless, these maps were the best sampling frame available, so the Ministry of Health team updated them.

A similar type of assessment of alternative sampling frames should be undertaken whenever LQAS is used to assess coverage adequacy. By no means will census maps always be the best option. In most developing nations they probably will not be optimal choices. Maps from the malaria campaigns, the World Fertility Survey, and the Demographic and Health Survey will provide adequate sampling frames.

Once the 1984 census maps were selected and updated using the hand-drawn maps of census takers, a team consisting of a map maker and a permanent member of the project staff visited each of the 60 Health Areas and, with the help of the CHW, delineated the portion of the map which represented his Health

---

Figure 5.2   A Hypothetical Map Constructed into a Sampling Frame

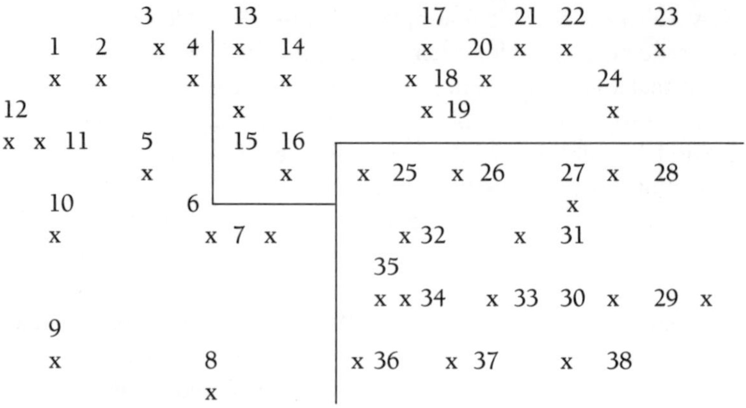

Area. The boundaries of these community areas were assessed for face validity by the CHW's supervisors. The team then updated the maps to ensure that all households, to the extent possible, were included in the maps. A combination of supplemental information sources was used for this task. Firstly, the hand-drawn maps, found in each Health Area, indicated houses visited by CHWs; some of these may have included houses that escaped census takers. Secondly, CHWs were interviewed since their maps were not always up to date. They sometimes knew a house existed although they had not entered it on their maps. Thirdly, the project team reconnoitered all 60 Health Areas to validate the map visually. New houses were added as necessary. On one occasion, a map produced by the malaria campaign near the Nicaraguan border was used since the map had been updated within the preceding month. Updating maps for all 60 Health Areas took one-and-a-half months.

After the maps were updated, they were organized into a sampling frame. Since these three steps are critical, I will explain them in detail using an example. Figure 5.2 contains a hypothetical map used in Costa Rica. We found that the political boundaries of communities rarely coincided with the catchment areas of Health Areas. Monitoring health programs could be facilitated if health planners used existing political boundaries or units of spatial division to define health unit catchment areas.

Table 5.1 Summary of Decisions Taken When Using a Sampling Frame

Map Section	Number of Houses	Cumulative Count	House Number Selected	Number of the Sampling Element
STEP 1	STEP 2	STEP 3	STEP 5*	STEP 6
1	88	88	10, 23, 37, 50, 63, 79	1 - 6
2	39	127	92, 106, 119	7 - 9
3	51	178	132, 145, 158, 172	10 - 13
4	43	221	185, 198, 211	14 - 16
5	69	290	224, 238, 251, 264, 277, 290	17 - 22
6	81	371	304, 317, 330, 343, 355, 370	23 - 28

* STEP 4 involves calculating the sampling interval.
13.25 = 371 households/28

The LQAS sampling elements were identified following an eight step procedure (Table 5.1). Firstly, the map was divided into sections using natural landmarks such as rivers, mountains, major roads or streets, and the like. In Figure 5.2, three sections of the map are indicated.

Secondly, each house within each block was counted and its number written onto the map next to the representation of the house.

Thirdly, all of the houses were counted. Although 39 houses are recorded in Figure 5.2, about 500 were found in each catchment area. For this example, we will assume the community consists of 371 households.

In step four, the sampling interval is calculated by dividing the cumulative number of houses by the sample size 28. In this example the sampling interval for the Health Area is 13.25. From here on, this calculation is expressed as a three digit whole number (132), rather than as a decimal.

A random number is selected between 1 and 132 to determine the first sampling element. The third digit is always truncated to determine the house selected. If the random number was 106, then the first house is 10. The interval 132 is added to 106 to identify the second house (132 + 106 = 238). House 23 is the next selection. The third sampling point is 37, as found through the calculation (238 + 132 = 370). Each of the other sampling elements are selected following the same procedure.

Steps five and six consist of identifying the correct house number to include in the sample, and indicating which of the 28 sampling elements it represents. It is important to maintain the fraction in the sampling interval rather than rounding. Otherwise the last interval would include less than 13 houses, thus making the houses in that interval have a higher probability of being included in the sample than the houses in any other sampling interval.

Table 5.1 summarizes the house numbers and the sampling elements which they represent. The advantage of using this summary format is that it aids the interviewer to rapidly locate the house on the map. Once the block is identified on a large map, finding a house is relatively simple.

Seventh, each house selected for the sample is identified on the map, such as by drawing a circle around it.

Eighth, since one cannot expect to find a child in the target population in every house, the sampler should devise a systematic method for identifying which houses near the sampling element to visit next. In the project several methods were tried such as choosing the house to the right, selecting subsequent houses by moving clockwise, choosing the closest door, or circling the block clockwise. None of these methods survived the pretest. Houses found in slums and rural areas are neither geometrically organized nor regular. None of these methods were usable in the field.

The most simple method to use and to verify was to mark on the map itself the order in which the houses were to be searched. This order was indicated by drawing arrows from one house to the next. This sequence always followed the order in which the houses were included in the sampling frame. Although we were not sure how many houses would have to be searched before finding one in which a child under three years of age resided, the 1984 census indicated that approximately 33% of Costa Rican families had children in this age group.

In instances in which more than one child under three years of age resided in the household, one of the children was randomly selected by the data collector with the aid of a random number table.

Alternative LQAS Designs

A census, however, is not necessary for constructing a sampling frame. Various less labor intensive alternatives exist that could be sufficient for use with LQAS. For example, consider the example of a village depicted in Figure 5.3. Although the village used in this example is organized on a grid system, the principles for sampling are applicable to villages with different types of organization. An LQAS user could organize a group of people to count the number of doors on each street. Children, or anyone who can count, or who can put a stone in a bucket for every doorway he passes, could do this task. In Figure 5.3 the number of doorways for each street is represented on the left of the grid and immediately below it. The cumulative count of households appears on the right side. In total there are 510 households in the village. Assuming an LQAS

Figure 5.3   A Village Grid with the Number of Doors Found on Each Street List on the X and Y Axes

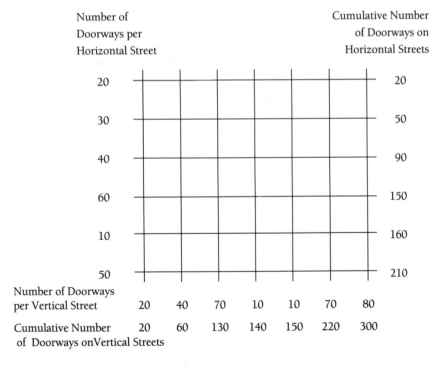

Number of Doorways per Horizontal Street		Cumulative Number of Doorways on Horizontal Streets
20		20
30		50
40		90
60		150
10		160
50		210

Number of Doorways per Vertical Street	20	40	70	10	10	70	80
Cumulative Number of Doorways on Vertical Streets	20	60	130	140	150	220	300

Total Number of Doorways on Horizontal and Vertical Streets = 200 + 310 = 510

of 19 families, the sampling fraction would be 510/19 = 27.23. With the first house being a random number between one and 27, say 13, the second house would be 40, the fifth house 67, and so forth. Should more than one family reside behind the doorway, then one could be chosen randomly. This method for constructing a sampling frame may be used in urban areas or in villages of some indigenous cultures that are organized around plazas. Alternatives would need to be considered for rural areas. Although many innovative approaches were considered by the work teams in Costa Rica and elsewhere, a full discussion of them would be beyond the scope of this section.

Another method of rapidly creating a sampling frame is useful for villages with dispersed clusters of housing in which it is difficult to use the preceding method. For purposes of discussion, I will call this method "Coordinates Sampling." The investigator measures the width and length of the village either by pacing it out or using a jeep. These measures compose the values on the x- and y-axes, as represented in Figure 5.4. Using a random number table, the investigator selects two numbers to identify each sampling element (or household). These values determine the values of the x and y coordinates. Two additional random numbers determine the sign of the coordinate values. This procedure is performed by placing a decimal in front of the random number. If the number is under .5 then the sign is positive; otherwise it is negative. The third

Figure 5.4 Coordinate Sampling Design for Villages with Dispersed Housing

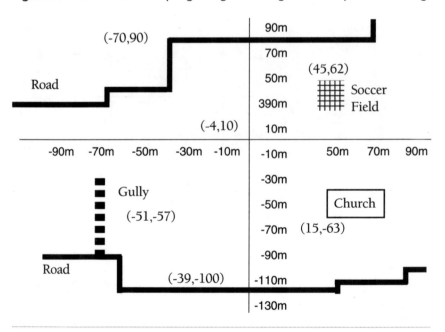

random number is the sign for the x value and the fourth one is for the y value. For each coordinate, the investigator locates the closest household. This method can be made easier if landmarks such as rivers, soccer fields, churches, roads, and the like are located on the map as points of reference. The number of coordinates should be equal to the sample size. Several random numbers are represented in Figure 5.4 to demonstrate this method.

Collecting Reliable Data

Coverage data for several interventions were collected in Costa Rica, including vaccinations, household visits, referrals of pregnant women and neonates, growth monitoring, and mothers' competency in using ORT. Whenever possible, the questionnaire relied on data recorded in the household rather than on the memory of mothers. The vaccination data were recorded in the household on vaccination cards. Household visit data were recorded on a household registry, posted on the back of the door, that the CHW signed every time he visited the house. Additional questions compared the data recorded in the households with the corresponding data noted in the Health Area's Family Health Records. For example, if the information system was working, at least its records of vaccination dates on Family Health Records and those on vaccination cards had to correspond, as would dates of the last visit to the household, and the number of individuals in the household.

All pretesting occurred in periurban areas of San José, but never in the catchment area of a Health Area selected for assessment. The main focus of the pretest was to assess whether the questions could be asked comfortably, whether they were clear to the mothers being interviewed, and whether the data could be easily recorded on questionnaire forms.

Interviewers followed the maps to locate the selected homes. If no child under the age of three was found in the indicated house, the interviewer followed the direction indicated by the arrows on the map until a household with a child in the proper age range was located.

After the mother in each of the 28 households of an area was interviewed, the questionnaires were taken to the archives of that Health Area to check correspondence of household data with the data for the same variables in the records of the Health Area. These variables included: all polio, DPT, and measles vaccination dates; the number of individuals residing in the household; the date of the last household visit; and whether the child under study was included in the Health Area's family health records.

In order to determine the reliability of the data, a separate quality control team was formed by the Director General of Health. Using the same questionnaire, the team re-interviewed slightly more than 10% of the mothers previously interviewed.

Although these reliability studies may not be feasible for other LQAS users, they are reported here to inform readers of additional procedures to improve data quality. Results of ≥90% reliability for a Health Area were considered acceptable. The data obtained for the weight and height of the children were of such a low quality that they were excluded from the study. Mothers tended not to remember when their children were weighed and measured, and CHWs tended not to record the dates they performed these activities. These data were neither reliable nor verifiable. Interventions with such wide-spread problems do not require quality control procedures to determine the need for Health Area specific improvements. National level reforms were necessary.

If the quality of any subset of questions was less than 100% for a Health Area, the supervisor of the appropriate interview team was notified. She was instructed to contact the appropriate interviewer and explain the error. The goal was to prevent the same error from being committed in subsequent interviews. Some 11 Health Areas exhibited data reliability scores less than 90%. The quality control group then returned to these 11 Health Areas to collect the appropriate data a second time. In all cases the faulty data consisted of those portions of the questionnaire in which family health records were compared with interview data.

After the data were entered twice to identify data entry errors, these same data were checked to ensure that values of all the variables were in appropriate ranges and were logical. For example, variables with values from a data set of one through five could not have a value of six in the database. Vaccination dates could not antedate a child's birth, and so forth.

The database was then sampled to measure the remaining error. A sample of 1111 observations was taken of all of the cells forming the database. The size of the universe of data points was 169,680 (N = 101 questions x 1680 questionnaires). The expected level of reliability between the questionnaire responses and the database was 97% ($\pm$1%) with a 95% level of confidence. Two errors were found, indicating .2% remaining error.

The sample size was calculated using the following standard formula recommended by the Centers for Disease Control (CDC):

$$n = \frac{t^2 pq}{d^2} = \frac{1.96^2 \times .97 \times .03}{.01^2} = 1,118$$

where n = the sample size
     t = z score for the 95% level of confidence
     p = the expected level of reliability
     q = 1 − p
     d = the precision.

The final sample size was determined by correcting the value of n for the size of the universe being sampled, N, using the following formula:

$$nf = \frac{n}{1 + \dfrac{n}{N}} = \frac{1,118}{1 + \dfrac{1,118}{169,680}} = 1,111$$

where n = the sample size with a correction for a finite population
     n = the sample size.
     N = the population size

This formula was also recommended by the CDC.

In summary, the following 11 steps were taken to field test LQAS:

1. Sixty Health Areas were randomly selected from throughout Costa Rica for the study.

2. A sampling frame based on the 1984 census was constructed and then updated by the LQAS team. Three procedures were used. Firstly, each of the 60 CHWs defined the boundary of the communities for which he was supposed to deliver PHC services. Secondly, a map maker inspected each CHW's hand-drawn map to transfer houses that appeared there but not on the census map. Thirdly, all catchment areas were reconnoitered to detect additional houses to add to the sampling frame and to verify whether houses that were on the CHWs' maps existed.

3. All houses on the updated map were numbered in order to construct a sampling frame.

4. The 28 households were systematically identified.

5. Interviewers were selected and trained.

6. Questionnaires were developed and pretested.

7. Interviewers visited the 28 randomly selected households and implemented the questionnaire.

8. The interviewers took the questionnaires to the Health Area to compare the information possessed by the mother (such as vaccination dates written on vaccination cards) with the information recorded in the Family Health Record located in the Health Area archives. They should have been identical.

9. Ten percent of all of these data were assessed for quality by a separate data collection team.

10. The data from 11 Health Areas which were less than 90% reliable were collected a second time. These data were also checked for their quality as in step 9.

11. All data were then double entered into a computerized database and edited to remove data entry errors.

A Review of the Information System

In order to interpret the results in the following section the reader must have a clear understanding of the data used to construct numerators and denominators. Therefore, I recapitulate the sources from which these data were recorded. All of these sources and their interrelations are recorded in Table 5.2. For the sake of clarity all locations from which data were obtained for analysis in a quantitative form are referred to as Data Recording Units (DRUs). DRUs were used to classify all Health Areas and to form the denominators for calculating

Table 5.2   Reference Chart of the Information Used in This Study

Services	Sources	Data Recording Units	Links and Redundancies	Numerators	Denominators
Information System	Family Health Records found in Health Areas	Family Health Records found in Health Area	Vaccination Cards Visual Verification by Interviewer	Dates Correctly Entered in Family Health Records	1680 Children and their Mothers in the Household Survey
Vaccinations	Vaccination Cards found in Homes	Vaccination Cards found in Homes	Family Health Records found in Health Areas	Vaccinated Children	1680 Children in the Household Survey
Home Visits	Household Register found in Homes	Household Register found in Homes	Family Health Records found in Health Areas	Dated Household Registers	1680 Children in the Household Survey
ORT	Mothers' Responses in their Homes	LQAS Questionnaire carried by Interviewer	None	Mothers Responding Correctly	1680 Mothers in the Household Survey
Referrals	Mothers' Responses in their Homes	LQAS Questionnaire carried by Interviewer	None	Mothers Responding Correctly	1680 Mothers in the Household Survey

proportions. This concept is used here to distinguish variables that are based on the memory of mothers versus the recording of a date or event by a CHW.

I suggest that the reader refer to this chart from time to time so as to remember that the source of all denominator information was the 1680 observations of 28 families in each of 60 Health Areas throughout Costa Rica.

Vaccination Coverage and Service Adequacy

Assessments of the vaccination interventions are presented first because they are the most complex. It is for these analyses that the distinction between measures of coverage and service adequacy will be made clear.

A *coverage* measure assesses whether an adequate proportion of children under three years have been vaccinated against five vaccine preventible communicable diseases (polio, diphtheria, pertussis, tetanus, and measles) according to a particular standard. BCG is not included in this assessment since in Costa Rica CHWs do not participate in this service. Therefore, it would be improper to classify CHWs for coverage with a service for which they are not responsible.

A *service adequacy* measure is used to assess whether the targeted individuals obtained services at the appropriate age. In this instance, the Ministry of Health considered children who were too young to receive an intervention, but did receive one, as not having been adequately served. For example, children who are one month of age should not have received polio, DPT, or measles vaccinations. If they have received one and are, therefore, presumed to be immunized, they have not been adequately served by their CHW since the likelihood that an immunization resulted is low. Also, the CHW should not vaccinate with the next dose children who have been vaccinated with polio or DPT within the past month. These are important decisions made by the CHW that district managers should monitor.

Both coverage and service adequacy measures will be discussed in turn. The main difference between them is in the construction of the numerators and denominators.

The standards by which polio and DPT vaccination coverages are assessed are based both on those promulgated by the Pan American Health Organization and the Ministry of Health. The polio and DPT service standard is three vaccinations within the first year of life with at least a one month interval between doses. We have added the additional stipulation that children vaccinated younger than 45 days would be counted as not vaccinated since the dose would have been neutralized by maternal antibodies.

The standard for measles vaccination was complicated. The Pan American Health Organization standard of vaccination between nine and 12 months of age was never used in Costa Rica. Prior to May 31, 1986, the norm was to vaccinate children after their first birthday. After that date, children were supposed to be vaccinated between six and 11 months of age. Therefore, two norms were used to assess CHWs, depending on the age of the child. As for polio and DPT, children vaccinated earlier than the norm were counted as not vaccinated.

For all three assessments of coverage only the children between 12 and 35 months of age were included since all these children should have been vaccinated. They form the denominator. Numerators consisted of children vaccinated according to the standard.

Data always consisted of dates recorded on vaccination cards. This decision was discussed with the Pan American Health Organization and the Director General of the Ministry of Health. Both concurred that vaccination card data only should be used. Studies that base conclusions on maternal recall of the number of doses their children have received (Rosero et al. 1990) are making improper assumptions about the reliability of mothers' memories. Mothers with children who have few vaccinations overestimate and those whose children have most of their vaccinations tend to underestimate (Valadez and Weld 1991).

Table 5.3   Number of Adequate and Inadequate Health Areas by Polio, DPT, and Measles Vaccination and Weighted Coverage Proportions: Assessments Performed Using World Health Organization and Ministry of Health Standards

Key: Ad. = Number of adequate areas
       Inad.= Number of inadequate areas

Vaccinations	Rural Ad.	Rural Inad.	Urban Ad.	Urban Inad.	National Ad.	National Inad.	Total	Weighted Coverage	Confidence Interval
Polio:WHO	34	5	18	3	52	8	60	82%	2%
DPT:WHO	34	5	19	2	53	7	60	82%	2%
Measles:MOH	37	2	19	2	56	4	60	83%	2%

As reported in Table 5.3, national coverage for the complete polio series was 82% ($\pm$2%). Coverage for the DPT series was also 82% ($\pm$2%). Coverage by measles vaccination was 83% ($\pm$2%). Health Areas with inadequate coverage were found in equivalent magnitudes in both rural and urban areas.

An LQAS report for Health Areas in Region Huetar Atlántica is found in Table 5.4. Three of the six Health Areas listed exhibited inadequate polio and DPT coverage, thereby indicating to local managers where to input their assistance. In this Region none of the Health Areas exhibited inadequate measles vaccination coverage.

The standards used to calculate coverage can vary depending on the manager's needs. For example, he may want to calculate coverage even if the vaccination occurred at an older age than stipulated by the standards. This proportion would indicate the children susceptible to a vaccine preventible disease and yet to be vaccinated in the Health Area. Another way to assess vaccination coverage is by each individual dose. Such an analysis would aid the manager to determine whether the breakdown in the system was dose specific. For example, if the first dose of polio or DPT was delivered when the child was already older than 10 months, the regimen could not possibly be completed

Table 5.4 Full Coverage with Polio, DPT, and Measles Vaccination Coverage in Six Health Areas According to World Health Organization and Ministry of Health Standards

Key: 0 = Adequate   1 = Inadequate

Health Areas:	3 Doses Polio	3 Doses DPT	1 Dose Measles
Region Huetar Atlántica			
Palmitas de Pococi	0	0	0
Colonia San Rafael	0	0	0
Los Angeles de Pococi	0	0	0
Penhurst de Limón	1	1	0
Barra de Parismina	1	1	0
La Bomba de Limón	1	1	0

during the first year of life. This finding would prompt the manager to improve procedures for identifying infants and for promoting with their mothers the importance of early vaccination.

Measures of vaccination **service adequacy** serve a different purpose from **coverage**. They are used to assess whether CHWs identify the appropriate services for children depending on their age. For example, a child who is too young to receive polio 1, and has not been vaccinated, has received the proper service by the CHW. A child who has received DPT 2 at 11.5 months of age, but has not yet been vaccinated with DPT 3, has been treated appropriately by the health worker if the minimum interval between doses has not lapsed. The CHW has made a proper decision even though the child will be older than one year of age by the time he receives the third dose.

The numerator for a **service adequacy** consists of children of all ages who have received proper service delivery. Adequacy was defined using the administrative norms of the Ministry of Health. According to Ministry of Health standards, all children should receive three doses of DPT vaccination, three doses of polio vaccination, and one dose of measles vaccination according to the following schedules: for DPT and polio, the first dose should be received at two months of age; the second and third doses should be received at two month intervals thereafter. These norms are slightly different from those used in the assessment of DPT and polio coverage discussed earlier since they indicate the months in which the vaccination should be given.

In all cases the numerators consist of children old enough to be vaccinated who were vaccinated during the proper age interval, and individuals too young to be vaccinated who were not vaccinated. The denominators consist of all of the children in the LQA sample who have the potential of being vaccinated. For measles, DPT 1, and polio 1, the denominators consist of all children in the LQA sample. For DPT 2 and polio 2, the denominators are all children who have received DPT 1 and polio 1. For DPT 3 and polio 3 assessments, the denominator includes all children who have received DPT 2 and polio 2.

Polio and DPT Doses

The Ministry norms were modified for the assessment since one cannot expect a dose of polio 1 or DPT 1 to be administered exactly at two months of age. One of the problems we encountered in this analysis was that the Ministry norms could not be used for monitoring the vaccination program. They were not practical. Few, if any, children are vaccinated at exactly two months of age. To overcome this deficiency the standards were modified slightly.

The modification consisted of defining a 1.5 month interval around the two month Ministry norm (-0.5 months to +1 months). The lower end of the range was defined as the minimum age at which a child should receive the first vaccination, 1.5 months of age. The upper end was defined arbitrarily by Ministry administrators who assumed that one month was a sufficiently long grace period to vaccinate a child who required one. The same interval is used for assessing the period of time between doses 1 and 2, and doses 2 and 3 of DPT and polio. Children who were within the 1.5 month interval and not yet vaccinated were counted as receiving adequate service since time still remained for the CHW to deliver the service.

This standard to assess service adequacy was considered by Ministry of Health officials to be administratively meaningful and practical. The CHW was allowed 1.5 months to deliver services. All service adequacy proportions reported have been weighted by the number of children in a given Health Area. National vaccination adequacy with polio 1 was 68% ($\pm$2%); 33 of 60 Health Areas were defective. DPT service adequacy was 68% ($\pm$2%); 31 Health Areas were substandard (see Table 5.5).

Table 5.5 Numbers of Adequate and Inadequate Health Areas by Polio and DPT Vaccinations and Weighted Service Adequacy Proportions.

Key: Ad.   = Number of adequate areas
        Inad.= Number of inadequate areas

	Rural		Urban		National		Total	Weighted Service Adequacy	Confidence Interval
	Ad	Inad.	Ad.	Inad.	Ad.	Inad.			
Polio									
1	15	24	12	9	27	33	60	68%	2%
2	24	15	18	3	42	18	60	72%	2%
3	18	21	14	7	32	28	60	68%	3%
DPT									
1	16	23	13	8	29	31	60	68%	2%
2	28	11	17	4	45	15	60	74%	2%
3	21	18	15	6	36	24	60	68%	3%

The service adequacy proportions for the first doses are different from coverage measures since both the numerator and the denominator include children under 1.5 months of age. The adequacy measures for the second doses only include children who have received the first dose. Children included in the adequacy assessment of the third dose include children who have received the second dose.

Vaccination service adequacy for DPT 2 and polio 2 was 74% (±2%) (15 Health Areas were inadequate), and 72% (±2%) (18 Health Areas were inadequate), respectively. Service adequacy for both DPT 3 and polio 3 was 68% (±3%); the corresponding number of inadequate Health Areas was 24 and 28. Further analysis of these results indicate that CHWs tended to vaccinate children for polio and DPT later than Ministry norms require.

Figure 5.5 Crude and Net Coverage Proportions with Measles Vaccination for Children According to Pre- and Post-May 1986 Ministry of Health Norms

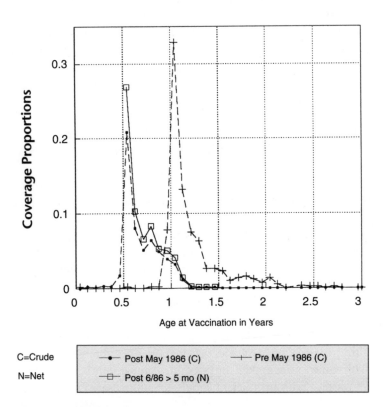

C=Crude   N=Net

Difference in Denominators:
Crude Proportions Include All Children
Net Proportion Includes Children >5 mo.

Measles

The service adequacy of measles vaccination nationally was 84% ($\pm$2%). Therefore, 16% of the population was either obtaining services too soon, too late, or not at all.

Relative to the adequacy proportions of DPT and polio vaccinations, measles vaccination service adequacy was higher. This result was probably due to the fact that the pre-May 31, 1986 norm permitted a year long interval in which the child could be vaccinated. Further analyses were performed to identify whether children living under the post-May 31, 1986 norm were also receiving adequate services.

Three age distributions for measles vaccinations are given in Figure 5.5. One represents the cohort of children old enough to be vaccinated under the norm in effect prior to May 31, 1986. A second one includes children living under the norm in force after May 31, 1986. The third one is the second cohort of children excluding children under six months of age. Several characteristics of the distributions require attention.

Firstly, approximately 10% of the children of the post-May 1986 cohort were vaccinated prior to their sixth month of life and, therefore, are counted as inadequately vaccinated since there is a low chance that they were protected. Quite probably, some CHWs vaccinated against measles too early in life since they were confusing the measles vaccination norm with those of polio and DPT.

Secondly, CHWs also vaccinated about 10% of the pre-May 1986 cohorts earlier than stipulated by the norm. This pattern was also probably due to confusing measles norms with polio/DPT norms.

Thirdly, the greatest number of children were vaccinated as soon as they were eligible; the frequency diminishes sharply thereafter. Therefore, most CHWs were knowledgeable about the vaccination norm and delivered the service to a child ready to receive it.

Fourthly, about 5% of the vaccines were delivered late to both cohorts. This was probably due to the work load and logistical problems of CHWs and should be expected.

Fifthly, the relative height of the two peaks indicates that a smaller proportion of children in the post-May 1986 cohort are receiving adequate services. This tendency led the Ministry of Health to investigate current operational problems of CHWs. They found that under the newer norm 10 dose vials of vaccines were being used, whereas one dose vials had been used during the earlier norm. CHWs tended to waste substantial numbers of doses when using the 10 dose vials since they seldom could find 10 children within 24 hours in their Health Areas needing a measles vaccination. Even though these vials are ordered with some wastage taken into account, it apparently was not sufficient. Therefore, wastage with insufficient supply to compensate for the loss, is an explanation for this observation.

Quality of the Health System Information
Quality of Family Health Records

These analyses were performed to determine the quality of the information recorded in the Family Health Records of Health Areas. The results are important for two reasons. Firstly, they measure the coverage of households and of children by CHWs. Secondly, they indicate whether or not health records could act as a substitute sampling frame in subsequent applications of LQAS. If health records could be sampled instead of households, then LQAS, or any other monitoring system, would be substantially cheaper and easier to perform. The results presented in this section indicate that at the time of the study health records were not adequate substitutes for a household survey.

This assessment included two measures. Firstly, Health Areas were classified according to whether an adequate proportion of households in their target population had health records. This measure would determine whether children under three were adequately identified for service delivery.

Secondly, Health Areas were classified according to whether vaccination dates on the Family Health Records matched those recorded in vaccination cards. This assessment is broken down by type of vaccination. A detailed analysis is performed for both BCG and polio 1 vaccinations.

The main indicator of whether a household was included in the PHC system was whether it had a Family Health Record in the Health Area. In Costa Rica, health records are organized by household. Every member is recorded on a single form along with each person's health data such as the services they have received.

A typical report to health managers using LQAS data about the quality of the information system is presented in Table 5.6. The quality of six CHWs from Health Areas in Region 5, Huetar Atlantica, is recorded using binary notation. "Zero" indicates the Health Area CHW who is functioning adequately and "one" indicates inadequacy. These reports can be quickly read and interpreted to determine the quality of any Health Area as well as the relative quality across

Table 5.6 Assessment of Six Health Areas According to the Proportion of Families and Children Under Three Years Recorded in Family Health Records

Key: 1 = inadequate   0 = adequate

Health Area	Family Health Record Exists	Child from family Included in Health Record
Palmitas de Pococi	0	0
Colonia San Rafael de Pococi	0	0
Penhurst de Limón	0	0
Barra de Parismina	0	0
La Bomba de Limón	1	0

them. In this case, one CHW (Health Area La Bomba de Limón) has identified an inadequate proportion of families in his catchment area and recorded them in Family Health Records, whereas all CHWs have adequately recorded in the Family Health Records the children under three years living in the families they have identified.

Table 5.7 shows another type of LQAS report that summarizes classifications of Health Areas for all six health regions. These data are also summarized as coverage proportions with 95% confidence intervals. On a regional level the percentage of households that had ever been visited by a CHW and, therefore, had a Family Health Record, ranged from 82% (±3%) coverage to 95% (±4%) coverage. On a national level 84% (±2%) of the households had Family Health Records. Most Health Areas performed the task of coverage according to the study's norm (adequate: ≥80% of all households are included in Health Area archives; inadequate: ≤50%).

Numerators consisted of households that had a Family Health Record in the Health Area, and the denominator consisted of the LQAS random sample of households contacted during the study.

Table 5.7 Assessments of Family Health Record System: Numbers of Health Areas with Adequate and Inadequate Proportions of Their Populations with Representative Family Health Records and Coverage Proportions

Key: Ad.   = Number of Adequate Health Areas
　　　 Inad. = Number of Inadequate Health Areas

	Family Health Record Exists		Weighted Coverage	Confidence Interval	Child from LQA Sample Included in Health Record		Weighted Coverage	Confidence Interval	Children Known to Health System
	Ad.	Inad.			Ad.	Inad.			
Region 1: South Central	12	4	82%	±3%	14	2	84%	±3%	69%
Region 2: North Central	8	0	86%	±4%	8	0	90%	±4%	77%
Region 3: North Huetar	6	0	87%	±5%	6	0	90%	±4%	78%
Region 4: Chorotega	13	1	95%	±4%	12	2	98%	±3%	93%
Region 5: Huetar Atlántica	5	1	88%	±6%	6	0	94%	±5%	83%
Region 6: Brunca	10	0	88%	±7%	10	0	89%	±6%	81%
National	**54**	**6**	84%	±2%	**56**	**4**	86%	±2%	72%

Stricter criteria could have been used to assess the presence and accuracy of Family Health Records. One could argue that health records should be more than 80% accurate since they are an important source of data through which health systems are evaluated. Nevertheless, since no existing baseline information existed about the quality of the information system, the Ministry of Health used an 80%:50% standard or triage system.

The second portion of the analysis consists of determining whether children in the target population (i.e., children <3 years of age) were recorded by CHWs in the health records. The denominator consisted of households in the LQAS sample with Family Health Records. Numerators consisted of LQAS sampled households with family records in which the child selected for the study was listed.

Any child whose family had no health record was not included in the denominator. In order to assess whether CHWs were updating the existing record system by accurately recording the number of children in the households, only those children whose households were already represented in the archives could be studied. In order to judge whether Family Health Records accurately list children living in their community, we studied only those families with records.

Here we include a subset of observations from these data. The implication of including the subset of observations in this portion of the analysis is that the sample size changed for several Health Areas since fewer than 28 children had households with health records. Hence, the corresponding operating characteristic curve also changed. Assuming that the same alpha and beta errors should be minimized, alternative decision rules were formulated by inspecting diverse OC curves and by varying the sample size and the number of defectives permitted in the sample. These alternative LQAS rules, formulated with the tables included in the Appendix, are summarized in Table 5.8.

Table 5.8 Decision Rules on Maximum Number of Children Uncovered by CHWs Permitted for Varying Sample Sizes

Assuming Alpha and Beta Errors of about 5%

Sample Size	Maximum Number of Uncovered Children Permitted
28 to 27	9
26 to 24	8
23 to 22	7
21 to 19	6
18 to 16	5
15 to 14	4
13 to 11	3

Table 5.7 reports two categories of coverage among Health Areas of the six Health Regions. Firstly, households in the community with children under three years of age that have Family Health Records, and secondly, children residing in households with Family Health Records that are also listed in them and are, therefore, known to the CHW. On a regional basis between 84% ($\pm$3%) and 98% ($\pm$3%) of all children under three years of age were included in the Family Health Records. Nationally, some 86% ($\pm$2%) of all children in households with Family Health Records were represented in the health information system. Of the 60 Health Areas investigated only four were defective. Of the defective Health Areas, two are located in South Central and another two are located in Chorotega. The former is a highly urbanized area whereas the latter is highly rural.

Having analyzed the representativeness of the health record system, and the children within the record system, it is now possible to create a measure of the proportion of children in a Health Region that are included in the health records and are, therefore, known to the CHWs. This proportion can be estimated as follows:

$$\text{Child}_{FHR} = \text{HH}_{FHR} \times \text{HH}_{\text{Child/FHR}}$$

where Child_{FHR} = proportion of children in a Health Area community represented in the Family Health Records and therefore known to the Health system

HH_{FHR} = proportion of households with children that have Family Health Records

$\text{HH}_{\text{Child/FHR}}$ = proportion of these households in which children are listed in the Family Health Record.

Table 5.7 exhibits the result of this analysis. The coverage, or proportion, of children represented in the PHC information system ranged in 1987 from 68.9% to 93% on a regional basis, and was 72% nationally. Hence, any LQAS that sampled health records rather than households for PHC data would exclude, on average, 28% of the children nationally. The implication of this result is that 72% of the children of Costa Rica are covered by the national PHC program.

Quality of Vaccination Data Recorded in a Health Area's Family Health Records

Family Health Records are supposed to document accurately the vaccination dates found on the vaccination cards of their clients. Since individual clients can receive vaccinations at any facility in the health system, it is essential that these dates be accurately recorded in family records if administrators want to monitor health care status in their Health Area communities. The Family Health Records are a prime source of data for monitoring health interventions. Therefore, the Health Areas were classified according to the accuracy of vaccination dates in their health records.

All 28 observations in each Health Area were used in this analysis. The goal was to determine whether the proportion of vaccinations in each Health Area community was reflected in the information system. Numerators consisted of children whose vaccination dates appeared in the Health Area's health records. Denominators consisted of all children in the LQA sample. This proportion, therefore, indicated the proportion of vaccination dates accurately recorded in the Family Health Records. Three decision rules were followed. Firstly, for a household with a Family Health Record, vaccination information was judged to be acceptable if the vaccination date recorded in the child's vaccination card matched the date recorded in the Family Health Record. Otherwise, it was inadequate. Secondly, if a household or child did not have a Family Health Record, but the child's vaccination card indicated a vaccination, a deficiency was judged since the Family Health Record lacked that information. Thirdly, if a household or child did not have a Family Health Record and the child's vaccination card indicated no vaccination, a deficiency was not judged since the information system did not lack the recording of the event of interest.

The results aggregated on a national basis are recorded in Table 5.9. These results suggest a relationship between the prevalence of a vaccination and the number of deficiencies in the information system. For example, BCG vaccination coverage is virtually universal since 95% of births occur in hospitals. Because the vaccinations occur after birth, the vaccination dates are recorded in the vaccination card alone. The CHW subsequently records that date of vaccination in the Health Area Family Health Records. Of the 60 Health Areas observed, some 26 were judged inadequate in relation to BCG vaccination. Thus, CHWs inadequately copied the vaccination date from vaccination cards onto the Family Health Records.

The next most frequent vaccinations by CHWs are DPT 1 and polio 1. For these events 16 of 60 and 15 of 60 Health Areas were classified as inadequate, respectively. The number of inadequate Health Areas diminishes with the expected prevalence of the vaccination. For example, more Health Areas are inadequate for DPT 2 than for DPT 3 while more Health Areas are inadequate for DPT 3 than for a DPT booster. Few Health Areas were classified as inadequate for the recording of measles vaccination dates. Therefore, there were few opportunities for CHWs to make an error when recording vaccination dates. These results may, therefore, suggest that CHWs are more likely to make errors in recording information about events in which they were not personally involved. Another possibility is that the act of inscribing two dates on two different record sheets (i.e., simultaneously on a vaccination card and on a health record) produces fewer errors than transferring dates from one record to another one (i.e., from a vaccination card to a health record).

With these data, health system managers can perform additional analyses. An example is presented for BCG and polio 1 vaccination dates. The former was selected since it is a universal activity and involves the transferring of data from a vaccination card to a health record. The latter was selected since it is an activity widely performed by the CHW himself.

Table 5.9   Classifications of 60 Health Areas by the Quality of Their Vaccination Data by the Specific Vaccinations Dichotomized into Adequate and Inadequate Health Areas

Vaccination	Adequate	Inadequate
BCG	34	26
DPT 1	44	16
DPT 2	48	12
DPT 3	52	8
DPT Booster	59	1
Polio 1	45	15
Polio 2	47	13
Polio 3	51	9
Polio Booster	59	1
Measles	59	1
Measles, Rubella	52	8

Table 5.10 indicates that the proportion of accurate information about BCG ranged from 65% ($\pm$4%) to 72% ($\pm$5%) regionally. The national proportion was 65% ($\pm$1%). The proportion of accurate recording of polio 1 dates ranged from 69% ($\pm$4%) to 84% ($\pm$4%) regionally. The national proportion was 73% ($\pm$1%). These results indicate substantial error in the Costa Rican health information system, and the need for refinement prior to using Health Area records as an LQA sampling frame.

Table 5.10   Proportion of Accurate BCG and Polio 1 Dates in Health Area Archives by Health Region; Weighted Coverage and Confidence Interval

	BCG Weighted Coverage	BCG Confidence Interval	Polio 1 Weighted Coverage	Polio 1 Confidence Interval
Region 1: South Central	65%	$\pm$4%	69%	$\pm$4%
Region 2: North Central	72%	$\pm$6%	77%	$\pm$6%
Region 3: North Huetar	71%	$\pm$7%	77%	$\pm$6%
Region 4: Chorotega	72%	$\pm$5%	84%	$\pm$4%
Region 5: Huetar Atlántica	68%	$\pm$7%	75%	$\pm$7%
Region 6: Brunca	65%	$\pm$9%	80%	$\pm$9%
National	65%	$\pm$1%	73%	$\pm$1%

Despite the level of error in the Family Health Record system, if samples of archives and of households produce similar assessments of CHW performance, then health records could potentially be used as an easily accessible and inexpensive sampling frame for regular quality control of the PHC system.

During the time in which the household survey was collected, the team of researchers that resampled 10% of the household data also took an LQA sample of 28 health records from the archives of the 60 Health Areas. The conclusions of the study were that measures of national coverage were about the same using the household sample and the health record sample. However, Health Areas were classified differently. Therefore, the Family Health Records were not as accurate as the household data for judging Health Areas; however, in aggregate they were accurate for measuring national or regional coverage (Valadez and Ulrich 1989).

Following a report by the Ministry of Health's Office of Quality Control concerning these findings, the Director General of Health ordered that all CHWs update their local Health Area maps to verify vaccination card and Family Health Record entries. Therefore, many of the problems reported in this section may no longer exist.

Quality of Integrated Health Interventions

Having established that the Family Health Records of the Health Areas underrepresent Costa Rican children, and that they reflect inaccurate vaccination coverage in Health Areas, the Ministry should doubt analyses that rely on those data. This situation is probably typical of the quality of information in many nations. Assessments of Integrated Health Programs should, therefore, consider using rapid LQAS collected data. The following analysis forms a comprehensive assessment since it is based on a representative LQA sample of children under three years of age and of Health Areas throughout the entire nation. The services under assessment included: home visits by CHWs, referral of pregnancies to a physician, referral of newborns to a physician, and Oral Rehydration Therapy (knowledge, use, and preparation). LQAS reporting systems for each of these five interventions are now discussed separately. All of the coverage proportions have been weighted as described in Chapter 4, namely, by the number of children in the catchment area of a Health Area.

Home Visits

An important result that affects the interpretation of the analysis is that 44% of the houses interviewed had no Household Register. This form is supposed to be located in each household so that it can be signed during a CHW home visit or by any Ministry of Health worker, such as a supervisor or member of the malaria campaign. It is the responsibility of the CHW to ensure that every household has one. Only 22% of the homes had a Household Register and had been visited more than four months prior to the interview. Given these results, several questions arose. It is not possible to determine whether the remaining

78% of the families were not covered for any of the basic health services by their CHW or simply did not have a Household Register in which the CHW could register the visit. Apparently, there is a grave problem with this information system. Table 5.11 stratifies the findings to throw some light on this problem. Is the Household Register not used or is it that no forms are available? These questions are answered in part in Table 5.11.

Table 5.11　Proportions of Home Visits as Indicated by the Household Register; Denominators Are All Households Identified by the Survey; Numerators as Indicated under Category of Household; Pooled Data from All 60 Sampled Health Areas in 1987

Category of Household	Percent Indicated by Household Register
Visited in the last 4 months	22%
Not visited in the last 4 months	34%
Household is known to the Health Area but it does not have a Household Register	28%
Household not known to the Health Area	16%
TOTAL	100%

Using the results of the previous section, we know that of the 44% of families that do not have the register, 16% had never been identified by a CHW, while the remaining 28% did not have the register even though the household had been identified by a CHW. Therefore, while 16% of all households in the Health Areas were not receiving basic services since they were unknown to the Health Area, one cannot make any conclusions about whether the remaining 28% of all households, who did not have household registries, had received three annual CHW visits for service delivery. As discussed in Chapter 3, this poor record keeping produced the internal validity problem called *instrumentation*. A result may be due to the way information is gathered and not reflect reality.

This particular dearth of information forced us to analyze the Home Visits data using the two criteria explained below. Two criteria were used instead of one, since our role as investigators was to produce alternative data analyses whenever policy guidelines were absent or sufficiently vague. This reinforces the fact that our role is to advise and assist administrators to make decisions concerning their own health system.

The first criterion was relatively liberal. Any home in which the Household Register indicated no visit during the four months preceding the interview was considered as not adequately covered by the health worker. The four month interval was selected as a decision rule since the Ministry required a minimum of three visits annually to each household. Households which did not have a

Household Register were not judged as deficient under this criterion. In other words, the CHW was "given the benefit of the doubt." National coverage by this activity was 78% (±2%). With this criterion, 13 of the 60 areas evaluated were operating below the Ministry standards.

The second criterion was conservative. For this set of Health Area classifications, any household that either had not been visited during a four month interval or that did not have a Household Register was considered deficient. The latter portion of this decision rule is justified on the grounds that it was the responsibility of the CHW to ensure that a Household Register was present in every household. The register is an essential part of the management information system since a CHW's supervisor uses it to determine whether CHW visits were being made on time. The results using this criterion were far worse. National Coverage was 34% (±5%). Fully 53 out of the 60 areas sampled were classified as inadequate.

Referral of Pregnancies and Young Children

If a mother had visited a physician at least once during the nine months of pregnancy, coverage was considered acceptable. Otherwise it was inadequate. Hence, referral is being judged operationally by whether a consultation resulted. Whether a message was conveyed by the CHW to the mother that she should visit a physician is less important than whether the women for whom the CHW was responsible actually visited a physician during their pregnancies. Numerators consist of all mothers who visited a physician at least once during their pregnancies. Denominators consisted of all mothers in the LQA sample.

Some 93% (±1%) of all pregnant women consulted a physician. In addition, not one of the 60 Health Areas analyzed were deficient in this service (Table 5.12).

Two standards were used to assess referral of young children. Standard 1 assesses referral during the neonate period. According to Pan American Health Organization standards, all infants should visit a health professional within 30 days of birth. Those who had actually visited a health professional within the first month of birth were considered as receiving adequate coverage. For this assessment numerators consisted of infants who had visited a health professional within the first 30 days of birth. Denominators consisted of all children more than 30 days of age in the LQA sample.

Standard 2 expands the interval for a consultation to the first 60 days of life. The denominators are the same as for the preceding standard although additional children are included in the numerator. Additional standards could be created depending on the interests of local managers.

By standard 1, some 52 of 60 Health Areas were inadequate. National coverage was 49% (±2%). Using standard 2, coverage increased to 67% (±2%). Of the 60 Health Areas studied, 25 were deficient.

Table 5.12   Number of Health Areas with Adequate Visits by Pregnant Women and Young Children to a Physician

Key: Ad.   = Number of Adequate Areas
      Inad.   = Number of Inadequate Areas
      Child.   = Children

Visit to a Physician	Rural Ad.	Rural Inad.	Urban Ad.	Urban Inad.	National Ad.	National Inad.	Total	Weighted Coverage	Confidence Interval
Pregnancies	39	0	21	0	60	0	60	93%	±1%
Child.<30 days	3	36	5	16	8	52	60	49%	±2%
Child.<60 days	18	21	17	4	35	25	60	67%	±2%

As is the case for all assessments, the results can be presented in reports for individual Health Areas. Table 5.13 tracks the adequacy of all referrals for local facilities in Region Huetar Atlántica located on the Atlantic Coast of Costa Rica. As is evident, the referral of young children is adequate in four of the six Health Areas during the second month of life of the child, but is universally low in quality during the neonate period. This negative result occurred in spite of the fact that all six Health Areas were visited regularly by CHWs. Therefore, the intervention intended to create incentives for mothers to bring their infants to a health professional within the first 30 days probably needs to be redesigned since the expected outcome did not take place.

Table 5.13   LQAS Report of Adequate Coverage of Six Health Areas through Home Visits by CHWs, Pregnancy Referral, and Young Children Referral

Key: 0 = Adequate
      1 = Inadequate

Health Area	Home Visits	Pregnancy Referral	Referral Children < 30 days	Referral Children ≤ 60 days
Region Huetar Atlántica:				
Palmitas de Pococi	0	0	1	1
Colonia San Rafael	0	0	1	0
Los Angeles de Pococi	0	0	1	0
Penhurst de Limón	1	0	1	0
Barra de Parismina	0	0	1	0
La Bomba de Limón	0	0	1	1
Total Inadequate	**1**	**0**	**6**	**2**

Oral Rehydration Therapy

The service adequacy was assessed using several Ministry standards. According to the Primary Health Care Program, CHWs are required to distribute packages of oral rehydration salts to all of the households in their Health Area in which children under six years of age reside. They are also supposed to educate mothers about the importance of oral rehydration therapy in the treatment and prevention of dehydration, and teach the preparation of the ORT solution.

Four indicators were used for judging CHWs. These consisted of the proportion of mothers who were knowledgeable about the existence of oral rehydration salt envelopes; the proportion of them who had used ORS envelopes during the child's last episode of diarrhea; the proportion who correctly recited the recipe for the "home ORT" mixture; and the proportion of mothers who correctly prepared the ORT solution using the envelope mixture. This last indicator was subdivided into three distinct judgments: whether a mother added an extra ingredient that contained salt, whether she diluted the mixture with the proper amount of water, and whether she mixed the preparation to dissolve the salts. This last indicator was measured only in one part of the country, Region Central Sur, using a separate team of two interviewers.

At the national level, 91% ($\pm$1%) of the mothers knew that ORS envelopes existed. Some 72% ($\pm$2%) had actually used these packets during their child's last case of diarrhea. However, only 3% ($\pm$1%) knew how to prepare the household solution.

None of the 60 Health Areas were defective with respect to the first indicator. Most mothers knew ORT packets existed. Some 17 Health Areas were inadequate in the use of oral rehydration therapy during their child's last diarrhea episode. All 60 were deficient in regard to the mother's knowledge of how to prepare the household mixture.

The inadequacy of mothers preparing the home mixture may be due to CHWs concentrating on the envelope preparation. The data tend to support this hypothesis. In Region Central Sur, 49% ($\pm$ 3%) of the mothers prepared the envelope mixture correctly when asked to do so by the interviewer. Seven of the 12 Health Areas were judged inadequate. The factors contributing to this inadequacy included the facts that 20% ($\pm$4%) of the mothers added a pernicious ingredient to the preparation; 40% ($\pm$3%) did not add the proper amount of water and, thereby, rendered the solution either dangerous or ineffective; and 27% ($\pm$4%) did not mix the preparation sufficiently. Some mothers committed more than one type of error when preparing the envelope mixture.

In conclusion, this chapter demonstrates how to use LQAS for assessing both the coverage and the adequacy of health services. Although the case of Costa Rica was used, the analyses and reporting forms should be applicable for most developing nations.

The next chapter concerns the use of LQAS for assessing the technical quality of service delivery by CHWs. In my experience the technical quality of service delivery is information that can be collected regularly, several times a year, by the Ministry of Health as part of its supervision system. The assessments of coverage and adequacy can be taken at longer intervals, such as every two years or longer. The pros and cons of each method will be discussed again in Chapter 8 concerning new directions for improving assessments of integrated health projects. ✧

6

Assessing Technical Quality of Service Delivery

The previous chapter discussed assessment of coverage and service adequacy in integrated health programs. As pointed out in Chapter 2, managers are often only concerned with these indicators to the extent that they do not really know whether the intervention has been properly implemented. Improperly implemented programs cannot be expected to have an impact. The 83% measles vaccination coverage of children under three years will convert into lower immunizational coverage if 20% of the time the cold chain did not function. The current chapter describes a quality control procedure based on LQAS procedures for assessing the technical competency of CHWs in service delivery. It was field tested during 1988-1990 in Costa Rica, in Guatemala during 1990, and in Trinidad during 1991. It has proven to provide rapid, precise, and useful information to local and national managers. The basic aim of the method is to identify substandard practices which might produce low quality service delivery.

The first step in the assessment involves constructing a model (as discussed in Chapter 3) of the various activities comprising the service. As an example, this chapter will consider the vaccination system only. However, during 1989-91 these methods were also used to assess other services: anthropometry, maternal education for preparation of oral rehydration therapy, and perinatal care. The information used to construct the model of the vaccination system was obtained from several sources: focus groups consisting of health workers from national and regional levels of organization, interviews of key officials at the regional and national levels, the experience of the assessment team members, and a careful review of the Ministry of Health manuals and pamphlets in circulation defining the norms and procedures for the administration of the vaccination program.

The different vaccination subsystems include: maintenance of the cold chain (i.e., refrigerators, condition of thermoses, and knowledge of how to maintain the cold chain), technical knowledge regarding the norms and procedures for administration of the vaccination system, education of mothers, quality of service delivery (i.e., hygiene, preparation of the syringe, injection technique, and disposal of the syringe), supervision, use and management of information, and availability and distribution of materials and equipment necessary for conducting the vaccination program.

In the end, the vaccination system is divided into 15 categories of essential materials or activities; these categories are referred to as subsystems. Each category or subsystem consists of one or more activities. The individual activities of a subsystem are referred to as components. In this section we will only be concerned with the eight subsystems that involve the CHWs' service delivery in the household and the preparation to do so in the Health Area and in the household (see Valadez et al. 1988 for a more complete assessment of the 15 subsystems).

Each subsystem comprises several essential tasks or components. All of them must operate correctly for the subsystem to function. For example, maintaining a cold chain requires that the temperature of the vaccine be regulated and that essential equipment, such as a refrigerator or thermos, is present and operating effectively. If any component is faulty, the cold chain fails. Therefore, all of the components included in the assessment can be thought of as steps in the critical pathway in the system. None of them are expendable. For example, the cold chain subsystem consists of three components after the CHW leaves the Health Area for the field. Firstly, the vaccine should be taken from the thermos only at the time when a child is to be vaccinated. Secondly, the top of the thermos should be kept shut except when vaccines or ice are put in or when vaccines are taken out. Thirdly, the thermos should be kept at least one third filled with ice. If any of these components fails the vaccines could be destroyed. This portion of the cold chain subsystem is modeled in Figure 6.1.

Figure 6.1 Model of a Portion of the Cold Chain Subsystem of the Vaccination System

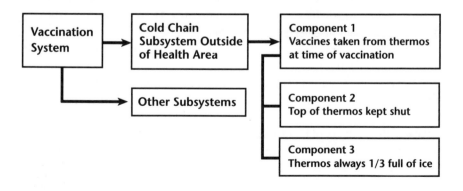

If one or more of the components is not maintained, the system is judged to be faulty. For example, Table 6.1 lists a hypothetical set of observations of six children for each of the three components of the cold chain discussed above.

Table 6.1   Observations of Six Children to Judge the Adequacy of Three Components of the Cold Chain

Key: 0 = Adequate
         1 = Inadequate

Components				Child Observed			
	1	2	3	4	5	6	Total
1	0	0	1	0	0	0	1
2	1	0	1	0	1	0	3
3	0	0	0	0	1	1	2
Totals	1	0	2	0	2	1	6

In four of the six vaccinations of children, at least one of the three components was violated. Therefore, the cold chain subsystem failed for four children, albeit for different reasons. Component 2 was violated three times, component 3 was violated twice, and component 1 was violated once. Overall, of the 18 opportunities to use the Cold Chain correctly, on six occasions errors were made. To improve the subsystem, a manager would focus on all three components, with special emphasis on the most frequently violated components.

LQAS Sampling

Assessments of technical quality have two objectives. The first one is to identify the subsystems and components which any CHW performs inadequately. The second is to determine whether any subsystem has a problem existing throughout the health system. The first problem could be addressed by the local manager of the problematic Health Area. However, a widespread problem indicates that higher level management should become involved in problem resolution since reform of the training system for CHWs would need to be planned.

Both objectives can be achieved in a two stage sampling design. In the first stage a representative sample of CHWs is selected; judgments of their subsystems are representative of conditions on a national basis. The production unit for this assessment is the Ministry of Health CHW training unit. The second stage classifies each CHW's performance as either adequate or inadequate. The production unit for this assessment is the CHW.

The first stage sampling was to be carried out as in previous applications of LQAS. The manager defines the thresholds of a triage system for identifying priorities and then selects acceptable provider and consumer risks. Following these decisions, a manager could select a sample size and the number of inadequate performances that were permitted before judging the subsystem as below standard.

The Director General of Health selected an 80%:50% triage system for this assessment. He expected that at least 80% of the CHWs would perform adequately the tasks of each subsystem. Subsystems in which 50% or fewer of the CHWs performed up to the standard were considered priorities for national reform. Since the national training unit may be deficient in their training of CHWs to perform relevant tasks.

The selection of provider and consumer risks was performed under the following constraints. The available funding for this assessment indicated that a total of 18 CHWs could be assessed nationally. The operating characteristic curve for a sample of 18 with the smallest producer and consumer risks is the one which permits five inadequate performances per subsystem or component. Any activity for which more than five CHWs were judged inadequate was considered to be a national problem. Table 6.2 exhibits the probabilities for accepting subsystems with differing levels of performance. With an 18:5 decision rule, this LQAS design will be 87% specific (provider risk 13%) in identifying adequate subsystems and 95% sensitive for identifying inadequate ones (consumer risk 5%) in an 80%:50% triage system.

Table 6.2   Probabilities for Classifying a Subsystem as Acceptable or Substandard When a Sample of 18 Unrelated Community Health Workers Is Used to Assess the Quality Nationally of CHW Service Delivery Technique: Five Defects Permitted

Quality of Subsystem	Probability to Classify a Subsystem as Acceptable	Probability to Classify a Subsystem as Substandard
.95	1.00	.0
.90	.99	.01
.85	.96	.04
.80	.87	.13
.75	.72	.28
.70	.53	.47
.65	.36	.64
.60	.21	.79
.55	.11	.89
.50	.05	.95
.45	.02	.98
.40	.01	.99
.35	.001	.99
.30	.0	1.00

The second stage sampling uses binomials to classify CHWs' performance by their adequacy. The triage system and provider and consumer risks were selected in the following way. Since the assessment of technical quality should take place as a regular supervisory activity, about one day should be budgeted for observing each CHW. It was not feasible to observe a CHW delivering services to more than six children on a single day. With this constraint, a 95%:60% triage system was selected. With one inaccurate performance in six permitted, this small sample is 97% specific in identifying adequate tasks and 77% sensitive to inadequate performance at the two thresholds of the triage system.

During the course of performing the sampling we discovered another reason for using a small sample size, namely, on any day few children require certain services, such as a vaccination. Observing a larger number of children being vaccinated is often not possible because of too few children needing the target service.

Table 6.3 Probabilities for Classifying a Health Area as Acceptable or Substandard When a Sample of Six Unrelated Children Is Used to Assess the Quality of a CHW's Work: One Defect Permitted

Quality of Subsystem	Probability to Classify a Health Area as Acceptable	Probability to Classify a Health Area as Substandard
.95	.97	.03
.90	.89	.11
.85	.78	.22
.80	.66	.34
.75	.53	.47
.70	.42	.58
.65	.32	.68
.60	.23	.77
.55	.16	.84
.50	.11	.89
.45	.07	.93
.40	.04	.96
.35	.02	.98
.30	.01	.99
.25	.005	.99
.20	.002	.99
.15	.0	1.00

The rationale for the selection of the 95%:60% triage system is as follows. Each CHW selected was judged on the basis of his performance. We assumed that any CHW had to perform his activities correctly 95% of the time for them to be classified as adequate. Performance less than that would indicate, for example, that at least five in 100 children were being vaccinated incorrectly, and thus, that the problem was too frequent. Many tasks performed at less than 95% quality are useless. For example, a cold chain that is maintained less than 95% of the time may result in damaged vaccines.

The probabilities appear in Table 6.3 from which the OC curve for this sampling design can be constructed. The lower the quality of the subsystem, the greater the probability it will be correctly classified as dysfunctional.

Selecting probabilities that exhibit higher specificity is recommended over a higher sensitivity for two reasons. Firstly, we expected to find many problems in the quality of CHW service delivery. Therefore, managers should be sure that resources were being invested into improving activities that really needed reform. Secondly, since supervision occurs on a regular basis, several times a year, the probability of twice misclassifying as adequate an activity that is performed properly 60% of the time is:

$$(1 - .77) \times (1 - .77) = .05$$

Therefore, there is only a small likelihood that a CHW who was erroneously classified as adequate for an activity during one round of supervision will be similarly misclassified during a second round. Figure 6.2 exhibits the classification error of CHWs with technical quality ranging from 5% to 75% inadequate performance. During five supervision sessions the error decreases by progressively greater amounts.

Regular supervision of health worker performance represents the largest potential use of LQAS. Health systems throughout much of the world are currently not equipped to perform this function reliably. The use of a 6:1 LQAS design addresses this need in the following way. As the following sections demonstrate, because this design is 97% specific to identifying activities that were performed adequately, supervisors can be certain of the deficiencies they have detected. However, as Figure 6.2 indicates, the cost of high specificity in this design is lower sensitivity to inadequate performance. As reported in the above discussion, LQAS is 77% sensitive to activities performed adequately 60% of the time. It is 58% sensitive to activities performed adequately 70% of the time. The worse the performance, the greater the sensitivity.

As is clear from this discussion, the cost for high specificity is lower sensitivity. In our experience, we have found that this trade-off is worthwhile. As the following sections of this chapter show, during a single round of supervision, numerous performance errors were detected. A substantial amount of work by the Ministry of Health's supervisors and continuing education unit was required to address these problems. All of these individuals agreed that because a large number of problems had been encountered, a low provider risk was desirable. The Ministry needed assurance for investing into the amelioration of these problems.

This need was met with the 6:1 LQAS design. Since the specificity was 97%, they could be sure that only a small number of false positives had occurred.

Figure 6.2 Classification Errors for 1 through 5 Supervision Sessions

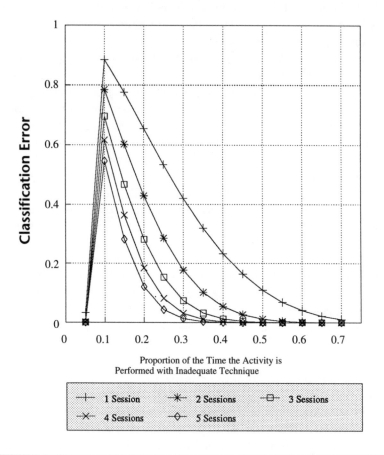

However, a larger proportion of false negatives probably did occur. Nevertheless, since supervision is performed frequently during the year, the sensitivity of the method improves during longitudinal applications. The likelihood of misclassifying the same health worker for the same task, regardless of the performance level, continuously decreases over time. Within one year most of the problem activities should be detected. Over time, through regular supervision, misclassifications should reduce to zero, as suggested by Figure 6.2.

Data Collection of Community Health Worker Technical Quality

In the example given in this chapter, data about the technical quality of service delivery were collected with four instruments. The principal source of information was an observation checklist of a CHW's service delivery in the households of six children.

Other information was collected through interviews of six mothers of children under three years of age who had been vaccinated during the previous

12 months. The goal was to find out whether the mother knew the disease against which her child had been vaccinated, if she had a vaccination card for her child, and if the child had been vaccinated at home or in another health facility, such as in a different Health Area. Health system managers also wanted to find out if the mother was aware of the number of vaccinations her child was supposed to receive. This information indicates the retention of CHW educational messages by mothers.

A third instrument obtained information for making binary or yes/no judgments. These components were not repetitive acts. Since only one observation was possible, CHWs were classified as either adequate or inadequate using the available information. This instrument was a checklist to assess the availability and condition of equipment (e.g., thermos) and material (e.g., vaccine and syringes) needed by the CHW to carry out the vaccination program. CHWs were also observed maintaining their Health Area's cold chain.

In each of the 18 randomly selected Health Areas, supervisors assessed the physical condition of equipment and supplies, and performed the required observations. The six households were chosen in the following manner.

The CHW was asked the number of localities (a unit division of land in rural areas) or manzanas (a unit division of land in urban areas) for which he was responsible. Next, a locality or manzana was randomly selected as a starting point. Six families in which children under three years of age needed a measles or DPT vaccination were identified from the health records. These families were selected as the sites to observe the quality of the CHW's service delivery. In the instances in which we could not identify at least six children needing a vaccination, an adjoining locality or manzana was selected and the same procedure already outlined was followed to identify the remaining children.

In this stage of sampling it is not necessary that the six households be randomly selected. Since the focus is to observe a CHW performing six repetitions, almost any set of households will do. Presumably, the quality of performance is associated with the CHW's competency and not with the characteristics of the family. It is worthwhile to use the above procedures for randomly selecting a first household to minimize the interference that could arise from the CHW's own preferences.

It is also worthwhile to select four additional families in addition to the six required. In many cases a selected child had already been vaccinated in the Health Center, in the Social Security clinic, in a private establishment, or in a Health Area by another CHW. At times CHWs had not entered vaccination dates into the Family Health Record although they had recorded them on the vaccination card. At other times, upon the CHW's arrival at the home of a selected family, the particular child in question was either not at home, or the family had moved away.

In addition to selecting households in which to observe the work of the CHW, we also selected another six Family Health Records in order to identify six mothers to interview. The children of these women had been vaccinated within the last 12 months.

After selecting the Family Health Records for the household visits, and after completing the interview of the CHW, the interviewer gives the Family Health Records to the CHW to prepare the household visits for the purpose of vaccinating children under three years of age.

After the CHW has prepared the vaccination equipment, the supervisor reviews the preparations for each selected family record to ensure that they are in accordance with the established norms. If established norms have been violated, the CHW is asked to explain the violation. If the justifications are valid (e.g., no vaccine was prepared for family "X" since they no longer reside in the area), the family is eliminated and another one is selected and given to the CHW. The substitution ensures that the observer has had the six observations necessary to perform the analysis.

Following this preparation the CHW begins the household visits in any order he prefers.

Judging Technical Quality

All of the following results were produced by first classifying each of the randomly selected 18 CHWs as having either adequate or inadequate performance for a particular subsystem. Then the subsystem is judged to determine whether a sufficient number of CHWs are substandard to indicate a national problem. As discussed in the previous section, a CHW fails when more than one of six observations indicates incorrect performance of a component. Some components can only be observed once since they are not repeatable (e.g., whether a sufficient number of ice packets are present in the refrigerator). In these cases an LQAS 6:1 rule is not relevant. Instead, a binary rule is used. The component either functions adequately or it does not. A component failed nationally when more than five CHWs were classified as inadequate. A subsystem is judged to be substandard if any one of its components fails to operate adequately. Several examples of vaccination subsystems are now presented for which technical quality can be assessed.

The Health Area refrigerator is an essential component of the cold chain. Three of the eleven components that compose this subsystem were inadequate. A typical report is exhibited in Table 6.4. Firstly, vaccine vials tended to be arranged too close together to permit an unobstructed flow of cool air. Secondly, ice packets and bottles of water had not been placed in refrigerators to conserve the cool temperature in the event of a power outage. Thirdly, vaccine vials had not been placed in trays nor placed in the center of the refrigerator. Therefore, they tended to be scattered in the refrigerator rather than placed in a location to preserve the appropriate temperature.

Probably the most important characteristic of this subsystem failure is that all of the inadequate components of this portion of the cold chain are preventative measures to preserve the vaccine in the event of a power shortage. The other characteristic of these inadequacies concerns the hygiene or management of the vaccines within the refrigerator. Each of these deficiencies should have

Table 6.4   Subsystem 1 of the Vaccination System

Cold Chain: Refrigerator	Number of Failed Health Areas	Substandard Component?: Yes or No
1. In good physical condition	3	No
2. Ice packets present	4	No
3. Protected from the sun	1	No
4. Located 15 cm from the wall	3	No
5. Refrigerator shelves are horizontal	2	No
6. Vaccine vials have a space of 2.5 cm or more between them	14	Yes
7. Refrigerator is used for vaccines only	4	No
8. Ice packets and bottles of water have been placed in the refrigerator to conserve the cold temperature in case of emergency	8	Yes
9. A thermometer is located in the center of the refrigerator	5	No
10. The interior refrigerator temperature was recorded both in the morning and afternoon in the center of the refrigerator	5	No
11. The vaccine vials have been placed in trays in the center of the refrigerator	9	Yes

been detected and corrected through normal supervision. The fact that they were not suggests that the supervision is not being performed adequately.

The second subsystem assessed was also a part of the cold chain and consisted of the thermos used by the CHW to transport vaccines from the Health Area to households. Three of the eight components of this subsystem, exhibited in Table 6.5, failed to be performed adequately. CHWs did not fill their thermoses with a sufficient quantity of ice. CHWs failed to secure the top of the thermos after withdrawing vaccines from it to vaccinate children. CHWs did not replenish the thermos with a sufficient quantity of ice once they were in the field.

The three problems identified in this subsystem are very important since they destroy the vaccine. As in the previous instance, the substandard components of the subsystem should have been detected and resolved through normal supervision.

The next subsystem concerns the availability of official documents or circulares in the Health Area that the CHW can use to verify vaccination norms. Five of the six components of this subsystem were not present. Several important circulares were not present: the dose specific ages at which children should be vaccinated, the time interval between doses, the vaccination technique (e.g., the portion of the body in which to insert the needle, angle of the

Table 6.5 Subsystem 2 of the Vaccination System

Cold Chain: Thermos	Number of Failed Health Areas	Substandard Component?: Yes or No
1. Thermos was in good condition	4	No
2. CHW filled the thermos one-third full with ice	6	Yes
3. Vaccines were placed in the bag in the thermos that does not contact the ice	4	No
4. CHW withdrew the vaccines directly from the refrigerator and placed them in the thermos	1	No
5. Vaccines vials were taken from the thermos only when being given to a child	2	No
6. CHW always ensured that the thermos' top was tight after removing vaccines	11	Yes
7. CHW maintained the thermos with sufficient ice	7	Yes

Table 6.6 Subsystem 3 of the Vaccination System

Documentation: Availability of the following circulares:	Number of Failed Health Areas	Substandard Component?: Yes or No
1. Age of child at vaccination	6	Yes
2. Number of doses	5	No
3. Time interval between doses	8	Yes
4. Vaccination technique	9	Yes
5. Contraindications to vaccinate	6	Yes
6. Cold chain procedures	10	Yes

needle, and the like), contraindications to vaccination, and procedures for maintaining the cold chain. Again, adequate supervision could have detected these inefficiencies. The fourth subsystem concerns education of mothers in households. All five components of this particular subsystem exhibited inadequacies.

Components two through five should have been detected through normal supervision since one responsibility of the head nurse is to observe the performance of the CHW. Inadequate performance in these components may help explain why component one was defective. It is unlikely that mothers would retain information they never possessed!

The fifth subsystem concerns appropriate use and updating of the information system by CHWs. Five technical errors were detected. The first two

Table 6.7   Subsystem 4 of the Vaccination System

Education:	Number of Failed Health Areas	Substandard Component?: Yes or No
1. Mothers remembered educational messages (the number of vaccines their children required)	18	Yes
2. CHW explained to mothers the protective advantages of vaccinating their children	15	Yes
3. CHW explained to mothers the number of doses their children should receive	14	Yes
4. CHW explained to mothers the potential reactions by their children to the vaccination	15	Yes
5. CHW questioned mothers to determine whether they had learned the above educational messages	18	Yes

problem techniques indicate that CHWs were not identifying adequately children who needed vaccinations. Therefore, CHWs may have contributed to lower than necessary vaccination coverage. Additional problems with this subsystem were that CHWs neglected to report dates on which vaccinations were given. They also did not record the vaccination date in the Family Health Record immediately after the vaccination was given. Nor did they record the vaccination date on the vaccination card immediately after the vaccination was given. Each of these problems in the information system has different implications. The failure to record the vaccinations correctly in the weekly report can lead to underestimation of national vaccination coverage.

The seventh, eighth, and ninth components can also introduce errors into the national information system. The Ministry norm is to record the vaccination date in the family record and on the vaccination card immediately after the vaccination is given. This procedure reduces the chance of the CHW forgetting to enter the information after returning to the Health Area. Another less likely reason for this norm is to prevent the CHW from recording the date of a planned vaccination and then either forgetting to vaccinate the child or being unable to do so.

These problems should also have been detected by the technical supervision. Therefore, these results point again to improving supervision as a possible solution.

A sixth subsystem concerns service delivery itself. One of four components was inconsistent with Ministry norms. As exhibited in Table 6.9, children tended to be vaccinated through other health facilities, rather than through the home outreach program. An objective of the Primary Health Care Program has been to deliver services, including vaccinations, to individuals in their homes. Since children are not receiving their vaccinations in the home, one must ask,

Table 6.8 Subsystem 5 of the Vaccination System

Information System: Use and Updating	Number of Failed Health Areas	Substandard Component?: Yes or No
1. CHW correctly identify children who are recorded in Family Health Records who need vaccinations	1	No
2. CHW reviewed children's vaccination cards to determine whether they needed vaccination	7	Yes
3. CHW correctly interpreted the information on the vaccination card	9	Yes
4. Vaccination dates in the Family Health Records and on personal vaccination cards matched	3	No
5. CHW recorded the vaccination date in the Family Health Record	1	No
6. CHW recorded the vaccination date on the vaccination card	3	No
7. CHW recorded the vaccination date in the weekly report to the Primary Health Care Program	10	Yes
8. CHW recorded the vaccination date in the Family Health Record in the household immediately after the vaccination	13	Yes
9. CHW recorded the vaccination date on the vaccination card in the household immediately after the vaccination was given	13	Yes

Table 6.9 Subsystem 6 of the Vaccination System

Service Delivery	Number of Failed Health Areas	Substandard Component?: Yes or No
1. Mothers report they have been visited by CHWs	0	No
2. Mothers possessed vaccination cards	0	No
3. Mother's child was vaccinated in the household	17	Yes
4. CHWs correctly identify children who are recorded in that Health Area who need a vaccination	1	No
5. CHWs vaccinate children once they have been identified	1	No

"Why not?" Do parents not have confidence in the ability of CHWs to provide vaccinations and, therefore, look elsewhere? Or is it that because of insufficient resources, CHWs are advising parents to take their children to health facilities to be vaccinated? Or is it that mothers are well informed and take their children voluntarily to a Health Center when they require a vaccination?

Whether these or other alternatives explain the low proportion of children vaccinated in their own households is less important than what this problematic component implies. A large proportion of the children was vaccinated outside of the household. One would expect this reaction of mothers if CHWs were unable to vaccinate children at home. Follow-up investigations or diagnosis should investigate this possibility. LQAS identified the problem; other diagnostic methods identify the underlying causes.

The next subsystem, preparation prior to vaccination, contains seven components. Three were not performed adequately. CHWs tended to contaminate the syringe or vaccine. CHWs tended to contaminate the vaccine while filling the syringe. CHWs tended neither to wash their hands nor to repack their material after using it. All of the these program implementation problems should be classified as inadequate hygiene behavior of CHWs. Further, all of them should have been prevented or corrected through normal supervision.

Table 6.10 Subsystem 7 of the Vaccination System

Quality of Service Delivery: Preparatory Activities	Number of Failed Health Areas	Substandard Component?: Yes or No
1. CHW washed his hands before vaccinating children	3	No
2. CHWs kept the vaccination materials clean	5	No
3. CHWs did not contaminate either the syringe or vaccine	10	Yes
4. CHW filled the syringe without any contamination	14	Yes
5. CHW cleaned the work area where the vaccine is to be placed	3	No
6. CHW cleaned the body area where the vaccine is to be applied according to Ministry norms	4	No
7. CHW washed his hands and repacked the material after use	10	Yes

The eighth subsystem concerns the quality of the application of the vaccination by CHWs. Two of the three components were performed inadequately. The needle was introduced into the child incorrectly. The needle was either not aspirated or the vaccine was not injected sufficiently slowly. As with many of the implementation problems presented in preceding sections, these two problematic components could have either been prevented or corrected with an adequately functioning supervision system.

Table 6.11 Subsystem 8 of the Vaccination System

Quality of Service Delivery: Application	Number of Failed Health Areas	Substandard Component?: Yes or No
1. Introduced needle at the correct angle into the correct body location	14	Yes
2. Aspirated and injected the liquid slowly	11	Yes
3. Applied pressure and withdrew the needle	3	No

These analyses have revealed several problems with service delivery existing on a local and a national level. Many of them were probably due to inadequate supervision of CHWs. LQAS methods identified them rapidly and precisely. Additional subsystems and components could have been added; others could have been eliminated depending on national priorities.

The purpose of this chapter was to demonstrate how technical quality of service delivery can be measured, judged, and reported as part of regular supervision. Although discussion focused on the vaccination system, we have applied the same principles to growth monitoring, identification and referral of pregnant woman and neonates, and detection and follow-up of malnourished children.

Having uncovered numerous problems with service delivery, it may now be clearer why the higher specificity of the 6:1 LQAS design was desirable. We can be quite certain that the problems presented above are not false positives. Although all problematic CHWs may not have been identified in this round of supervision, the likelihood that the same CHWs will be misclassified as adequate during subsequent rounds of supervision continuously diminishes.

There are potential limitations to this method for which precautions should be taken. Firstly, there are two maturation effects, as discussed in Chapter 3. CHWs that are fatigued will perform at a lower than normal quality than those who are observed while they are still fresh. However, CHWs may also need to become accustomed to being observed. Taking the observations of the condition of the Health Area and allowing the CHW to prepare himself at a normal pace will help adjust himself to the observer.

Another potential influence to consider is a Hawthorne effect of CHWs performing at a higher quality than normal because they are being judged. This effect may be irrelevant if the manager is interested in identifying widespread performance problems. If inadequate quality is detected, although the CHW thinks he is performing well, that task is a clear area for improvement. ✧

7

A Cost Analysis of LQAS

This chapter analyzes the costs of two LQAS strategies. The first one assumes that the sampling is performed by a centralized data collection team from the Ministry of Health or a national university in San José. The second alternative assumes a decentralized data collection system in which local health managers or supervisors are data collectors. As discussed in Chapter 1, on average, one supervisor is responsible for nine Health Areas.

Additional analyses estimate the costs associated with classification errors. These results address the question of what is an optimal LQA sample size. Rather than choosing a specific number, this section attempts to determine the relative costs and, hence, the relative magnitude of errors that could be permitted using economic criteria. However, all costs are expressed as dollars using a 58.8 colones/dollar exchange rate. Optimal LQA samples will thus be defined in terms of the relative weight that can be given to alpha and beta errors.

All of the costs reported were taken directly from original receipts or from cost accounting reports of the LQAS field test of 1987, which measured coverage and service adequacy. I have tried to provide as complete a listing as possible to permit readers to estimate costs of using LQAS in their own countries, although the actual amounts will vary substantially from one country to another. For this same reason the assumptions of these current analyses are presented in as much detail as possible. Costs for measuring technical quality were about 33% less.

Costs of LQAS

The LQAS field test was centrally organized in the sense that the three data collection teams were organized and directed from San José, the capital of Costa Rica. The teams set out from a base office for all 60 Health Areas distributed throughout the country to perform the sampling and then returned to this location when finished. Future applications should be decentralized when possible.

Several cost categories are summarized in Table 7.1. The values are expressed either as a level of effort of personnel or in terms of the cost of materials. Preliminary costs are associated with the initial development phase of LQAS in a country. They concern planning the base office in San José and deciding on a sampling frame. These costs were unique to the field test and would not necessarily recur in future applications. For this reason I have not transformed the level of effort information into monetary terms.

Questionnaire development comprises the second category. In addition to the time of actually formulating the questionnaire, these costs included pretesting and refining it. Not reflected in these values are the days of preparatory and nonscheduled thinking that precede the actual task of writing a questionnaire. Printing the questionnaires cost $1,707.14. In my opinion, this expense was an extravagance. Although the questionnaires were exquisitely typeset and printed, mimeographed forms would have served well enough at a fraction of the price. A six page questionnaire at $.03 per page for 1680 observations costs about $342.86. Thus, the latter cost category is included in the analyses as a recurrent cost.

The third cost category covers updating the maps at the Census Department per the discussion presented in Chapter 5.

The next portion of Table 7.1 contains the costs of training interviewers. These costs will be repeated every time LQAS is used if different interviewers have to be trained on each occasion. The decentralized sampling alternative discussed in the next section would preclude or reduce this cost for two reasons. Firstly, the same individuals, barring attrition, namely, health supervisors, would collect the data, thereby reducing the time of identifying appropriate interviewers and training them. Secondly, the logistics of data collection would be simpler since all interviewers would know their area, even perhaps the actual location of many households.

The final cost category concerns the act of identifying on the maps the houses within the catchment area of each Health Area, thus indicating the eligible households for the sample. This cost could be substantially reduced. After LQAS procedures are routinized, the consultant hired by the project would be an unnecessary expense; a project supervisor should be able to oversee the actual selection of houses by trained technicians.

The next set of information, Table 7.2, calculates the cost per household of collecting LQAS data. These costs should be considered as the recurrent costs of LQAS that a Ministry of Health should budget for this activity if the Ministry of Health uses a centrally organized team configured as it was in this project. Probably the best analog for this approach to data collection is a private voluntary organization (PVO) that is commissioned by the Ministry of Health for data collection. These costs would be higher than if members of the Ministry of Health collected the data. Two reasons support this assumption. First, salaries for similar work tend to be higher outside the Ministry of Health than inside. Secondly, fringe benefits outside the Ministry of Health are 33% of the base pay,

Table 7.1 Costs Associated with LQAS Preparatory Activities

Cost Category	Preliminary Stage Time		Instrument Development Time		Update Maps Time		Train Interviewer Time		Organize Sampling Frame	
	Weeks	Dollars	Weeks	Dollars	Weeks	Dollars	Weeks	Dollars	Weeks	Dollars
PERSONNEL:										
Principal Investigator	4.4		2.0		0.04		0.2		1	
Coprincipal	1.32		2.64		2.64		1.6		1	
Assistant 1	1.4		2.8		2.8		0.4		0	
Assistant 2	0.2				5.08		0.2		0	
Map Maker					6					
Trainer							0.25			
Consultant										2420
TRAVEL:										
Miscellaneous		79.17				198.80				
Jeep Rental						993.98				
Mileage:										
@ $.26/km						669.64	6.47			
Gas and Oil						350.00				
Per Diems						147.96				
OFFICE SUPPLIES:										
Miscellaneous		728.60						149.66		
Printing				342.86						
TOTALS	7.32	807.77	7.44	342.86	16.56	2360.38	9.12	149.66	2	2420

Dollar amounts created from Costa Rican colones used a 1987 exchange rate of 58.8 colones = $1 US.

while they are only 9% for Ministry of Health personnel. Overhead is 5% of salary and fringe benefits.

Data collection for the LQAS field test using 1680 observations took 2.11 months. Jeeps average $.26 per km to maintain. Gas and oil efficiency was 5.68 km per liter. Gas and oil costs were $.099/km. The total distance traveled by three jeeps during the course of the project was 21,424.5 km.

The 1680 LQAS questionnaires took, on average, 22.46 minutes to administer; each interviewer administered 3.4 daily.

The average cost per household for a PVO to administer LQAS when using a centralized form of organization was therefore:

$$\frac{\$32,631.26}{1680} = \$19.42.$$

Table 7.2   Costs in Dollars of Household LQAS Data Collection
$1 = 58.8 Colones

Cost Categories	Salary/Mo. Fringes Overhead Total	Travel Costs Total	Per Diems Total	Time Worked Months	People Number	Allocated Costs Dollars
Field Supervisor	380.96 125.71 25.33 532.00			2.11	1	1,122.52
Interviewers	270.73 89.34 18.00 378.07			2.11	9	7,179.55
Drivers	270.73 89.34 18.00 378.07			2.11	3	2,393.18
Team Supervisors	285.87 94.34 19.01 399.22			2.11	3	2,527.06
Group Expenses			11,562.88			11,562.88
Gas and Oil: @ $.099/km		2,121.03				2,121.03
Mileage: @$.26/km		5,570.37				5,570.37
Sick Time: 9 days						154.67
Total Costs						32,631.26

Data Collection through a Centralized Approach

These costs are lower when Ministry of Health personnel, rather than a specialized team or PVO, use LQAS. As mentioned earlier, all Ministry of Health personnel costs are average salaries that were obtained from the Ministry of Health personnel office. All salaries include 9% benefits. The assumptions for this estimation are that: the field supervisor would be a nurse-level professional from the Ministry of Health, whose average monthly salary is $383.50; the three team supervisors would be regional supervisors whose monthly salary is $259.35; and the nine interviewers would be local supervisors whose monthly salary is $245.75. Ministry of Health drivers earn $203.23 monthly.

Using Ministry of Health salaries as the base, LQAS would cost 11% less than if it were organized as a vertical program or contracted to PVOs to perform. Through this strategy the average cost per household is:

$$\frac{\$29,027.45}{1680} = \$17.28$$

Based on experience, it would be difficult to reduce the expenses any further except through negotiating salaries and per diems. Yet, since both of these are established by Ministry of Health norms, these costs should be viewed as stable.

Data Collection through a Decentralized Approach

Decentralized administration of LQAS envisages that local supervisors of the CHWs perform the LQAS sampling. Supervisors normally travel to and from a Health Area on a daily basis. No per diem expenses are incurred unless they intentionally stay in the catchment area overnight. Also, the average distance that supervisors travel to a Health Area is 30 km. The following analysis uses the following assumptions.

Firstly, a local supervisor could perform the LQAS about 33% more efficiently than the PVO interviewers since they would be more likely to know the households in which children lived. Therefore, they could perform 5.15 interviews per day. Thus, 5.44 days would be required for 28 observations in the catchment area of one Health Area.

A second assumption is that during these 5.44 days a supervisor would travel 163.06km. Also, gas costs are the same as in the centralized study. LQAS fuel costs for one Health Area are:

$$\frac{163.06 \text{ km}}{5.68 \text{ km per } \ell} \times \$.41 \text{ per } \ell = \$11.77$$

Operating a jeep costs: $.26 per km x 163.06 km = $42.40. Another assumption is that the salary of a local supervisor is about $245.75 per month, or $11.70 per day. Finally, for every 60 Health Areas, nine sick days will continue to be experienced, as in the previous analysis. This reduces to .15 days per Health Area.

Total costs for a 28 observation LQAS of one Health Area performed by a local CHW supervisor are estimated to be:

($11.77 gas) + ($42.40 jeep) + (5.44 days x $11.70 salaries) + (.15 sick days x $11.70 salaries) = $119.57.

Therefore, the cost per observation is:

$$\frac{\$119.57}{28} = \$4.27$$

per household. Thus, a decentralized data collection procedure would cost approximately 75% less than the cheapest centralized form of data collection.

Table 7.3 LQAS Data Collection Costs

Organization	Dollars per Household
Centralized: PVO	19.42
Centralized: MOH	17.28
Decentralized: MOH	4.27

These three reports contain what may be the highest costs for using LQAS. Results are summarized in Table 7.3. To each of these estimates the costs of printing questionnaires should be added. In the case of Costa Rica, this amount was $.03 per mimeographed sheet or $.18 for each six-page questionnaire. With the tables provided, readers should be able to use their own assumptions to calculate budgets pertinent to their own conditions.

Other cost savings could be realized by reducing the number of questions asked in the questionnaire. Potentially, the 22.46 minute questionnaire could be reduced to 15 minutes by asking fewer questions. About one third of the questions were included for research purposes and could be eliminated.

An Economic Assessment of Risk and its Association with Sample Size

Thus far both provider and consumer risks have been defined conceptually. This section applies economic data collected during the course of the field test to recommend sample sizes. If both provider and consumer risks are of equal importance, one could argue that the magnitude of the errors should also be similar. Such has been the assumption throughout this book. Yet, one could also argue that the magnitude of errors should be a function of the costs associated with making those errors. For example, if a consumer risk of .05 results in costs that are twice as high as those produced by a provider risk of the same magnitude, one could argue that provider risk could be increased by a factor of two in order to make it commensurate to the consumer risk.

One could also argue that consumer costs should always be lower than provider risks on the basis of ideological grounds, namely, that reducing the risk of disease to a population is inherently more important than the political and economic risks to the health system incurred by incorrectly labelling a Health Area as defective. Therefore, provider risks should be incremented by a factor to reflect this value.

This section estimates economic costs associated with both provider and consumer risks and the sample sizes that they imply. Additional discussion focuses on ideological influences on risk estimation, but this issue is of secondary importance since ideological decisions are not necessarily based on empirical analyses.

The main thrust of the next section consists of estimating both provider and consumer risks, and then expressing their relative cost as a ratio. The concluding portion of this section exhibits OC curves suggested by that ratio. Two sets of estimates are presented for both provider and consumer risks.

The first model assumes that the diagnosis and training activities are performed by Costa Rican Ministry of Health personnel. These costs were based on the salary scales of Ministry of Health personnel who would perform activities associated with provider risk. The second model assumes a developing country with poorer health conditions than those found in Costa Rica. This model is intended to help other nations select their own LQA sample sizes. The differences between the two models will become clear in the discussion.

The Costs Associated with Provider Risk:
Costa Rican Ministry of Health Model

The cost of false positives (i.e., classifying an adequate Health Area as inadequate) consists of two costs: diagnosis of a Health Area that really did not need it, and implementation of a Health Area improvement program that really did not need it. Both costs can be estimated on the basis of data already reported.

Table 7.4 shows both the diagnosis and treatment costs. Diagnosis costs consist of all expenses required to visit a Health Area and use a set of instruments that are intended to identify the problem in the Health Area with substandard PHC service delivery. The diagnosis team is centrally organized. Hence, everyone works directly for the Ministry of Health in the capital city, San José. The team consists of two diagnosticians and one driver. The diagnosticians are one nurse and one primary health care evaluator. Both of their salaries are equivalent to a nurse trainer with five years experience. The driver's salary has already been reported.

Experience has shown that a travel time of two days, on average, is required for diagnosis of a Health Area. Of these two days, only one is for a diagnosis; the other one is for travel.

The CHW normally accompanies the team during the diagnosis since observational instruments are used for data collection. It is for this reason that one full day of their salary is considered as a cost. Both the CHW's supervisor and the chief nurse of the Health Center are interviewed, which explains the one hour of their time that is attributed as a cost. Per diems are budgeted for the three person diagnosis team (i.e., two diagnosticians and one driver). Jeep and gas costs are the average daily expenditures experienced during the LQAS data collection. The printing costs refer to the 63 pages of questions used during the diagnosis of a Health Area. The total of all of these items equals $372.24.

Treatment costs refer to the costs of retraining the CHW. Thus, the main expenses are those associated with the five salary days and per diem that are typically paid during the retraining. One complete day of travel is also budgeted in terms of a jeep and gas.

Table 7.4 Estimates of Costs Associated with Provider Risks: Costs for Misclassifying One Acceptable Health Area as Defective

Cost Category	Unit Cost (Dollars)	Number of Units	Quantity	Total (Dollars)
I. DIAGNOSIS				
Per Diem	17.70	2 days	3 people	106.20
Jeep	33.11	2 days	1 jeep	66.22
Gas	12.87	2 days	1 jeep	25.74
Diagnosticians	34.86	2 days	2 people	139.44
Driver	9.24	2 days	1 person	18.48
CHW	10.55	1 day	1 person	10.55
Supervisor	11.17	1 hour	1 person	1.40
Chief Nurse	16.58	1 hour	1 person	2.07
Printing	2.14	1 packet	1	2.14
Subtotal				372.24
II. TREATMENT				
Per Diem	17.70	5 days	1 person	88.50
Jeep	33.11	1 day	1 jeep	33.11
Gas	12.87	1 day	1 jeep	12.87
Driver	9.24	1 day	1 person	9.24
CHW	10.55	5 days	1 person	52.75
Trainer	17.43	5 days	1/50th	1.74
Printing	2.14	1 packet	1	2.14
Subtotal				200.35
Total in Dollars				572.59

The development of the training course is not considered as part of the provider risk cost since the course would have to be planned even if provider risk was 0%. Of course this assumes that some Health Areas will in reality be substandard and some CHWs will require the course. Hence, developing the course is independent of the provider risk. Some of the trainer's time, however, is included in this calculation of provider risk. This cost was derived in the following way: training courses organized in Costa Rica through the Pan American Health Organization have included as many as 50 trainees. For each student, one fiftieth of the trainer's time is budgeted. The salary of a trainer is assumed to be equivalent to that of a diagnostician. Printing costs are associated with the course materials. All of the treatment costs amount to $200.35. The diagnosis and treatment costs total $572.59.

These costs could be reduced if the diagnosis involved staff from the regional offices rather than the central office in San José. One could reasonably assume that all of the diagnosis could take place in a single day since less travel would be involved. Thus, both jeep and gas costs could be reduced by 50% and the per diem expenses reduced by 75% since only one day of meals would need to be included in the budget.

The Costs Associated with Consumer Risk:
Costa Rican Ministry of Health Model

These costs result from having misclassified a substandard Health Area as an acceptable one. As displayed in Table 7.5, six costs are considered. Lost earnings were estimated using the following assumptions. The average catchment area of a Health Area has 500 households. Both the 1984 census and our own experience in sampling indicate that about 33% of the households have children under three years of age. Therefore, at least 165 children reside in a catchment area. There are probably more children since some households have more than one child under three years. Since a defective Health Area has ≤ .50 coverage, we further assume that half of the children (82.5) are not vaccinated against measles.

The second assumption is that 33% of the nonvaccinated children (27.23) contract measles in a year. The third assumption concerns the proportion of mothers in Costa Rica who work. We estimated that in local low income rural communities about 40% of the young women who have children work. This estimate was based on a case study William Vargas and I carried out in the community of San Joaquín de Las Flores near San José.

Based on findings from the Ghana Health Assessment Project Team (1981), we assume that 21 days of temporary disability for a child result from measles. Half of these days are sufficiently severe for 50% of working mothers to stay with their child rather than work.

A fifth assumption is that the daily salary of working women is $5.41. This figure is derived from salaries of banana plantation workers in Costa Rica.

Table 7.5   Estimates of Costs Associated with Consumer Risks in Costa Rica: Costs for Misclassifying One Inadequate Health Area as Adequate*

Cost Category	Number in Category	Proportion Affected	Number Affected	Totals
I. LOST EARNINGS:				
Children Not Vaccinated Who Contract Measles	82.50 A	0.33 B	27.23 AB	
Mothers with Infected Children Who Work	27.23 AB	0.40 C	10.89 ABC	
Days of Mothers' Work Lost per Infected Child	10.50 D	0.50 E	5.25 DE	
Daily Salary	$5.41 F	1.00 G	$5.41 FG=X	
Mothers' Foregone Earnings	10.89 ABC	1.00 G	10.89 ABCG=Y	$309.30 DEXY
Foregone Earnings of Unvaccinated Children Who Die of Measles	27.23 AB	0.000025 H	0.0007 ABH	$5.23 $(PV_{65} - PV_{13})$ ABH
II. TREATMENT				
Cost of Physician	$15.67 I			
Cost of Physician Treating Children	27.23 AB	0.33 J	8.99 ABJ	$140.81 IABJ
III. VACCINATION SAVINGS				
Doses Never Given	82.50 A	0.33 K	27.23 AK	
Savings due to One Dose Never Given	$2.00 L	0 M	0 LM	$0 AKLM
TOTAL IN DOLLARS				**$455.34**

* *Letters in columns 2–5 are cell references to aid readers to construct their own spreadsheets.*

The final set of assumptions concerns the foregone earnings of children who died of measles. These were calculated using the following four assumptions: (1) The annual income of adults is $1862.24 per year. This salary was based on the fact that the two children whose deaths in 1987 were suspected as being attributable to measles came from working class Costa Rican families who earn approximately 109,500 colones per year. (2) Life expectancy is 73 years as based on the State of the World's Children for 1986. (3) Active wage earning years are 13 to 65. (4) The discount rate for years is 8.5% (Shepard et al. 1986:373).

The foregone earnings of children who die of measles in Costa Rica are $371.58, which was calculated as follows:

$$(PV_{65} - PV_{13})(Pr_{death} \times Child_{measles})$$

PV_{65} = Present Value of Earnings at 65

PV_{13} = Present Value of Earnings at 13

Pr_{death} = Probability of Dying of Measles

$Child_{measles}$ = Children in One Health Area with Measles.

The cost of treatment by a physician for measles, $15.67, was estimated using 1980 estimates for the Ivory Coast (Shepard et al. 1986). The ensuing assumption was that 33% of the children are sufficiently ill to be treated by a physician. This particular assumption is conservative since the senior nurses of the Ministry of Health are convinced that mothers seldom bring their children for medical care attributable to measles. They mostly rely on home care.

Vaccination saving was estimated as being zero. Although a dose of measles vaccine costs about $2 (Shepard et al. 1986), and 33% of the children are not vaccinated, the doses not given should not be considered as a savings to the health system. Since all children in Costa Rica are required to have been vaccinated against measles prior to being admitted to school, there are no long term savings due to vaccinations never given.

The cost to the consumer was calculated as:

LOST EARNINGS + TREATMENT – VACCINATION SAVINGS =
$314.53 + $140.81 – 0 = $455.34.

Therefore, the ratio of Consumer Costs to Provider Costs when assuming personnel from San José is:

$$\frac{\$455.34}{\$572.29} = .8.$$

This we will call Alternative 1.

If personnel from the Regional offices are used in the Diagnosis and Treatment phases, as discussed in the preceding section, we assume a $5.09 savings to the consumer and a 14% savings to the provider due mostly to re-duced transportation costs. The ratio of Consumer costs to Provider costs is

$$\frac{\$450.25}{\$492.17} = .92, \text{ or Alternative 2.}$$

Therefore, in Alternative 1, with a consumer risk (CR) of .05, the corresponding provider risk (PR) when using a consumer:provider cost ratio of .8 is:

$$\frac{.05}{PR} = .8 \text{ or } \frac{.05}{.8} = .06.$$

A provider risk of .05 results in a consumer risk of:

$$\frac{CR}{.05} = .8 \text{ or } .8 \times .05 =. 04.$$

If a higher consumer risk of .10 was used then the corresponding provider risk is:

$$\frac{.10}{.8} = .125;$$

conversely, a provider risk of .10 indicates a consumer risk of .08.

The results differ for Alternative 2. When the ratio is based on the assumption of employing regional personnel, a consumer risk of .05 results in a provider risk of .06. A provider risk of .05 would lead to a consumer risk that also is .05.

The data presented in this and previous chapters, together with the probability tables in the Appendix, can be used to calculate optimal sample sizes for different countries using economic criteria. Although that actual calculation is rather complex and beyond the scope of this volume, I will indicate how it should be performed. Economic analysis should be conducted to minimize the cost due to alpha and beta errors and due to sampling cost. The data in this volume can be used to determine the sample size based on social costs. The following function should be used:

(Cost of Sample N) + (Cost of Alpha Error) + (Cost of Beta Error)

with the constraint of determining what levels of cost were possible for both alpha and beta.

The next section analyzes provider and consumer risks for a hypothetical developing country that has severe health conditions. The main purpose of this section is to demonstrate how the background public health conditions are related to LQA sample size and to the cost of quality control. Health systems like that of Costa Rica, in which children tend to have less severe cases of measles, are less burdened by the caseload of measles. Therefore, they represent a real savings. These savings have a direct impact on health care management: they result in a small consumer risk and hence a small Consumer:Provider Cost ratio. As the severity of measles increases in a country, the Consumer:Provider ratio increases.

Costs Associated with Consumer Risk
in a Hypothetical Developing Country

Discussion focuses on consumer risk alone since no changes in provider risk are produced by poor public health conditions. The costs of diagnosis and treating a Health Area we assume are constant.

The major changes in consumer costs in comparison with the Costa Rica situation are in lost earnings and vaccination savings. The economic and health data assume a nation similar to Bolivia or Ivory Coast (Shepard et al. 1986). Life expectancy is 51 years. Annual earnings are $510. Three percent of the measles specific child deaths could be averted with adequate vaccination. The discount rate is still assumed to be 8.5%. Active wage earning years are 13 to 51. Other costs used in the above section were also used for this calculation, with only a few exceptions.

The assumptions for this developing country model that differ from the Costa Rican model are:

1. 100% of the children contract measles.

2. The probability of a child dying from measles is .03.

3. 33% of children who had not been vaccinated will never become vaccinated, thus producing a net savings.

As Table 7.6 suggests, the cost of the consumer's risk is $6,328.80. The CP ratio differs from the preceding model of Costa Rica. The CP ratio is:

$$\frac{\$6,328.20}{\$572.29} = 11.06.$$

Consumer costs are about 11 times higher than those of the provider. Thus, sample sizes and values of "d" should take into account the higher consumer costs.

Throughout most of this book, I have assumed that provider and consumer risks are of equal importance and in practice I have not used the economic procedures just presented. I have found that Ministry of Health decision makers tend to have their own weighting systems that conform to their own values or to the political pressures they experience. At this point, I am certain that although the relative balance of provider and consumer risks can vary using the above procedures, they may vary within a limited threshold only. In my experience, policy makers are not willing to embrace increasingly higher provider risks because of a high cost to the consumer due to inadequate ser–vices. Therefore, economic research should focus on identifying the thresh-old at which providers cease to embrace additional risk by decreasing the specificity of LQAS designs while simultaneously increasing the sensitivity. If this ceiling effect can be identified, it would aid immensely the selection of LQA sample sizes and decision rules. ✧

Table 7.6   Estimates of Costs Associated with Consumer Risks in a Developing Nation with High Infant Mortality: Costs for Misclassifying One Inadequate Health Area as Adequate*

Cost Category	Number in Category	Proportion Affected	Number Affected	Totals
I. LOST EARNINGS:				
Children Not Vaccinated Who Contract Measles	82.50 A	1.00 B	82.50 AB	
Mothers with Infected Children Who Work	82.50 AB	0.40 C	33.00 ABC	
Days of Mothers' Work Lost per Infected Child	10.50 D	0.50 E	5.25 DE	
Daily Salary	$5.41 F	1.00 G	$5.41 FG=X	
Mothers' Foregone Earnings	33.00 ABC	1.00 G	33.00 ABCG=Y	$937.28 DEXY
Foregone Earnings of Unvaccinated Children Who Die of Measles	82.50 AB	0.03 H	2.475 ABH	$4,910.45 $(PV_{51}-PV_{13})ABH$
II. TREATMENT				
Cost of Physician	$15.67 I			
Cost of Physician Treating Children	82.50 AB	0.33 J	27.23 ABJ	$426.62 IABJ
III. VACCINATION SAVINGS				
Doses Never Given	82.50 A	0.33 K	27.23 AK	
Savings due to One Dose Never Given	$2.00 L	1.00 M	2.00 LM	$54.45 AKLM
TOTAL IN DOLLARS				**$6,328.80**

* *Letters in Columns 2-5 are cell references to aid readers to construct their own spreadsheets.*

8

Aiding Policy Makers to Maintain Decentralized National Health Services[1]

The Pan American Health Organization (PAHO) and the World Health Organization (WHO) recommend decentralized service delivery as a strategy to reduce infant, child, and maternal mortality and morbidity. Such systems place greater decisionmaking autonomy in the hands of local managers rather than in central offices of Ministries of Health (PAHO 1988). As discussed throughout this book, decentralized decisionmaking allows for adaptation of the national program to local epidemiological and environmental conditions.

This chapter describes the structure of a management information system that facilitates decentralized management of Primary Health Care service delivery in Third World countries through regular assessment of health services. This management information system achieves this effect by establishing a control system comprising two components. The first one links decentralized health facilities with the local communities for which they are responsible. It determines whether local demand for services has been satisfied and what constraints impede service delivery. The second one links central Ministry of Health offices with decentralized facilities to ensure quality control of their service delivery and to measure whether national and regional policy objectives have been reached. The first portion of this chapter analyzes implications of decentralized PHC in organizational terms in order to demonstrate the relevance of this information system. The second part describes the role of Lot Quality Assurance Sampling in management information systems.

Conceptualizing a Control System
The premise of this chapter is that the transition of the health system to a decentralized form of organization produces a division of labor between central

and peripheral health units. Each level of organization has a specialized and necessary role. This division of labor supports two control or administrative systems. The first one consists of a feedback loop at the local level through which Community Health Workers (CHWs) respond to local conditions when organizing their health service delivery. Local conditions include local community demand and needs for family planning, perinatal care, vaccination, malaria control, and diarrheal disease control. Through this loop, decentralized facilities serve a control function that establishes an equilibrium between them and their local environments. Management behaviors subsumed by this role are steering, adjustment, and adaptation of health service delivery to local conditions. These activities are basic cybernetic control processes described by Ashby (1956).

A second feedback loop links the central Ministry of Health and local facilities. Through this loop the Ministry of Health determines whether decentralized local facilities, when responding to local pressures, violate national quality standards. This loop is similar to the first one since, through it, centralized units like the Ministry of Health perform the control functions of steering, adjustment, and adaptation. However, the equilibrium they establish is between themselves and local peripheral facilities (Steinbruner 1974: Chapters 1 and 2).

The first feedback loop is maintained by managers of peripheral health facilities who respond to local pressures. The second loop is used by central managers to monitor the quality of local responses to ensure that national or regional standards are maintained. The first loop we refer to as a "management control function" since information is gathered for local decision making concerning specific personnel, infrastructure, and communities. The second loop serves a "bureaucratic control function" since information is gathered for central Ministry officials to assess whether local management is occurring adequately and needs additional support. Both of these control functions require the formulation of a management information system to monitor each decentralized unit.

Decentralizing Health Systems

Although centralized decision making has been traditionally associated with both higher efficiency and higher productivity (Weber 1947), modern studies question this assumption. They conclude that either centralized or decentralized organizations can be effective (Lawrence and Lorsch 1967, Pennings 1973). The trend in developing nations has been toward decentralization of management to increase efficiency and productivity. Although no conclusive studies have adequately identified incentives for decentralized health system management, several suggestions have been presented. Mangelsdorf (1988: 67) proposed that decolonization and populist movements favoring democratization and local community participation during the 1970s and 1980s created political conditions favoring decentralization. Others conclude that decentralized management in some development organizations may be a consequence of international pressures and Western influences (Mansfield and Alam 1985). Regardless of the accuracy of these studies, recent policies promulgated by Ministries of Health in Latin America (PAHO 1988) tend to contradict hypotheses that decentralization "may be more of a political symbol than a reality" (Mangelsdorf 1988:68, van Putten 1978).

Although historical and political factors may help explain decentralization movements, such social changes can also be understood in functional terms. Among the pressures facing new governments is the need to implement social programs to improve education, health, sanitation, and water systems for low income urban and rural communities. Decentralized administration of these programs has been viewed favorably for logistical and other practical reasons (Villegas 1978, Keare and Parris 1982) rather than ideological ones. Managers of local health programs face complex decisions arising from a variety of environmental and social pressures affecting local program management. For example, national program strategies do not take into account the different conditions and needs that local managers find in communities. In some locations the program could be implemented as planned while in others it would need to accommodate local pressures.

This adaptive pressure, which occurs in local health systems, is also found in analyses of Western companies (Hage 1980: 394). In those cases, as in health systems, decentralization is associated with the number of decision issues managers need to consider. Certainly, social programs consider a large number of decisions (UN 1982, Rondinelli et al. 1984:7).

Two reasons explain why managers of integrated health programs address a large number of decisions. Firstly, each PHC service facility provides several preventive services such as those assessed in Chapter 5 (e.g., vaccinations, oral rehydration therapy, growth monitoring, neonatal referral). Secondly, service delivery, when organized through local health systems, is affected by social and ecological conditions of local communities. For example, due to poor roads the CHW in a northern Costa Rican Health Area, San Joaquín, often delivered PHC by horseback rather than by motorcycle. Nevertheless, even on horseback he still had to overcome logistical problems such as wet, boggy terrain, a dispersed rural population, and, prior to 1990, military operations along the Nicaraguan border. The administrative decisions that this CHW must make regarding, say, home visits to vaccinate children under one year of age with polio, DPT, and measles vaccines are very different from those that the CHW at the Health Area Aserrí, a semi-urban area near the national capital, must take. In the former Health Area, the CHW decided to reduce the number of home visits in his catchment area to, at most, one per year rather than the three visits required by the Ministry of Health. He reasoned that in order to vaccinate children against polio with the three dose regimen during the first year of life, he had to modify the Ministry's service delivery norms. He decided to change the home visit program since he could not visit all homes in his catchment area three times a year, as well as vaccinate every child under one year of age with three doses of polio. The terrain was too difficult and transportation was too slow to accomplish both objectives; he therefore rank ordered his tasks rather than assume they were of equal priority.

The CHW at Aserrí had different local pressures affecting her delivery. Roads were good. However, an influx of Nicaraguan and Honduran refugees resulted in dozens of new marginal housing areas and required her to update regularly the local census to identify high risk families. This task was not only time consuming but also made tentative most of her planned activities since she would have to reorder her tasks to serve newly discovered households.

In the above examples, both CHWs had the same health service responsibilities; however, diverging social and environmental conditions produced different pressures affecting management of service delivery to their local communities. Following this reasoning, we conclude that local health system management is similar to other decentralized complex organizations. Decentralization of health service activities is associated with a larger number of decisions than centralized systems. The assumption is that health professionals working in the latter type of organization may be unaware of local conditions. Therefore, they do not realize that service delivery should be adapted to local conditions. Instead, they deliver standardized health services. In formal terms, the number of decisions is calculated as an interaction of the number of PHC services and the number of local health facilities (Edmunds and Paul 1984). Therefore, in a centralized management system, a national or regional manager has numerous decisions to make since he is responsible for the catchment area of several Health Areas. Through decentralizing management the number of decisions for a manager or supervisor decreases since the "number of local health facilities" for which he is responsible is much fewer.

Coordination and Policy Making

The preceding section argued that decentralization requires local health system managers to steer, adjust, or adapt to local constraints or local pressures. Through local management, the health system establishes an equilibrium between what a program is designed to produce and what is feasible at a local level (Ashby 1956).

However, there is another level of control to consider in this model. Health programs (and potentially other social programs) must conform to national performance standards. In public health this constraint is essential because deviations from national standards can lead to epidemics, medical malpractice, and suboptimal health for members of the community.

The relation between national standards and medical practices can be reduced to a simple set of examples. If CHWs do not maintain a vaccine's cold chain, the vaccine will lose its potency and become useless. If CHWs contaminate syringes, they can produce additional infections. If mothers are uneducated in preparation of oral rehydration solutions or the reasons for using them, children may die or fail to thrive. National standards of approved medical practices should prevent these problems occurring if CHWs embrace them.

Therefore, although decentralized public health systems rely on CHWs (or other local managers) to respond to local pressures, another level of control is also essential — but at a central level. This level is the bureaucratic control function of PHC organizations.

March and Simon (1958) and Thompson (1967) recommended control either through a system of reward and punishment, or through detection and correction of errors by providing new information, such as through additional training (also see Hage 1980: 352). However, this type of system management cannot be performed in a decentralized organization other than through the formulation of *an additional feedback loop* that allows the Ministries of Health to monitor performance at the local level to detect and solve problems in the decentralized units.

Examples of problems and possible solutions are now presented to demonstrate central bureaucracy decisions. Although incentives and penalties are feasible solutions for each of these problems, discussion focuses on other organizational adjustments that are probably more suitable and appropriate for local health system management.

Problem 1: The CHW is not able to deliver health services in a specific Health Area due to inadequate logistics because communities are too dispersed to be covered by currently assigned personnel. Transportation is also inadequate due to insufficient fuel and poor maintenance.

Solution 1: Assign additional personnel to the Health Area. Resolve problems at higher levels of organization to provide for adequate shipping of fuel and transport repair at the local level. Resolve problems at higher levels that produce delays in repair of transport. Consider alternative transportation systems such as bus, bicycle, or animal.

Problem 2: The Health Area has an inadequate supply of syringes, vaccines, oral rehydration salts.

Solution 2: Improve management information systems at all levels of organization for monitoring inventories, requisitions, shipment, receipt, and wastage of materials.

Problem 3: CHWs exhibit inadequate knowledge of existing procedures for maintenance of the cold chain; they also do not know service delivery standards, such as vaccination of all children with three doses of polio vaccine within the first year of life with a minimum of a one month interval between doses.

Solution 3: Retrain and supervise personnel to perform existing procedures and to adhere to existing production standards; train them to perform new tasks to accommodate local constraints.

Such a bureaucratic feedback mechanism in a decentralized health system aids national managers to control both the quality and impact of the multiple decisions made at the periphery, and it may lead to improved services. The solutions just presented are difficult to implement and can be costly. However, the resources for supporting them are seldom available at the periphery. National program managers tend to have more flexible budgets or better access to donors for obtaining the required funding and expertise than do local managers. This reasoning comprises another role for bureaucratic feedback.

How Much Decentralization?

The view that decentralized organizations have two control mechanisms — local management that responds to local pressures, and central bureaucratic monitoring that assesses local responses and that controls the production quality of services — marks a departure from Rondinelli's (1984) definition of decentralization. For him decentralization consists of a three point continuum ranging from least to most decentralized. At the first point, **deconcentration** shifts some work from central offices to field offices. The second one consists of **delegation**, which shifts decisionmaking authority to field managers who are only indirectly responsible to the center. The third point is **devolution**, which also shifts programmatic responsibility away from the center to the field units.

As noted by others, Rondinelli's continuum (Smith 1979, Carter and Cullen 1984) is not useful for understanding decentralized system reforms. The main reason for rejecting Rondinelli's framework is that it focuses on the peripheral organizational units and their response to local forces without considering the role of the central Ministry of Health as the chief national policy making body. Therefore, it obscures the policymaking role of both central and peripheral components of national organizations.

In the earlier examples of the decisions made by CHWs at the Health Areas of San Joaquín and Aserrí, Rondinelli's most decentralized motif, devolution, was evident. Both CHWs changed their programmed activities, probably with the approval of the rural supervisor who was their local manager. However, the decisions of neither CHW were monitored by the Ministry of Health's central office. Only the impact of service delivery was monitored to determine whether intervention by central management was required.

Contrary to Price (1972:43), decentralization involves more than deconcentration of power. In public health, the process of decentralizing an organization involves creating a division of labor between peripheral and central organizational units in which the former exercises local control to respond to local pressures, and the latter ensures the coordination of those local responses to achieve national policies.

Heretofore, few analyses have described methods that facilitate local control. Similarly, there have been few discussions of the bureaucratic role of central Ministry of Health officials in a decentralized system. Ostensibly, CHWs and Ministries of Health have been unable to carry out adequately their control functions. Although Ministries of Health have tried to assess health service delivery at a national level, such as by measuring coverage of the national population with health services (Chapter 5), they have not been able to assess the performance of peripheral facilities (Chapter 5 and Chapter 6).

The earlier chapters of this book presented LQAS instruments for assessing decentralized health systems that make feasible the cybernetic model of health system management. The discussion will now elaborate how management and bureaucratic control based on LQAS can aid the Costa Rican health reform through quality control of health service delivery at the community level of organization.

Thresholds of Health System Success and Failure

The final component of this cybernetic model concerns information gathering and decisionmaking for management and bureaucratic control. Similar to Steinbruner (1974), managers of health systems need not be sensitive to exact outputs of health facilities. Rather, they should determine whether control standards or thresholds for production of service delivery have been reached. For example, assume that a national vaccination standard mandates that children receive three doses of polio during their first year of life. The control system needs only to detect whether the threshold that marks minimum vaccination coverage has been reached. Little more is learned from control systems that measure exact production (e.g., 8%, 83.5%, 90%) than those that measure whether thresholds have been reached (e.g., 80%). The conclusions for decisionmaking may be the same. As demonstrated in Chapter 5, because LQA samples permit rapid classification of priority health areas, both local and central managers are able to direct attention and resources where they are most needed. Once the LQAS decision rules are established the method is easy to use, quick to provide results, and inexpensive.

Management and Bureaucracy in a Decentralized Health System

The management and bureaucratic control functions perform at least two activities. They screen Health Areas for inadequate coverage with health services and they identify improper technical procedures that negate services that are delivered. For both activities performance standards need to be established. Both control systems aim to maintain these standards. Together they comprise the means for assessing decentralized integrated health systems.

Both management and bureaucratic control functions do not measure the exact performance of CHWs. They need only to determine whether critical thresholds of a variable have been exceeded. Therefore, they identify whether any Health Area is below a critical performance standard in a critical task.

According to the decision rules of this control system, local managers and bureaucrats do not interfere with a CHW unless a certain proportion of the children under one year of age have not been vaccinated. At that point the community for which the CHW is responsible is at risk, thereby requiring intervention by the local manager and oversight of that intervention by the central bureaucracy.

Decentralized integrated health programs provide services at the community level of organization. If local managers are to recognize where problems in implementation arise, they must measure coverage, service adequacy, and technical quality of providers at that level. As discussed in Chapter 1, only by assessing services at the lowest or most peripheral level of organization can administrators identify health units contributing to low coverage, service adequacy or technical quality of a specific program.

LQAS, when applied to health units, identifies those with adequate coverage ($\geq$80%), and distinguishes them from units operating below a critical standard of coverage ($\leq$50%). Chapter 5 demonstrated how LQAS results can also be aggregated to measure coverage and service adequacy proportions within regions of nations with a precision not usually possible with conventional approaches, namely, $\pm$2% instead of $\pm$10%. Thus, LQAS can be used for both the management and bureaucratic control functions because it produces information that is applicable to the administrations at various levels of health system: nation, region, and community. Table 8.1 summarizes the results of the assessment of coverage adequacy discussed in Chapter 5. All Health Areas included in the investigation are listed. Of the thirteen services assessed, Table 8.1 records the number found to be inadequate. This summary report is typical of the information that either local mangers or central bureaucrats can receive. They can rapidly identify the Health Areas that have the greatest number of inadequacies, and they can compare the performance of any Health Area with any other one. A similar type of report can be developed for assessment of service adequacy and CHW technical quality.

With these rapid assessments local managers can focus on their specific problems and adapt the national program to local conditions. Simultaneously, central offices of the Ministry can track each facility to determine which communities are at risk to health problems due to inadequate services. Such information may also help decision makers appraise the viability of national health policies.

To date, few methods have been available for performing both control functions. LQAS can be used for these purposes. The model of decentralized health system reform envisaged in this paper would persist even if LQAS had not been developed. As in the case of Costa Rica, Ministries need to monitor performance at the periphery. However, as Chapter 6 demonstrated, local problems escape the attention of supervisors. Therefore, equilibrium would not be maintained between the decentralized units and central decision makers. Health reforms could be implemented, but their goals not achieved. Local CHWs may be motivated and their populations willing to participate, but poor service delivery technique and retention of inaccurate information by CHWs and their supervisors could neutralize the beneficial effects of PHC. Cold chains may not be maintained; children may not be vaccinated at the correct age; health information may be incorrectly entered in the record system; educational messages on the preparation of oral rehydration therapy may be incorrectly conveyed.

Table 8.1 List of Health Facilities by Total Number of Services Found to be Inadequate of 13 Services Assessed during 1987

Health Center	Total Number of Services Found Inadequate of 13 Assessed	Health Center	Total Number of Services Found Inadequate of 13 Assessed
Region Brunca		**Region Chorotega**	
Rivas de Perez Zeledon	2	Santa Cruz	2
Agua Buena de Coto Brus	2	Puntarenas	3
Palmar Norte De Osa	3	Puntarenas	3
Sierpe De Osa	3	Puntarenas	3
Tinoco De Osa	3	Belen De Carrillo	3
San Rafael De Coto Brus	3	Fortuna De Bagaces	3
La Uvita De Osa	4	San Isidro De Aguas Claras	3
Platanillo De Perez Zeledon	4	Mansion De Nicoya	3
Los Reyes De Coto Brus	4	Quebrada Honda De Nicoya	3
Golfito	4	Colorado De Abamgares	3
		Las Juntas De Abangares	3
Region Central Norte		San Buenaventura De Abangares	3
Valverde	2	Esparza	4
Heredia	2	Bocas De Nossara	6
Heredia	2		
Barva	2	**Region Huetar Atlántica**	
Turrucares De Alajuela	2	Colonia San Rafael De Pococi	2
Heredia	3	Los Angeles De Pococi	3
Carrizal De Alajuela	3	La Bomba De Limón	3
Sabanilla De Alajuela	4	Palmitas De Pococi	4
		Pemhurst De Limón	4
Region Central Sur		Barra Del Parismina	4
Guayabo De Mora	1		
Santa An	2	**Region Huetar Norte**	
Cristo Rey	2	Union De Rio Frio	2
Paraiso	2	Buenos Aires De Sarapiqui	3
Turrialba	2	San Miguel De Sarapiqui	3
Turrialba	2	Coopevega	3
Curridabat	2	Santa Rosa De San Carlos	3
Palmichal De Acosta	3	San Joaquín De San Carlos	3
Vuelta De Jorco	3		
Aserrí	3		
Cristo Rey	3		
Pacayas De Alvarado	3		
Cristo Rey	4		
Corralillo	4		
Cachi De Paraiso	4		
Turrialba	4		

LQAS lends credibility to the administrative division of labor proposed in this chapter because it is the tool with which the work can be performed. Qualitative measures such as those produced by LQAS can be destructive to institutional reform if they are used to interfere in local decision making, rather than support it (Campbell 1984:26). Although our methods are still in an early state of development, our knowledge about how to apply them adequately lags further behind. I have tried to address the first issue (crude methodology) by indicating that the bureaucratic control function should only detect whether critical thresholds have been violated. The second issue (problems for health services research), I can address briefly in the following, and final, chapter of this book. Although the Costa Rican experience has given us insight into how to assess integrated health systems, additional cross national applications of LQAS are needed to establish an externally valid and generalizable model. ✧

1 *This chapter was prepared originally for a conference on "International Policy Reforms" organized by the Harvard Institute for International Development in Marrakech, Morocco in 1988.*

9

Epilogue: Limitations and Needed Improvements to Health Services Research

Preceding chapters have explained the importance of assessing levels of organization, and they have demonstrated a strategy for doing it. Chapter 1 pointed out that the success of the primary health care system may, in part, depend on maintaining the adequacy of services of peripheral health units. Lot Quality Assurance Sampling (LQAS) was proposed as a rapid assessment method that can be used for three types of health services quality control: coverage, service adequacy, and health worker technique. Chapter 2 indicated how program evaluation activities should fit into a regular management cycle as a means of ensuring quality control. Chapter 3 pointed out several measurement problems specific to assessing programs in developing nations that need to be resolved by managers using any empirically based instrument. Chapter 4 explained, for its intended users, principles of LQAS. Chapter 5 demonstrated LQAS procedures in a field setting. It exhibited applications of LQAS in a system reporting coverage or service adequacy of 13 different health services, both at decentralized and centralized levels of Ministries of Health. Chapter 6 explained uses of LQAS in a regular supervision system of community health workers (CHWs). Chapter 7 analyzed the costs of LQAS to the Costa Rican health system and provided a spreadsheet for estimating costs in other nations. Chapter 8 explained for health system policy makers the different roles of local and central managers in a health services quality control system.

This book has demonstrated an important feature of LQAS methods, namely, that they can be used to screen and classify community health units according to the quality of health services in the communities they serve. As a tool for regular program assessment, LQAS produces precise information about the coverage or service adequacy of virtually all PHC interventions and the technical quality with which they were delivered. Probably the most important feature of LQAS for practitioners is that it can be used to monitor services in the specific community for which an individual CHW undertakes responsibility. Although these community based data can be aggregated at national, regional, and other administrative levels, a main utility of LQAS is that it can be used to rapidly classify CHWs as either having performed their tasks adequately or inadequately.

Chapter 7 demonstrated that an LQAS can cost less than $5.00 per household for assessing one Health Area. However, this cost varies with the organization of the data collection team. A decentralized team consisting of local supervisors would cost this amount, but a centralized team consisting of staff from the Ministry could cost about $19 for a similar survey. Therefore, costs of LQAS can be reduced substantially in a decentralized management system. Although LQAS is inexpensive, if its total costs are compared with EPI cluster sampling, LQAS would be more expensive. This result is because LQAS should be used to assess, say, coverage in each of 60 Health Areas, whereas EPI cluster sampling would be used to assess coverage across all 60 Health Areas. However, since the incentive for developing this LQAS was to screen individual Health Areas, this comparison is artificial. If EPI cluster sampling were used at the community level using its typical sample of 210, it could be more expensive than LQAS. Also, if low coverage in a large area was detected with an EPI cluster sample, one would not know if all health units or only some of them were responsible for the low coverage. Therefore, either a diagnosis of all health units would have to be undertaken or all health facilities would have to be the target for remediation. Therefore, potentially two steps and two sets of costs are necessary for management decision making with EPI cluster sampling. With LQAS the second step would not be necessary since one would know which health centers were performing below the ministry standard.

This chapter addresses three questions. Firstly, now that LQAS has been field tested, what is its role vis-à-vis other existing sampling methods currently in use by public health practitioners throughout the world to control the quality of health programs?

Secondly, once LQAS results are available for national or regional directors of health facilities, what are the steps to detect the determinants of those defects, implement interventions to resolve them, monitor the implementation, and evaluate their impacts?

Thirdly, should public health practitioners be satisfied with LQAS in its current state of development? If not, what procedural changes should be made?

LQAS Vis-à-Vis Other Monitoring Methods

Chapter 4 discussed EPI cluster sampling and suggested that because it does not easily measure coverage at the level where services are delivered, a method such as LQAS was necessary. However, in some circumstances EPI cluster sampling is more appropriate than LQAS.

Health program directors may not always be interested in measuring the quality of health services delivered by local facilities. If they want to measure coverage within a region or nation only, and are not concerned with linking it with any particular health facility, then an EPI cluster sample would be a reasonable method to use. It is rapid, uncomplicated, and does not require a sampling frame as does LQAS. However, it often does require a separate team to be organized to collect the data and, therefore, in general it must be organized as a vertical program.

Such a measure of coverage could be required for reporting national vaccination coverage to the World Health Organization or to international agencies requesting national coverage statistics. However, if LQAS had already been implemented as a regular component of the national primary health care program, then data would already be available for aggregate studies, thereby removing the need for an EPI cluster sample for vaccinations. The same LQAS system could be used to monitor many other problems of health and development.

In theory alternatives to LQAS can be devised. For example, ministries of health having a high quality management system could use indicators of service delivery similar to the following one used for assessing vaccination coverage:

$$\frac{\text{number of age specific vaccinations}}{\text{number of individuals in the same age groups}}$$
$$\text{of the same population}$$

Wherever the data for this indicator are available and accurate, they would probably be better than LQAS for measuring the quality of a health unit's service delivery. However, in practice such data are rarely accessible.

The ability of any society to undertake useful data collection on a national scale depends, among other things, on its ability to train its field staff in proper data collection methods and on their understanding of the principles upon which they are based. Until they achieve these capabilities, health practitioners need to use methods such as LQAS as an alternative for estimating coverage of populations by health facilities. Countries with such data collection and analysis abilities are generally not "less developed."

Post LQAS Activities

LQAS identifies the level of adequacy with which a health facility delivers services to the community for which it is responsible. Although its immediate contribution to public health practice stops there, LQAS lays the foundation for other necessary diagnostic and surveillance functions of a PHC service.

Ministries of health cannot stop once they have classified the quality of their service delivery units. They have several other activities to perform, each of which requires developing additional field methods. Firstly, they must identify the determinants of the service delivery problems LQAS has identified. Secondly, they must formulate feasible interventions to resolve these problems. Thirdly, they must implement these interventions as planned. Fourthly, they must monitor the interventions to determine whether they have been implemented as planned, and resolve operational problems when encountered. Fifthly, they must evaluate these interventions to determine their impact.

The host of activities implied by these tasks is governed by similar methodological principles of reliability and validity discussed in Chapter 3. From 1987 through 1990 the Ministry of Health of Costa Rica focused its attention on improving the vaccination technique of CHWs. This was accomplished by systematic application of LQAS by supervisors during their visits to CHWs. During 1988, CHWs performed inadequately 38 tasks related to vaccinating children. By May 1990, CHWs performed 36 of these 38 tasks adequately (Valadez 1990). This higher quality work is probably attributable to improved local management and regular supervision of CHWs using LQAS procedures reported in Chapter 6.

Considerations for the Next Applications of LQAS

Three issues are discussed in this section: selection of sample size for the subsequent applications of LQAS, identification of sampling frames, and questionnaire development.

Sample sizes selected for this field test of LQAS were based on the need to keep both producer and consumer risks <.05. They had to provide a large enough sample size to ensure a precise estimate of the adequacy of the 60 Costa Rican health facilities studied. However, the reader should not assume that LQAS always requires such a sample size. Chapter 5 demonstrated that a sample size of 19 could result in nearly the same number of misclassified Health Areas as a sample of 28. Chapter 7 presented economic criteria for sample size selection so that in future applications of LQAS, the user can choose samples based on estimated costs. The model used for estimating costs could be expanded. For example, the disease specific death rate for measles in Costa Rica is now nearly zero. In other nations it could be quite high. The foregone earnings of dead children could, therefore, be entered in the functions of Chapter 4 as a consumer cost. This and other factors particular to the conditions of the user nation need to be considered when selecting a sample size, rather than simply using this project's sample size.

The next issue concerns the selection of a sampling frame. Constructing a sampling frame is a limitation of LQAS when it is used for measuring coverage adequacy. As explained earlier, no sampling frame is necessary when assessing the technical quality of CHWs. Observing them deliver services to any child or woman is permissible, since the technical quality of a CHW in a repeated action is probably associated more with his own competency than with the characteristics of the family receiving the service. In other applications of LQAS, a sampling frame is necessary. However, this is an expensive and time consuming activity. Nevertheless, once it is completed that same sampling frame can be updated and used again at a much smaller cost. In the case of the Costa Rican assessment, the team used maps produced by the national census since it was the best sampling frame available. Alternative Costa Rican sampling frames were discussed in Chapter 5. Other LQAS users should seek out sampling frames appropriate to their own conditions.

Although an accurate national census is not a prerequisite for using LQAS, a sampling frame of some kind is necessary. Numerous alternative sampling frames exist other than census maps. Consider the following possibilities and their sources:

1. Maps: malaria campaign, ground water or sanitation system development companies, real estate planners, military;
2. Photographs: aerial, satellite, or military (these options for many countries are not viable or practical);
3. Lists: voter registration, baptismal or birth registries, membership lists of mothers clubs;
4. Two rapid approaches for developing local sampling frames, presented in Chapter 5: constructing a village grid (Figure 5.3) and coordinate sampling (Figure 5.4).

The bottom line in selecting any of these sampling frames is that if the program director wants to monitor the program accurately at any level, he must have a sampling frame appropriate to that level. If the central administrators using LQAS do not need to know aggregate coverage proportions across several Health Areas since these statistics are not a required output from their study, they could take a completely different approach. For example, they could sample a section of the community consisting of houses within a predetermined radius of a health area, say, 5 kilometers. In this instance they could assume that health service coverage should be associated with the distance a family lives from the health facility; families that live closer to a Health Area should have more contact with it than families living further away. Therefore, health facilities could be classified on the assumption that if coverage is unacceptable within subsections of their community that have greater access to health service, then it is likely to be unacceptable outside of that area as well. This approach requires developing a smaller sampling frame than if a larger area is used for the assessment. Also, since health units are often located in villages, maps may already exist for them. Nevertheless, since the individuals studied in this modified application of LQAS would not include the rural poor, who may be dispersed over a large area, LQAS data collection should be expedited.

The limitation of this abbreviated approach is that while Health Areas can be assessed individually, the information cannot be aggregated to create a meaningful coverage statistic, as was done in Chapter 5 for all of Costa Rica. The reason is that because the sample of each Health Area is not representative of its catchment area, the synthesis of the data from all Health Areas is not indicative of coverage of the region under study.

Although constructing a sampling frame is a requirement for LQAS, it is a reasonable cost, especially for public health practitioners advocating that local health workers develop community lists and maps, which would be used for identifying families needing service. These same maps can also be used for performing LQAS.

The third issue concerns questionnaire development. The cost of using LQAS could be further reduced if the number of questions asked was reduced. Users need to determine how many questions are needed to assess coverage adequacy with PHC services. If any two services turn out to be highly correlated, then only one of the services may have to be monitored; a measure of one of them could reflect the performance of the other.

Analysis of the Costa Rica LQAS data is given in Table 9.1. It shows the covariance of service delivery by listing correlation coefficients for eight services. With the exception of two of these correlations in which r > .90 (i.e., polio 1 and DPT 1, polio 3 and DPT 3), the correlation coefficients are unimpressive. Less than 75% of the variance of the performance of any activity is explained by its association with any other variable. With the possible exception of the first and third DPT and polio vaccinations, the performance of all of these variables should be included in an LQAS since no PHC activity can be used as a proxy measure for any other activity.

Another point to consider is that despite the strong correlations between vaccination coverage of children with polio 1 and DPT 1, polio 1 should not be used as a proxy for DPT 1. Although these cross sectional measures indicate strong covariance, the methods of delivery of polio and DPT differ. Administration of DPT requires a syringe whereas polio does not. Therefore, a shortage of syringes would lower DPT vaccination coverage while not affecting polio coverage. CHWs perform many activities once they are in a household. Therefore, they would vaccinate children against polio, instruct mothers to prepare ORT, and the like. Despite the covariance of polio and DPT vaccination coverage in this cross sectional study, the relationship is likely to be unstable over time or across different countries.

Further Needed Developments of LQAS

LQAS has its roots in industry. Early papers were written by the technical staff of the Bell Telephone Laboratories (Dodge and Romig 1959) during the first half of the twentieth century. Although the application of LQAS to assessment of integrated health interventions has maintained the original assumptions used in industry, there are differences between public health services and industrial conditions that are worth noting.

In industry, a machine's calibrations can be adjusted. It is much more difficult to adjust the work procedures of the staff of a Health Area. There are no knobs to turn or gauges to set. This difference raises the issue of how to

Table 9.1 A Matrix of Correlation Coefficients Examining the Association Among 8 PHC Services

	Polio 1	Polio 2	Polio 3	DPT 1	DPT 2	DPT 3	Measles	Home Visits
Polio 1	1.00							
Polio 2	.4939**	1.00						
Polio 3	.3786*	.5747	1.00					
DPT 1	.9504**	.4828**	.4155**	1.00				
DPT 2	.2846	.4170**	.3153*	.2849	1.00			
DPT 3	.3736*	.5425**	.9197**	.4398**	.3063*	1.00		
Measles	.4048**	.3392*	.2274	.4052**	.0389	.2097	1.00	
Home Visits	.3717*	.3071*	.1627	.3735*	.2742	.1734	.0218	1.00

One Tailed Significance: * p < .01, ** p < .001

define normal production standards. As Dodge and Romig (1959) demonstrate, a production standard in industry is established by measuring the average quality of the lots of items produced by a precise machine. Should the quality of subsequent products deviate from that norm by a factor, say, of one or two standard deviations, then the inspector would judge the machine to be producing at an unacceptable quality. Next, the inspector would identify the cause of the poor production and remedy it.

In public health there is seldom any backlog of performance of Health Areas. As a field, international public health is still at an early stage of developing methods to measure performance. Therefore, there are no measurements of average coverage of empirically identified excellent Health Areas which may establish an appropriate production standard. Public health is still in the process of trying to develop Health Areas to reach a level of performance which their administrators can then help them maintain. For this reason, the formula which has been used for calculating the probability tables in the Appendix assumes no average production standard.

The priority future task in the development of LQAS is to compile a database of performance for a set of Health Areas, say, in Costa Rica, for which an empirically based average performance standard can be established. Then industrial quality control statistics should be studied to determine how they can be adapted to the quality control of Child Survival services delivery.

Another difference between the uses of LQAS by industry and by public health practitioners is revealed in the level of training required for users. Dodge and Romig (1959) report that quality assurance procedures have been used successfully by industry foremen with little education. It is not clear whether local managers with little training would be equally successful users of LQAS.

Firstly, in industry a randomly selected item from a lot can be identified by the identification number. A particular light bulb can be identified as being in the ith box and in the jth cell of that box. Houses on maps of developing countries are much more difficult to identify. Any public health user of LQAS in a developing country should understand basic random sampling principles so he can appreciate the importance of ensuring a proper selection of households rather than selecting a convenient sample of households.

For example, since maps are imperfect, it is feasible that interviewers could find in the field two or more houses which could be the predetermined sampling element. In this case, the staff should use some randomized procedure to select the alternative houses. A training manual should be developed that presents random sampling principles in a simple form that instructs local managers about the importance of adhering to LQAS procedures and how to select reliably according to the principles. The manual should also illustrate a set of potential problems that can be encountered in the field and their solutions. This material should aim to guide practitioners through complicated field settings without violating LQAS procedures.

A third difference between the LQAS application discussed in this book and others used in industry is that the latter use both single and double sampling procedures. Single sampling only was considered in the application in Costa Rica since all 28 observations were collected at the same time. Double sampling procedures are based on the following rationale.

Let us assume that the 28 observations were collected in two stages. The first one would consist of 19 households in each Health Area and the second of nine. If all 19 children observed in the first wave of sampling exhibited, say, adequate vaccinations, then the second wave would not have to be collected. Even if all nine children observed in the second sample were defective, vaccination, coverage in that Health Area would be judged adequate since the 28:9 rule classifies as inadequate a Health Area in which more than nine children exhibit substandard vaccinations coverage. Therefore, regardless of the vaccination status of the last nine children, sufficient information is known from the first 19 observations to classify that Health Area.

Conversely, if the first 19 children included 10 who have not been adequately vaccinated, the Health Area would be classified as substandard regardless of the adequacy of the vaccination coverage of the nine children observed in the second wave. Therefore, once again the second wave of sampling would yield no more useful information for the purpose of assessing vaccination coverage.

The only reason to collect the data in the second wave of sampling would be if less than 10 observations but more than zero observations in the first wave of sampling indicated substandard performance. In that case, the nine additional children would have to be observed in order to be able to classify the Health Area.

If a double sampling scheme were used, then approximately a 33% savings could result when sufficient information is collected in the first wave to preclude the need for the second wave of data collection. The next segment of work on LQAS should concentrate on developing the probability tables and methodology associated with double sampling (Lemeshow and Stroh 1986, 1989).

Double sampling will be most useful in assessments of one intervention alone. When more than one service is investigated, the local manager would be forced to keep track simultaneously of the number of inadequate households or techniques observed for all services being assessed. Some interventions may need the second stage sample while others may not. During the field test of LQAS for assessing CHW technique (Chapter 6), the assessment team found this tracking to be a great burden and a potential source of error. Therefore, while double sampling may be applicable to vertical programs or to single service monitoring, it may be less useful for Child Survival Programs.

Analyses of the application of other industrial quality control procedures to assessments of Child Survival Programs may have a higher priority. For example, if average quality production standards could be developed for use in public health, then it may be possible to apply the more advanced industrial quality control procedures that replaced LQAS several years ago in industry. Control charts and sequential sampling methods may also have application to public health as Reinke (1988) recently suggested.

There are also directions from which it may be worthwhile to discourage further work. Recently some researchers suggested use of hypergeometric distributions rather than binomials (Rosero et al. 1990). Such applications could make LQAS more difficult to use by local managers. The hypergeometric assumes that the population size is known. Therefore, a separate sample size would have to be calculated for each Health Area. Because hypergeometrics approximate binomial distributions, except in very small populations, little precision would be gained at the expense of potentially adding considerable complexity and error to the procedure.

This book has presented a rationale for using LQAS and exhibited its application for assessing Child Survival Programs. In addition to responding to the request of Dr. Jaramillo Antillón, the former Minister of Health of Costa Rica, to participate with the Ministry in the development of a monitoring and evaluation system for the National Primary Health Care System, this work has produced a body of information which can be scrutinized to help determine both the limitations and advantages of LQAS vis-à-vis other more traditional methods for measuring coverage in primary health care programs. I have attempted to identify some limitations of the LQAS approach and to chart needed future work.

During the 1980s considerable attention was given by international public health policy makers to identifying priority interventions for their countries. During the 1990s these decisions may be modified as local epidemiologies change or as interventions improve. However, greater attention by both local and central public health managers will probably be focused on understanding why mortality and morbidity in local communities are not decreasing as quickly as expected even though the relevant interventions are being implemented. The answer, in part, lies in the likelihood that services have not been implemented properly. The sources of these problems could be due to difficult logistical conditions, low incentives for consumers or providers, or inadequate CHW training. Chapter 5 presented various reports to demonstrate that pockets of inadequate coverage and service adequacy may persist in some communities, thereby maintaining their health risks. Chapter 6 showed that inadequate service delivery technique may place the health of communities at risk by rendering delivered services ineffective. Since both of these categories of problems occur at the local level, the challenge of the 1990s, and potentially beyond, will be to target these priority Health Areas.

Although we should expect that material resources will continue to be scarce in the foreseeable future, a priority for the developing countries will be to use more efficiently those resources that are currently available and already being invested. To accomplish this goal, administrators and local managers will have to actively and regularly search for the operational problems in their programs. Achieving this management style will depend as much on the development of an experimental attitude (Campbell 1969) by policy makers and managers as it will on developing technical solutions. This book attempted to address both issues although it emphasized the latter. Now, we need to apply LQAS and other methods in diverse country settings to understand better the problems affecting integrated health programs that diminish their impacts. Although the nations of the world may not ensure Health For All By The Year 2000, we may at least by then understand the impediments. ✧

Appendix

LQAS Probability Tables for Selecting Sample Size and Consumer/Provider Risks for n = 5 to n = 50

d Cumulative Probabilities for Values of p with d Defects   n = 5

d	.05	.10	.15	.20	.25	.30	.35	.40	.45	.50	.55	.60	.65	.70	.75	.80	.85	.90	.95
0	.000	.000	.000	.000	.001	.002	.005	.010	.018	.031	.050	.078	.116	.168	.237	.328	.444	.590	.774
1	.000	.000	.002	.007	.016	.031	.054	.087	.131	.188	.256	.337	.428	.528	.633	.737	.835	.919	.977
2	.001	.009	.027	.058	.104	.163	.235	.317	.407	.500	.593	.683	.765	.837	.896	.942	.973	.991	.999
3	.023	.081	.165	.263	.367	.472	.572	.663	.744	.813	.869	.913	.946	.969	.984	.993	.998	1.000	1.000
4	.226	.410	.556	.672	.763	.832	.884	.922	.950	.969	.982	.990	.995	.998	.999	1.000	1.000	1.000	1.000
5	1.000	1.000	1.000	1.000	1.000	1.000	1.000	1.000	1.000	1.000	1.000	1.000	1.000	1.000	1.000	1.000	1.000	1.000	1.000

d Cumulative Probabilities for Values of p with d Defects   n = 6

d	.05	.10	.15	.20	.25	.30	.35	.40	.45	.50	.55	.60	.65	.70	.75	.80	.85	.90	.95
0	.000	.000	.000	.000	.000	.001	.002	.004	.008	.016	.028	.047	.075	.118	.178	.262	.377	.531	.735
1	.000	.000	.000	.002	.005	.011	.022	.041	.069	.109	.164	.233	.319	.420	.534	.655	.776	.886	.967
2	.000	.001	.006	.017	.038	.070	.117	.179	.255	.344	.442	.544	.647	.744	.831	.901	.953	.984	.998
3	.002	.016	.047	.099	.169	.256	.353	.456	.558	.656	.745	.821	.883	.930	.962	.983	.994	.999	1.000
4	.033	.114	.224	.345	.466	.580	.681	.767	.836	.891	.931	.959	.978	.989	.995	.998	1.000	1.000	1.000
5	.265	.469	.623	.738	.822	.882	.925	.953	.972	.984	.992	.996	.998	.999	1.000	1.000	1.000	1.000	1.000
6	1.000	1.000	1.000	1.000	1.000	1.000	1.000	1.000	1.000	1.000	1.000	1.000	1.000	1.000	1.000	1.000	1.000	1.000	1.000

d Cumulative Probabilities for Values of p with d Defects   n = 7

d	.05	.10	.15	.20	.25	.30	.35	.40	.45	.50	.55	.60	.65	.70	.75	.80	.85	.90	.95
0	000	.000	.000	.000	.000	.000	.001	.002	.004	.008	.015	.028	.049	.082	.133	.210	.321	.478	.698
1	.000	.000	.000	.000	.001	.004	.009	.019	.036	.063	.102	.159	.234	.329	.445	.577	.717	.850	.956
2	.000	.000	.001	.005	.013	.029	.056	.096	.153	.227	.316	.420	.532	.647	.756	.852	.926	.974	.996
3	.000	.003	.012	.033	.071	.126	.200	.290	.392	.500	.608	.710	.800	.874	.929	.967	.988	.997	1.000
4	.004	.026	.074	.148	.244	.353	.468	.580	.684	.773	.847	.904	.944	.971	.987	.995	.999	1.000	1.000
5	.044	.150	.283	.423	.555	.671	.766	.841	.898	.938	.964	.981	.991	.996	.999	1.000	1.000	1.000	1.000
6	.302	.522	.679	.790	.867	.918	.951	.972	.985	.992	.996	.998	.999	1.000	1.000	1.000	1.000	1.000	1.000
7	1.000	1.000	1.000	1.000	1.000	1.000	1.000	1.000	1.000	1.000	1.000	1.000	1.000	1.000	1.000	1.000	1.000	1.000	1.000

d Cumulative Probabilities for Values of p with d Defects   n = 8

d	.05	.10	.15	.20	.25	.30	.35	.40	.45	.50	.55	.60	.65	.70	.75	.80	.85	.90	.95
0	.000	.000	.000	.000	.000	.000	.000	.001	.002	.004	.008	.017	.032	.058	.100	.168	.272	.430	.663
1	.000	.000	.000	.000	.000	.001	.004	.009	.018	.035	.063	.106	.169	.255	.367	.503	.657	.813	.943
2	.000	.000	.000	.001	.004	.011	.025	.050	.088	.145	.220	.315	.428	.552	.679	.797	.895	.962	.994
3	.000	.000	.003	.010	.027	.058	.106	.174	.260	.363	.477	.594	.706	.806	.886	.944	.979	.995	1.000
4	.000	.005	.021	.056	.114	.194	.294	.406	.523	.637	.740	.826	.894	.942	.973	.990	.997	1.000	1.000
5	.006	.038	.105	.203	.321	.448	.572	.685	.780	.855	.912	.950	.975	.989	.996	.999	1.000	1.000	1.000
6	.057	.187	.343	.497	.633	.745	.831	.894	.937	.965	.982	.991	.996	.999	1.000	1.000	1.000	1.000	1.000
8	.337	.570	.728	.832	.900	.942	.968	.983	.992	.996	.998	.999	1.000	1.000	1.000	1.000	1.000	1.000	1.000
8	1.000	1.000	1.000	1.000	1.000	1.000	1.000	1.000	1.000	1.000	1.000	1.000	1.000	1.000	1.000	1.000	1.000	1.000	1.000

d Cumulative Probabilities for Values of p with d Defects   n = 9

d	.05	.10	.15	.20	.25	.30	.35	.40	.45	.50	.55	.60	.65	.70	.75	.80	.85	.90	.95
0	.000	.000	.000	.000	.000	.000	.000	.000	.001	.002	.005	.010	.021	.040	.075	.134	.232	.387	.630
1	.000	.000	.000	.000	.000	.000	.001	.004	.009	.020	.039	.071	.121	.196	.300	.436	.599	.775	.929
2	.000	.000	.000	.000	.001	.004	.011	.025	.050	.090	.150	.232	.337	.463	.601	.738	.859	.947	.992
3	.000	.000	.001	.003	.010	.025	.054	.099	.166	.254	.361	.483	.609	.730	.834	.914	.966	.992	.999
4	.000	.001	.006	.020	.049	.099	.172	.267	.379	.500	.621	.733	.828	.901	.951	.980	.994	.999	1.000
5	.001	.008	.034	.086	.166	.270	.391	.517	.639	.746	.834	.901	.946	.975	.990	.997	.999	1.000	1.000
6	.008	.053	.141	.262	.399	.537	.663	.768	.850	.910	.950	.975	.989	.996	.999	1.000	1.000	1.000	1.000
7	.071	.225	.401	.564	.700	.804	.879	.929	.961	.980	.991	.996	.999	1.000	1.000	1.000	1.000	1.000	1.000
8	.370	.613	.768	.866	.925	.960	.979	.990	.995	.998	.999	1.000	1.000	1.000	1.000	1.000	1.000	1.000	1.000
9	1.000	1.000	1.000	1.000	1.000	1.000	1.000	1.000	1.000	1.000	1.000	1.000	1.000	1.000	1.000	1.000	1.000	1.000	1.000

d Cumulative Probabilities for Values of p with d Defects   n = 10

d	.05	.10	.15	.20	.25	.30	.35	.40	.45	.50	.55	.60	.65	.70	.75	.80	.85	.90	.95
0	.000	.000	.000	.000	.000	.000	.000	.000	.000	.001	.003	.006	.013	.028	.056	.107	.197	.349	.599
1	.000	.000	.000	.000	.000	.000	.001	.002	.005	.011	.023	.046	.086	.149	.244	.376	.544	.736	.914
2	.000	.000	.000	.000	.000	.002	.005	.012	.027	.055	.100	.167	.262	.383	.526	.678	.820	.930	.988
3	.000	.000	.000	.001	.004	.011	.026	.055	.102	.172	.266	.382	.514	.650	.776	.879	.950	.987	.999
4	.000	.000	.001	.006	.020	.047	.095	.166	.262	.377	.504	.633	.751	.850	.922	.967	.990	.998	1.000
5	.000	.002	.010	.033	.078	.150	.249	.367	.496	.623	.738	.834	.905	.953	.980	.994	.999	1.000	1.000
6	.001	.013	.050	.121	.224	.350	.486	.618	.734	.828	.898	.945	.974	.989	.996	.999	1.000	1.000	1.000
7	.012	.070	.180	.322	.474	.617	.738	.833	.900	.945	.973	.988	.995	.998	1.000	1.000	1.000	1.000	1.000
8	.086	.264	.456	.624	.756	.851	.914	.954	.977	.989	.995	.998	.999	1.000	1.000	1.000	1.000	1.000	1.000
9	.401	.651	.803	.893	.944	.972	.987	.994	.997	.999	1.000	1.000	1.000	1.000	1.000	1.000	1.000	1.000	1.000
10	1.000	1.000	1.000	1.000	1.000	1.000	1.000	1.000	1.000	1.000	1.000	1.000	1.000	1.000	1.000	1.000	1.000	1.000	1.000

d Cumulative Probabilities for Values of p with d Defects   n = 11

	.05	.10	.15	.20	.25	.30	.35	.40	.45	.50	.55	.60	.65	.70	.75	.80	.85	.90	.95
0	.000	.000	.000	.000	.000	.000	.000	.000	.000	.000	.001	.004	.009	.020	.042	.086	.167	.314	.569
1	.000	.000	.000	.000	.000	.000	.000	.001	.002	.006	.014	.030	.061	.113	.197	.322	.492	.697	.898
2	.000	.000	.000	.000	.000	.001	.002	.006	.015	.033	.065	.119	.200	.313	.455	.617	.779	.910	.985
3	.000	.000	.000	.000	.001	.004	.012	.029	.061	.113	.191	.296	.426	.570	.713	.839	.931	.981	.998
4	.000	.000	.000	.002	.008	.022	.050	.099	.174	.274	.397	.533	.668	.790	.885	.950	.984	.997	1.000
5	.000	.000	.003	.012	.034	.078	.149	.247	.367	.500	.633	.753	.851	.922	.966	.988	.997	1.000	1.000
6	.000	.003	.016	.050	.115	.210	.332	.467	.603	.726	.826	.901	.950	.978	.992	.998	1.000	1.000	1.000
7	.002	.019	.069	.161	.287	.430	.574	.704	.809	.887	.939	.971	.988	.996	.999	1.000	1.000	1.000	1.000
8	.015	.090	.221	.383	.545	.687	.800	.881	.935	.967	.985	.994	.998	.999	1.000	1.000	1.000	1.000	1.000
9	.102	.303	.508	.678	.803	.887	.939	.970	.986	.994	.998	.999	1.000	1.000	1.000	1.000	1.000	1.000	1.000
10	.431	.686	.833	.914	.958	.980	.991	.996	.999	1.000	1.000	1.000	1.000	1.000	1.000	1.000	1.000	1.000	1.000
11	1.000	1.000	1.000	1.000	1.000	1.000	1.000	1.000	1.000	1.000	1.000	1.000	1.000	1.000	1.000	1.000	1.000	1.000	1.000

d Cumulative Probabilities for Values of p with d Defects   n = 12

	.05	.10	.15	.20	.25	.30	.35	.40	.45	.50	.55	.60	.65	.70	.75	.80	.85	.90	.95
0	.000	.000	.000	.000	.000	.000	.000	.000	.000	.000	.001	.002	.006	.014	.032	.069	.142	.282	.540
1	.000	.000	.000	.000	.000	.000	.000	.000	.001	.003	.008	.020	.042	.085	.158	.275	.443	.659	.882
2	.000	.000	.000	.000	.000	.000	.001	.003	.008	.019	.042	.083	.151	.253	.391	.558	.736	.889	.980
3	.000	.000	.000	.000	.000	.002	.006	.015	.036	.073	.134	.225	.347	.493	.649	.795	.908	.974	.998
4	.000	.000	.000	.001	.003	.009	.026	.057	.112	.194	.304	.438	.583	.724	.842	.927	.976	.996	1.000
5	.000	.000	.001	.004	.014	.039	.085	.158	.261	.387	.527	.665	.787	.882	.946	.981	.995	.999	1.000
6	.000	.001	.005	.019	.054	.118	.213	.335	.473	.613	.739	.842	.915	.961	.986	.996	.999	1.000	1.000
7	.000	.004	.024	.073	.158	.276	.417	.562	.696	.806	.888	.943	.974	.991	.997	.999	1.000	1.000	1.000
8	.002	.026	.092	.205	.351	.507	.653	.775	.866	.927	.964	.985	.994	.998	1.000	1.000	1.000	1.000	1.000
9	.020	.111	.264	.442	.609	.747	.849	.917	.958	.981	.992	.997	.999	1.000	1.000	1.000	1.000	1.000	1.000
10	.118	.341	.557	.725	.842	.915	.958	.980	.992	.997	.999	1.000	1.000	1.000	1.000	1.000	1.000	1.000	1.000
11	.460	.718	.858	.931	.968	.986	.994	.998	.999	1.000	1.000	1.000	1.000	1.000	1.000	1.000	1.000	1.000	1.000
12	1.000	1.000	1.000	1.000	1.000	1.000	1.000	1.000	1.000	1.000	1.000	1.000	1.000	1.000	1.000	1.000	1.000	1.000	1.000

d	Cumulative Probabilities for Values of p with d Defects																	n = 13	

	.05	.10	.15	.20	.25	.30	.35	.40	.45	.50	.55	.60	.65	.70	.75	.80	.85	.90	.95
0	.000	.000	.000	.000	.000	.000	.000	.000	.000	.000	.000	.001	.004	.010	.024	.055	.121	.254	.513
1	.000	.000	.000	.000	.000	.000	.000	.000	.001	.002	.005	.013	.030	.064	.127	.234	.398	.621	.865
2	.000	.000	.000	.000	.000	.000	.000	.001	.004	.011	.027	.058	.113	.202	.333	.502	.692	.866	.975
3	.000	.000	.000	.000	.000	.001	.003	.008	.020	.046	.093	.169	.278	.421	.584	.747	.882	.966	.997
4	.000	.000	.000	.000	.001	.004	.013	.032	.070	.133	.228	.353	.501	.654	.794	.901	.966	.994	1.000
5	.000	.000	.000	.001	.006	.018	.046	.098	.179	.291	.427	.574	.716	.835	.920	.970	.992	.999	1.000
6	.000	.000	.001	.007	.024	.062	.129	.229	.356	.500	.644	.771	.871	.938	.976	.993	.999	1.000	1.000
7	.000	.001	.008	.030	.080	.165	.284	.426	.573	.709	.821	.902	.954	.982	.994	.999	1.000	1.000	1.000
8	.000	.006	.034	.099	.206	.346	.499	.647	.772	.867	.930	.968	.987	.996	.999	1.000	1.000	1.000	1.000
9	.003	.034	.118	.253	.416	.579	.722	.831	.907	.954	.980	.992	.997	.999	1.000	1.000	1.000	1.000	1.000
10	.025	.134	.308	.498	.667	.798	.887	.942	.973	.989	.996	.999	1.000	1.000	1.000	1.000	1.000	1.000	1.000
11	.135	.379	.602	.766	.873	.936	.970	.987	.995	.998	.999	1.000	1.000	1.000	1.000	1.000	1.000	1.000	1.000
12	.487	.746	.879	.945	.976	.990	.996	.999	1.000	1.000	1.000	1.000	1.000	1.000	1.000	1.000	1.000	1.000	1.000
13	1.000	1.000	1.000	1.000	1.000	1.000	1.000	1.000	1.000	1.000	1.000	1.000	1.000	1.000	1.000	1.000	1.000	1.000	1.000

d   Cumulative Probabilities for Values of p with d Defects   n = 14

d	.05	.10	.15	.20	.25	.30	.35	.40	.45	.50	.55	.60	.65	.70	.75	.80	.85	.90	.95
0	.000	.000	.000	.000	.000	.000	.000	.000	.000	.000	.000	.001	.002	.007	.018	.044	.103	.229	.488
1	.000	.000	.000	.000	.000	.000	.000	.000	.000	.001	.003	.008	.021	.047	.101	.198	.357	.585	.847
2	.000	.000	.000	.000	.000	.000	.000	.001	.002	.006	.017	.040	.084	.161	.281	.448	.648	.842	.970
3	.000	.000	.000	.000	.000	.000	.001	.004	.011	.029	.063	.124	.220	.355	.521	.698	.853	.956	.996
4	.000	.000	.000	.000	.000	.002	.006	.018	.043	.090	.167	.279	.423	.584	.742	.870	.953	.991	1.000
5	.000	.000	.000	.000	.002	.008	.024	.058	.119	.212	.337	.486	.641	.781	.888	.956	.988	.999	1.000
6	.000	.000	.000	.002	.010	.031	.075	.150	.259	.395	.546	.692	.816	.907	.962	.988	.998	1.000	1.000
7	.000	.000	.002	.012	.038	.093	.184	.308	.454	.605	.741	.850	.925	.969	.990	.998	1.000	1.000	1.000
8	.000	.001	.012	.044	.112	.219	.359	.514	.663	.788	.881	.942	.976	.992	.998	1.000	1.000	1.000	1.000
9	.000	.009	.047	.130	.258	.416	.577	.721	.833	.910	.957	.982	.994	.998	1.000	1.000	1.000	1.000	1.000
10	.004	.044	.147	.302	.479	.645	.780	.876	.937	.971	.989	.996	.999	1.000	1.000	1.000	1.000	1.000	1.000
11	.030	.158	.352	.552	.719	.839	.916	.960	.983	.994	.998	.999	1.000	1.000	1.000	1.000	1.000	1.000	1.000
12	.153	.415	.643	.802	.899	.953	.979	.992	.997	.999	1.000	1.000	1.000	1.000	1.000	1.000	1.000	1.000	1.000
13	.512	.771	.897	.956	.982	.993	.998	.999	1.000	1.000	1.000	1.000	1.000	1.000	1.000	1.000	1.000	1.000	1.000
14	1.000	1.000	1.000	1.000	1.000	1.000	1.000	1.000	1.000	1.000	1.000	1.000	1.000	1.000	1.000	1.000	1.000	1.000	1.000

d   Cumulative Probabilities for Values of p with d Defects   n = 15

d	.05	.10	.15	.20	.25	.30	.35	.40	.45	.50	.55	.60	.65	.70	.75	.80	.85	.90	.95
0	.000	.000	.000	.000	.000	.000	.000	.000	.000	.000	.000	.000	.002	.005	.013	.035	.087	.206	.463
1	.000	.000	.000	.000	.000	.000	.000	.000	.000	.000	.002	.005	.014	.035	.080	.167	.319	.549	.829
2	.000	.000	.000	.000	.000	.000	.000	.000	.001	.004	.011	.027	.062	.127	.236	.398	.604	.816	.964
3	.000	.000	.000	.000	.000	.000	.000	.002	.006	.018	.042	.091	.173	.297	.461	.648	.823	.944	.995
4	.000	.000	.000	.000	.000	.001	.003	.009	.025	.059	.120	.217	.352	.515	.686	.836	.938	.987	.999
5	.000	.000	.000	.000	.001	.004	.012	.034	.077	.151	.261	.403	.564	.722	.852	.939	.983	.998	1.000
6	.000	.000	.000	.001	.004	.015	.042	.095	.182	.304	.452	.610	.755	.869	.943	.982	.996	1.000	1.000
7	.000	.000	.001	.004	.017	.050	.113	.213	.346	.500	.654	.787	.887	.950	.983	.996	.999	1.000	1.000
8	.000	.000	.004	.018	.057	.131	.245	.390	.548	.696	.818	.905	.958	.985	.996	.999	1.000	1.000	1.000
9	.000	.002	.017	.061	.148	.278	.436	.597	.739	.849	.923	.966	.988	.996	.999	1.000	1.000	1.000	1.000
10	.001	.013	.062	.164	.314	.485	.648	.783	.880	.941	.975	.991	.997	.999	1.000	1.000	1.000	1.000	1.000
11	.005	.056	.177	.352	.539	.703	.827	.909	.958	.982	.994	.998	1.000	1.000	1.000	1.000	1.000	1.000	1.000
12	.036	.184	.396	.602	.764	.873	.938	.973	.989	.996	.999	1.000	1.000	1.000	1.000	1.000	1.000	1.000	1.000
13	.171	.451	.681	.833	.920	.965	.986	.995	.998	1.000	1.000	1.000	1.000	1.000	1.000	1.000	1.000	1.000	1.000
14	.537	.794	.913	.965	.987	.995	.998	1.000	1.000	1.000	1.000	1.000	1.000	1.000	1.000	1.000	1.000	1.000	1.000
15	1.000	1.000	1.000	1.000	1.000	1.000	1.000	1.000	1.000	1.000	1.000	1.000	1.000	1.000	1.000	1.000	1.000	1.000	1.000

186 Assessing Child Survival Programs

d	Cumulative Probabilities for Values of p with d Defects																		n = 16
	.05	.10	.15	.20	.25	.30	.35	.40	.45	.50	.55	.60	.65	.70	.75	.80	.85	.90	.95
0	.000	.000	.000	.000	.000	.000	.000	.000	.000	.000	.000	.000	.001	.003	.010	.028	.074	.185	.440
1	.000	.000	.000	.000	.000	.000	.000	.000	.000	.000	.001	.003	.010	.026	.063	.141	.284	.515	.811
2	.000	.000	.000	.000	.000	.000	.000	.000	.001	.002	.007	.018	.045	.099	.197	.352	.561	.789	.957
3	.000	.000	.000	.000	.000	.000	.000	.001	.003	.011	.028	.065	.134	.246	.405	.598	.790	.932	.993
4	.000	.000	.000	.000	.000	.000	.001	.005	.015	.038	.085	.167	.289	.450	.630	.798	.921	.983	.999
5	.000	.000	.000	.000	.000	.002	.006	.019	.049	.105	.198	.329	.490	.660	.810	.918	.976	.997	1.000
6	.000	.000	.000	.000	.002	.007	.023	.058	.124	.227	.366	.527	.688	.825	.920	.973	.994	.999	1.000
7	.000	.000	.000	.001	.007	.026	.067	.142	.256	.402	.563	.716	.841	.926	.973	.993	.999	1.000	1.000
8	.000	.000	.001	.007	.027	.074	.159	.284	.437	.598	.744	.858	.933	.974	.993	.999	1.000	1.000	1.000
9	.000	.001	.006	.027	.080	.175	.312	.473	.634	.773	.876	.942	.977	.993	.998	1.000	1.000	1.000	1.000
10	.000	.003	.024	.082	.190	.340	.510	.671	.802	.895	.951	.981	.994	.998	1.000	1.000	1.000	1.000	1.000
11	.001	.017	.079	.202	.370	.550	.711	.833	.915	.962	.985	.995	.999	1.000	1.000	1.000	1.000	1.000	1.000
12	.007	.068	.210	.402	.595	.754	.866	.935	.972	.989	.997	.999	1.000	1.000	1.000	1.000	1.000	1.000	1.000
13	.043	.211	.439	.648	.803	.901	.955	.982	.993	.998	.999	1.000	1.000	1.000	1.000	1.000	1.000	1.000	1.000
14	.189	.485	.716	.859	.937	.974	.990	.997	.999	1.000	1.000	1.000	1.000	1.000	1.000	1.000	1.000	1.000	1.000
15	.560	.815	.926	.972	.990	.997	.999	1.000	1.000	1.000	1.000	1.000	1.000	1.000	1.000	1.000	1.000	1.000	1.000
16	1.000	1.000	1.000	1.000	1.000	1.000	1.000	1.000	1.000	1.000	1.000	1.000	1.000	1.000	1.000	1.000	1.000	1.000	1.000

d Cumulative Probabilities for Values of p with d Defects   n = 17

d	.05	.10	.15	.20	.25	.30	.35	.40	.45	.50	.55	.60	.65	.70	.75	.80	.85	.90	.95
0	.000	.000	.000	.000	.000	.000	.000	.000	.000	.000	.000	.000	.001	.002	.008	.023	.063	.167	.418
1	.000	.000	.000	.000	.000	.000	.000	.000	.000	.000	.001	.002	.007	.019	.050	.118	.252	.482	.792
2	.000	.000	.000	.000	.000	.000	.000	.000	.000	.001	.004	.012	.033	.077	.164	.310	.520	.762	.950
3	.000	.000	.000	.000	.000	.000	.000	.000	.002	.006	.018	.046	.103	.202	.353	.549	.756	.917	.991
4	.000	.000	.000	.000	.000	.000	.001	.003	.009	.025	.060	.126	.235	.389	.574	.758	.901	.978	.999
5	.000	.000	.000	.000	.000	.001	.003	.011	.030	.072	.147	.264	.420	.597	.765	.894	.968	.995	1.000
6	.000	.000	.000	.000	.001	.003	.012	.035	.083	.166	.290	.448	.619	.775	.893	.962	.992	.999	1.000
7	.000	.000	.000	.000	.003	.013	.038	.092	.183	.315	.474	.641	.787	.895	.960	.989	.998	1.000	1.000
8	.000	.000	.000	.003	.012	.040	.099	.199	.337	.500	.663	.801	.901	.960	.988	.997	1.000	1.000	1.000
9	.000	.000	.002	.011	.040	.105	.213	.359	.526	.685	.817	.908	.962	.987	.997	1.000	1.000	1.000	1.000
10	.000	.001	.008	.038	.107	.225	.381	.552	.710	.834	.917	.965	.988	.997	.999	1.000	1.000	1.000	1.000
11	.000	.005	.032	.106	.235	.403	.580	.736	.853	.928	.970	.989	.997	.999	1.000	1.000	1.000	1.000	1.000
12	.001	.022	.099	.242	.426	.611	.765	.874	.940	.975	.991	.997	.999	1.000	1.000	1.000	1.000	1.000	1.000
13	.009	.083	.244	.451	.647	.798	.897	.954	.982	.994	.998	1.000	1.000	1.000	1.000	1.000	1.000	1.000	1.000
14	.050	.238	.480	.690	.836	.923	.967	.988	.996	.999	1.000	1.000	1.000	1.000	1.000	1.000	1.000	1.000	1.000
15	.208	.518	.748	.882	.950	.981	.993	.998	.999	1.000	1.000	1.000	1.000	1.000	1.000	1.000	1.000	1.000	1.000
16	.582	.833	.937	.977	.992	.998	.999	1.000	1.000	1.000	1.000	1.000	1.000	1.000	1.000	1.000	1.000	1.000	1.000
17	1.000	1.000	1.000	1.000	1.000	1.000	1.000	1.000	1.000	1.000	1.000	1.000	1.000	1.000	1.000	1.000	1.000	1.000	1.000

d   Cumulative Probabilities for Values of p with d Defects   n = 18

d	.05	.10	.15	.20	.25	.30	.35	.40	.45	.50	.55	.60	.65	.70	.75	.80	.85	.90	.95
0	.000	.000	.000	.000	.000	.000	.000	.000	.000	.000	.000	.000	.000	.002	.006	.018	.054	.150	.397
1	.000	.000	.000	.000	.000	.000	.000	.000	.000	.000	.000	.001	.005	.014	.039	.099	.224	.450	.774
2	.000	.000	.000	.000	.000	.000	.000	.000	.000	.001	.003	.008	.024	.060	.135	.271	.480	.734	.942
3	.000	.000	.000	.000	.000	.000	.000	.000	.001	.004	.012	.033	.078	.165	.306	.501	.720	.902	.989
4	.000	.000	.000	.000	.000	.000	.000	.001	.005	.015	.041	.094	.189	.333	.519	.716	.879	.972	.998
5	.000	.000	.000	.000	.000	.000	.001	.006	.018	.048	.108	.209	.355	.534	.717	.867	.958	.994	1.000
6	.000	.000	.000	.000	.000	.001	.006	.020	.054	.119	.226	.374	.549	.722	.861	.949	.988	.999	1.000
7	.000	.000	.000	.000	.001	.006	.021	.058	.128	.240	.391	.563	.728	.859	.943	.984	.997	1.000	1.000
8	.000	.000	.000	.001	.005	.021	.060	.135	.253	.407	.578	.737	.861	.940	.981	.996	.999	1.000	1.000
9	.000	.000	.001	.004	.019	.060	.139	.263	.422	.593	.747	.865	.940	.979	.995	.999	1.000	1.000	1.000
10	.000	.000	.003	.016	.057	.141	.272	.437	.609	.760	.872	.942	.979	.994	.999	1.000	1.000	1.000	1.000
11	.000	.001	.012	.051	.139	.278	.451	.626	.774	.881	.946	.980	.994	.999	1.000	1.000	1.000	1.000	1.000
12	.000	.006	.042	.133	.283	.466	.645	.791	.892	.952	.982	.994	.999	1.000	1.000	1.000	1.000	1.000	1.000
13	.002	.028	.121	.284	.481	.667	.811	.906	.959	.985	.995	.999	1.000	1.000	1.000	1.000	1.000	1.000	1.000
14	.011	.098	.280	.499	.694	.835	.922	.967	.988	.996	.999	1.000	1.000	1.000	1.000	1.000	1.000	1.000	1.000
15	.058	.266	.520	.729	.865	.940	.976	.992	.997	.999	1.000	1.000	1.000	1.000	1.000	1.000	1.000	1.000	1.000
16	.226	.550	.776	.901	.961	.986	.995	.999	1.000	1.000	1.000	1.000	1.000	1.000	1.000	1.000	1.000	1.000	1.000
17	.603	.850	.946	.982	.994	.998	1.000	1.000	1.000	1.000	1.000	1.000	1.000	1.000	1.000	1.000	1.000	1.000	1.000
18	1.000	1.000	1.000	1.000	1.000	1.000	1.000	1.000	1.000	1.000	1.000	1.000	1.000	1.000	1.000	1.000	1.000	1.000	1.000

d Cumulative Probabilities for Values of p with d Defects   n = 19

d	.05	.10	.15	.20	.25	.30	.35	.40	.45	.50	.55	.60	.65	.70	.75	.80	.85	.90	.95
0	.000	.000	.000	.000	.000	.000	.000	.000	.000	.000	.000	.000	.000	.001	.004	.014	.046	.135	.377
1	.000	.000	.000	.000	.000	.000	.000	.000	.000	.000	.000	.001	.003	.010	.031	.083	.198	.420	.755
2	.000	.000	.000	.000	.000	.000	.000	.000	.000	.000	.002	.005	.017	.046	.111	.237	.441	.705	.933
3	.000	.000	.000	.000	.000	.000	.000	.000	.001	.002	.008	.023	.059	.133	.263	.455	.684	.885	.987
4	.000	.000	.000	.000	.000	.000	.000	.001	.003	.010	.028	.070	.150	.282	.465	.673	.856	.965	.998
5	.000	.000	.000	.000	.000	.000	.001	.003	.011	.032	.078	.163	.297	.474	.668	.837	.946	.991	1.000
6	.000	.000	.000	.000	.000	.001	.003	.012	.034	.084	.173	.308	.481	.666	.825	.932	.984	.998	1.000
7	.000	.000	.000	.000	.000	.003	.011	.035	.087	.180	.317	.488	.666	.818	.923	.977	.996	1.000	1.000
8	.000	.000	.000	.000	.002	.011	.035	.088	.184	.324	.494	.667	.815	.916	.971	.993	.999	1.000	1.000
9	.000	.000	.000	.002	.009	.033	.087	.186	.329	.500	.671	.814	.913	.967	.991	.998	1.000	1.000	1.000
10	.000	.000	.001	.007	.029	.084	.185	.333	.506	.676	.816	.912	.965	.989	.998	1.000	1.000	1.000	1.000
11	.000	.000	.004	.023	.077	.182	.334	.512	.683	.820	.913	.965	.989	.997	1.000	1.000	1.000	1.000	1.000
12	.000	.002	.016	.068	.175	.334	.519	.692	.827	.916	.966	.988	.997	.999	1.000	1.000	1.000	1.000	1.000
13	.000	.009	.054	.163	.332	.526	.703	.837	.922	.968	.989	.997	.999	1.000	1.000	1.000	1.000	1.000	1.000
14	.002	.035	.144	.327	.535	.718	.850	.930	.972	.990	.997	.999	1.000	1.000	1.000	1.000	1.000	1.000	1.000
15	.013	.115	.316	.545	.737	.867	.941	.977	.992	.998	.999	1.000	1.000	1.000	1.000	1.000	1.000	1.000	1.000
16	.067	.295	.559	.763	.889	.954	.983	.995	.998	1.000	1.000	1.000	1.000	1.000	1.000	1.000	1.000	1.000	1.000
17	.245	.580	.802	.917	.969	.990	.997	.999	1.000	1.000	1.000	1.000	1.000	1.000	1.000	1.000	1.000	1.000	1.000
18	.623	.865	.954	.986	.996	.999	1.000	1.000	1.000	1.000	1.000	1.000	1.000	1.000	1.000	1.000	1.000	1.000	1.000
19	1.000	1.000	1.000	1.000	1.000	1.000	1.000	1.000	1.000	1.000	1.000	1.000	1.000	1.000	1.000	1.000	1.000	1.000	1.000

d Cumulative Probabilities for Values of p with d Defects   n = 20

d	.05	.10	.15	.20	.25	.30	.35	.40	.45	.50	.55	.60	.65	.70	.75	.80	.85	.90	.95
0	.000	.000	.000	.000	.000	.000	.000	.000	.000	.000	.000	.000	.000	.001	.003	.012	.039	.122	.358
1	.000	.000	.000	.000	.000	.000	.000	.000	.000	.000	.000	.001	.002	.008	.024	.069	.176	.392	.736
2	.000	.000	.000	.000	.000	.000	.000	.000	.000	.000	.001	.004	.012	.035	.091	.206	.405	.677	.925
3	.000	.000	.000	.000	.000	.000	.000	.000	.000	.001	.005	.016	.044	.107	.225	.411	.648	.867	.984
4	.000	.000	.000	.000	.000	.000	.000	.000	.002	.006	.019	.051	.118	.238	.415	.630	.830	.957	.997
5	.000	.000	.000	.000	.000	.000	.000	.002	.006	.021	.055	.126	.245	.416	.617	.804	.933	.989	1.000
6	.000	.000	.000	.000	.000	.000	.002	.006	.021	.058	.130	.250	.417	.608	.786	.913	.978	.998	1.000
7	.000	.000	.000	.000	.000	.001	.006	.021	.058	.132	.252	.416	.601	.772	.898	.968	.994	1.000	1.000
8	.000	.000	.000	.000	.001	.005	.020	.057	.131	.252	.414	.596	.762	.887	.959	.990	.999	1.000	1.000
9	.000	.000	.000	.001	.004	.017	.053	.128	.249	.412	.591	.755	.878	.952	.986	.997	1.000	1.000	1.000
10	.000	.000	.000	.003	.014	.048	.122	.245	.409	.588	.751	.872	.947	.983	.996	.999	1.000	1.000	1.000
11	.000	.000	.001	.010	.041	.113	.238	.404	.586	.748	.869	.943	.980	.995	.999	1.000	1.000	1.000	1.000
12	.000	.000	.006	.032	.102	.228	.399	.584	.748	.868	.942	.979	.994	.999	1.000	1.000	1.000	1.000	1.000
13	.000	.002	.022	.087	.214	.392	.583	.750	.870	.942	.979	.994	.998	1.000	1.000	1.000	1.000	1.000	1.000
14	.000	.011	.067	.196	.383	.584	.755	.874	.945	.979	.994	.998	1.000	1.000	1.000	1.000	1.000	1.000	1.000
15	.003	.043	.170	.370	.585	.762	.882	.949	.981	.994	.998	1.000	1.000	1.000	1.000	1.000	1.000	1.000	1.000
16	.016	.133	.352	.589	.775	.893	.956	.984	.995	.999	1.000	1.000	1.000	1.000	1.000	1.000	1.000	1.000	1.000
17	.075	.323	.595	.794	.909	.965	.988	.996	.999	1.000	1.000	1.000	1.000	1.000	1.000	1.000	1.000	1.000	1.000
18	.264	.608	.824	.931	.976	.992	.998	.999	1.000	1.000	1.000	1.000	1.000	1.000	1.000	1.000	1.000	1.000	1.000
19	.642	.878	.961	.988	.997	.999	1.000	1.000	1.000	1.000	1.000	1.000	1.000	1.000	1.000	1.000	1.000	1.000	1.000
20	1.000	1.000	1.000	1.000	1.000	1.000	1.000	1.000	1.000	1.000	1.000	1.000	1.000	1.000	1.000	1.000	1.000	1.000	1.000

d	Cumulative Probabilities for Values of p with d Defects																	$n = 21$

d	.05	.10	.15	.20	.25	.30	.35	.40	.45	.50	.55	.60	.65	.70	.75	.80	.85	.90	.95
0	.000	.000	.000	.000	.000	.000	.000	.000	.000	.000	.000	.000	.000	.001	.002	.009	.033	.109	.341
1	.000	.000	.000	.000	.000	.000	.000	.000	.000	.000	.000	.000	.001	.006	.019	.058	.155	.365	.717
2	.000	.000	.000	.000	.000	.000	.000	.000	.000	.000	.001	.002	.009	.027	.075	.179	.370	.648	.915
3	.000	.000	.000	.000	.000	.000	.000	.000	.000	.001	.003	.011	.033	.086	.192	.370	.611	.848	.981
4	.000	.000	.000	.000	.000	.000	.000	.000	.001	.004	.013	.037	.092	.198	.367	.586	.803	.948	.997
5	.000	.000	.000	.000	.000	.000	.000	.001	.004	.013	.039	.096	.201	.363	.567	.769	.917	.986	1.000
6	.000	.000	.000	.000	.000	.000	.001	.004	.013	.039	.096	.200	.357	.551	.744	.891	.971	.997	1.000
7	.000	.000	.000	.000	.000	.001	.003	.012	.038	.095	.197	.350	.536	.723	.870	.957	.992	.999	1.000
8	.000	.000	.000	.000	.000	.002	.011	.035	.091	.192	.341	.524	.706	.852	.944	.986	.998	1.000	1.000
9	.000	.000	.000	.000	.002	.009	.031	.085	.184	.332	.512	.691	.838	.932	.979	.996	1.000	1.000	1.000
10	.000	.000	.000	.001	.006	.026	.077	.174	.321	.500	.679	.826	.923	.974	.994	.999	1.000	1.000	1.000
11	.000	.000	.000	.004	.021	.068	.162	.309	.488	.668	.816	.915	.969	.991	.998	1.000	1.000	1.000	1.000
12	.000	.000	.002	.014	.056	.148	.294	.476	.659	.808	.909	.965	.989	.998	1.000	1.000	1.000	1.000	1.000
13	.000	.001	.008	.043	.130	.277	.464	.650	.803	.905	.962	.988	.997	.999	1.000	1.000	1.000	1.000	1.000
14	.000	.003	.029	.109	.256	.449	.643	.800	.904	.961	.987	.996	.999	1.000	1.000	1.000	1.000	1.000	1.000
15	.000	.014	.083	.231	.433	.637	.799	.904	.961	.987	.996	.999	1.000	1.000	1.000	1.000	1.000	1.000	1.000
16	.003	.052	.197	.414	.633	.802	.908	.963	.987	.996	.999	1.000	1.000	1.000	1.000	1.000	1.000	1.000	1.000
17	.019	.152	.389	.630	.808	.914	.967	.989	.997	.999	1.000	1.000	1.000	1.000	1.000	1.000	1.000	1.000	1.000
18	.085	.352	.630	.821	.925	.973	.991	.998	.999	1.000	1.000	1.000	1.000	1.000	1.000	1.000	1.000	1.000	1.000
19	.283	.635	.845	.942	.981	.994	.999	1.000	1.000	1.000	1.000	1.000	1.000	1.000	1.000	1.000	1.000	1.000	1.000
20	.659	.891	.967	.991	.998	.999	1.000	1.000	1.000	1.000	1.000	1.000	1.000	1.000	1.000	1.000	1.000	1.000	1.000
21	1.000	1.000	1.000	1.000	1.000	1.000	1.000	1.000	1.000	1.000	1.000	1.000	1.000	1.000	1.000	1.000	1.000	1.000	1.000

d   Cumulative Probabilities for Values of p with d Defects   n = 22

d	.05	.10	.15	.20	.25	.30	.35	.40	.45	.50	.55	.60	.65	.70	.75	.80	.85	.90	.95
0	.000	.000	.000	.000	.000	.000	.000	.000	.000	.000	.000	.000	.000	.000	.002	.007	.028	.098	.324
1	.000	.000	.000	.000	.000	.000	.000	.000	.000	.000	.000	.000	.001	.004	.015	.048	.137	.339	.698
2	.000	.000	.000	.000	.000	.000	.000	.000	.000	.000	.000	.002	.006	.021	.061	.154	.338	.620	.905
3	.000	.000	.000	.000	.000	.000	.000	.000	.000	.000	.002	.008	.025	.068	.162	.332	.575	.828	.978
4	.000	.000	.000	.000	.000	.000	.000	.000	.000	.002	.008	.027	.072	.165	.323	.543	.774	.938	.996
5	.000	.000	.000	.000	.000	.000	.000	.000	.002	.008	.027	.072	.163	.313	.517	.733	.900	.982	.999
6	.000	.000	.000	.000	.000	.000	.000	.002	.008	.026	.071	.158	.302	.494	.699	.867	.963	.996	1.000
7	.000	.000	.000	.000	.000	.000	.002	.007	.024	.067	.152	.290	.474	.671	.838	.944	.989	.999	1.000
8	.000	.000	.000	.000	.000	.001	.006	.021	.062	.143	.276	.454	.647	.814	.925	.980	.997	1.000	1.000
9	.000	.000	.000	.000	.001	.004	.018	.055	.133	.262	.435	.624	.792	.908	.970	.994	.999	1.000	1.000
10	.000	.000	.000	.000	.003	.014	.047	.121	.246	.416	.604	.772	.893	.961	.990	.998	1.000	1.000	1.000
11	.000	.000	.000	.002	.010	.039	.107	.228	.396	.584	.754	.879	.953	.986	.997	1.000	1.000	1.000	1.000
12	.000	.000	.001	.006	.030	.092	.208	.376	.565	.738	.867	.945	.982	.996	.999	1.000	1.000	1.000	1.000
13	.000	.000	.003	.020	.075	.186	.353	.546	.724	.857	.938	.979	.994	.999	1.000	1.000	1.000	1.000	1.000
14	.000	.001	.011	.056	.162	.329	.526	.710	.848	.933	.976	.993	.998	1.000	1.000	1.000	1.000	1.000	1.000
15	.000	.004	.037	.133	.301	.506	.698	.842	.929	.974	.992	.998	1.000	1.000	1.000	1.000	1.000	1.000	1.000
16	.001	.018	.100	.267	.483	.687	.837	.928	.973	.992	.998	1.000	1.000	1.000	1.000	1.000	1.000	1.000	1.000
17	.004	.062	.226	.457	.677	.835	.928	.973	.992	.998	1.000	1.000	1.000	1.000	1.000	1.000	1.000	1.000	1.000
18	.022	.172	.425	.668	.838	.932	.975	.992	.998	1.000	1.000	1.000	1.000	1.000	1.000	1.000	1.000	1.000	1.000
19	.095	.380	.662	.846	.939	.979	.994	.998	1.000	1.000	1.000	1.000	1.000	1.000	1.000	1.000	1.000	1.000	1.000
20	.302	.661	.863	.952	.985	.996	.999	1.000	1.000	1.000	1.000	1.000	1.000	1.000	1.000	1.000	1.000	1.000	1.000
21	.676	.902	.972	.993	.998	1.000	1.000	1.000	1.000	1.000	1.000	1.000	1.000	1.000	1.000	1.000	1.000	1.000	1.000
22	1.000	1.000	1.000	1.000	1.000	1.000	1.000	1.000	1.000	1.000	1.000	1.000	1.000	1.000	1.000	1.000	1.000	1.000	1.000

d Cumulative Probabilities for Values of p with d Defects   n = 23

d	.05	.10	.15	.20	.25	.30	.35	.40	.45	.50	.55	.60	.65	.70	.75	.80	.85	.90	.95
0	.000	.000	.000	.000	.000	.000	.000	.000	.000	.000	.000	.000	.000	.000	.001	.006	.024	.089	.307
1	.000	.000	.000	.000	.000	.000	.000	.000	.000	.000	.000	.000	.001	.003	.012	.040	.120	.315	.679
2	.000	.000	.000	.000	.000	.000	.000	.000	.000	.000	.000	.001	.004	.016	.049	.133	.308	.592	.895
3	.000	.000	.000	.000	.000	.000	.000	.000	.000	.000	.001	.005	.018	.054	.137	.297	.540	.807	.974
4	.000	.000	.000	.000	.000	.000	.000	.000	.000	.001	.005	.019	.055	.136	.283	.501	.744	.927	.995
5	.000	.000	.000	.000	.000	.000	.000	.000	.001	.005	.019	.054	.131	.269	.468	.695	.881	.977	.999
6	.000	.000	.000	.000	.000	.000	.000	.001	.005	.017	.051	.124	.253	.440	.654	.840	.954	.994	1.000
7	.000	.000	.000	.000	.000	.000	.001	.004	.015	.047	.115	.237	.414	.618	.804	.928	.985	.999	1.000
8	.000	.000	.000	.000	.000	.001	.003	.013	.041	.105	.220	.388	.586	.771	.904	.973	.996	1.000	1.000
9	.000	.000	.000	.000	.000	.002	.010	.035	.094	.202	.364	.556	.741	.880	.959	.991	.999	1.000	1.000
10	.000	.000	.000	.000	.001	.007	.028	.081	.184	.339	.528	.713	.858	.945	.985	.997	1.000	1.000	1.000
11	.000	.000	.000	.001	.005	.021	.068	.164	.313	.500	.687	.836	.932	.979	.995	.999	1.000	1.000	1.000
12	.000	.000	.000	.003	.015	.055	.142	.287	.472	.661	.816	.919	.972	.993	.999	1.000	1.000	1.000	1.000
13	.000	.000	.001	.009	.041	.120	.259	.444	.636	.798	.906	.965	.990	.998	1.000	1.000	1.000	1.000	1.000
14	.000	.000	.004	.027	.096	.229	.414	.612	.780	.895	.959	.987	.997	.999	1.000	1.000	1.000	1.000	1.000
15	.000	.001	.015	.072	.196	.382	.586	.763	.885	.953	.985	.996	.999	1.000	1.000	1.000	1.000	1.000	1.000
16	.000	.006	.046	.160	.346	.560	.747	.876	.949	.983	.995	.999	1.000	1.000	1.000	1.000	1.000	1.000	1.000
17	.001	.023	.119	.305	.532	.731	.869	.946	.981	.995	.999	1.000	1.000	1.000	1.000	1.000	1.000	1.000	1.000
18	.005	.073	.256	.499	.717	.864	.945	.981	.995	.999	1.000	1.000	1.000	1.000	1.000	1.000	1.000	1.000	1.000
19	.026	.193	.460	.703	.863	.946	.982	.995	.999	1.000	1.000	1.000	1.000	1.000	1.000	1.000	1.000	1.000	1.000
20	.105	.408	.692	.867	.951	.984	.996	.999	1.000	1.000	1.000	1.000	1.000	1.000	1.000	1.000	1.000	1.000	1.000
21	.321	.685	.880	.960	.988	.997	.999	1.000	1.000	1.000	1.000	1.000	1.000	1.000	1.000	1.000	1.000	1.000	1.000
22	.693	.911	.976	.994	.999	1.000	1.000	1.000	1.000	1.000	1.000	1.000	1.000	1.000	1.000	1.000	1.000	1.000	1.000
23	1.000	1.000	1.000	1.000	1.000	1.000	1.000	1.000	1.000	1.000	1.000	1.000	1.000	1.000	1.000	1.000	1.000	1.000	1.000

d Cumulative Probabilities for Values of p with d Defects   n = 24

d	.05	.10	.15	.20	.25	.30	.35	.40	.45	.50	.55	.60	.65	.70	.75	.80	.85	.90	.95
0	.000	.000	.000	.000	.000	.000	.000	.000	.000	.000	.000	.000	.000	.000	.001	.005	.020	.080	.292
1	.000	.000	.000	.000	.000	.000	.000	.000	.000	.000	.000	.000	.000	.002	.009	.033	.106	.292	.661
2	.000	.000	.000	.000	.000	.000	.000	.000	.000	.000	.000	.001	.003	.012	.040	.115	.280	.564	.884
3	.000	.000	.000	.000	.000	.000	.000	.000	.000	.000	.001	.004	.013	.042	.115	.264	.505	.786	.970
4	.000	.000	.000	.000	.000	.000	.000	.000	.000	.001	.004	.013	.042	.111	.247	.460	.713	.915	.994
5	.000	.000	.000	.000	.000	.000	.000	.000	.001	.003	.013	.040	.104	.229	.422	.656	.861	.972	.999
6	.000	.000	.000	.000	.000	.000	.000	.001	.003	.011	.036	.096	.211	.389	.607	.811	.943	.993	1.000
7	.000	.000	.000	.000	.000	.000	.000	.002	.010	.032	.086	.192	.358	.565	.766	.911	.980	.998	1.000
8	.000	.000	.000	.000	.000	.000	.002	.008	.027	.076	.173	.328	.526	.725	.879	.964	.994	1.000	1.000
9	.000	.000	.000	.000	.000	.001	.005	.022	.065	.154	.299	.489	.687	.847	.945	.987	.999	1.000	1.000
10	.000	.000	.000	.000	.001	.004	.016	.053	.134	.271	.454	.650	.817	.926	.979	.996	1.000	1.000	1.000
11	.000	.000	.000	.000	.002	.012	.042	.114	.242	.419	.615	.787	.906	.969	.993	.999	1.000	1.000	1.000
12	.000	.000	.000	.001	.007	.031	.094	.213	.385	.581	.758	.886	.958	.988	.998	1.000	1.000	1.000	1.000
13	.000	.000	.000	.004	.021	.074	.183	.350	.546	.729	.866	.947	.984	.996	.999	1.000	1.000	1.000	1.000
14	.000	.000	.001	.013	.055	.153	.313	.511	.701	.846	.935	.978	.995	.999	1.000	1.000	1.000	1.000	1.000
15	.000	.000	.006	.036	.121	.275	.474	.672	.827	.924	.973	.992	.998	1.000	1.000	1.000	1.000	1.000	1.000
16	.000	.002	.020	.089	.234	.435	.642	.808	.914	.968	.990	.998	1.000	1.000	1.000	1.000	1.000	1.000	1.000
17	.000	.007	.057	.189	.393	.611	.789	.904	.964	.989	.997	.999	1.000	1.000	1.000	1.000	1.000	1.000	1.000
18	.001	.028	.139	.344	.578	.771	.896	.960	.987	.997	.999	1.000	1.000	1.000	1.000	1.000	1.000	1.000	1.000
19	.006	.085	.287	.540	.753	.889	.958	.987	.996	.999	1.000	1.000	1.000	1.000	1.000	1.000	1.000	1.000	1.000
20	.030	.214	.495	.736	.885	.958	.987	.996	.999	1.000	1.000	1.000	1.000	1.000	1.000	1.000	1.000	1.000	1.000
21	.116	.436	.720	.885	.960	.988	.997	.999	1.000	1.000	1.000	1.000	1.000	1.000	1.000	1.000	1.000	1.000	1.000
22	.339	.708	.894	.967	.991	.998	1.000	1.000	1.000	1.000	1.000	1.000	1.000	1.000	1.000	1.000	1.000	1.000	1.000
23	.708	.920	.980	.995	.999	1.000	1.000	1.000	1.000	1.000	1.000	1.000	1.000	1.000	1.000	1.000	1.000	1.000	1.000
24	1.000	1.000	1.000	1.000	1.000	1.000	1.000	1.000	1.000	1.000	1.000	1.000	1.000	1.000	1.000	1.000	1.000	1.000	1.000

d Cumulative Probabilities for Values of p with d Defects   n = 25

d	.05	.10	.15	.20	.25	.30	.35	.40	.45	.50	.55	.60	.65	.70	.75	.80	.85	.90	.95
0	.000	.000	.000	.000	.000	.000	.000	.000	.000	.000	.000	.000	.000	.000	.001	.004	.017	.072	.277
1	.000	.000	.000	.000	.000	.000	.000	.000	.000	.000	.000	.000	.000	.002	.007	.027	.093	.271	.642
2	.000	.000	.000	.000	.000	.000	.000	.000	.000	.000	.000	.000	.002	.009	.032	.098	.254	.537	.873
3	.000	.000	.000	.000	.000	.000	.000	.000	.000	.000	.000	.002	.010	.033	.096	.234	.471	.764	.966
4	.000	.000	.000	.000	.000	.000	.000	.000	.000	.000	.002	.009	.032	.090	.214	.421	.682	.902	.993
5	.000	.000	.000	.000	.000	.000	.000	.000	.000	.002	.009	.029	.083	.193	.378	.617	.838	.967	.999
6	.000	.000	.000	.000	.000	.000	.000	.000	.002	.007	.026	.074	.173	.341	.561	.780	.930	.991	1.000
7	.000	.000	.000	.000	.000	.000	.000	.001	.006	.022	.064	.154	.306	.512	.727	.891	.975	.998	1.000
8	.000	.000	.000	.000	.000	.000	.001	.004	.017	.054	.134	.274	.467	.677	.851	.953	.992	1.000	1.000
9	.000	.000	.000	.000	.000	.000	.003	.013	.044	.115	.242	.425	.630	.811	.929	.983	.998	1.000	1.000
10	.000	.000	.000	.000	.000	.002	.009	.034	.096	.212	.384	.586	.771	.902	.970	.994	1.000	1.000	1.000
11	.000	.000	.000	.000	.001	.006	.025	.078	.183	.345	.543	.732	.875	.956	.989	.998	1.000	1.000	1.000
12	.000	.000	.000	.000	.003	.017	.060	.154	.306	.500	.694	.846	.940	.983	.997	1.000	1.000	1.000	1.000
13	.000	.000	.000	.002	.011	.044	.125	.268	.457	.655	.817	.922	.975	.994	.999	1.000	1.000	1.000	1.000
14	.000	.000	.000	.006	.030	.098	.229	.414	.616	.788	.904	.966	.991	.998	1.000	1.000	1.000	1.000	1.000
15	.000	.000	.002	.017	.071	.189	.370	.575	.758	.885	.956	.987	.997	1.000	1.000	1.000	1.000	1.000	1.000
16	.000	.000	.008	.047	.149	.323	.533	.726	.866	.946	.983	.996	.999	1.000	1.000	1.000	1.000	1.000	1.000
17	.000	.002	.025	.109	.273	.488	.694	.846	.936	.978	.994	.999	1.000	1.000	1.000	1.000	1.000	1.000	1.000
18	.000	.009	.070	.220	.439	.659	.827	.926	.974	.993	.998	1.000	1.000	1.000	1.000	1.000	1.000	1.000	1.000
19	.001	.033	.162	.383	.622	.807	.917	.971	.991	.998	1.000	1.000	1.000	1.000	1.000	1.000	1.000	1.000	1.000
20	.007	.098	.318	.579	.786	.910	.968	.991	.998	1.000	1.000	1.000	1.000	1.000	1.000	1.000	1.000	1.000	1.000
21	.034	.236	.529	.766	.904	.967	.990	.998	1.000	1.000	1.000	1.000	1.000	1.000	1.000	1.000	1.000	1.000	1.000
22	.127	.463	.746	.902	.968	.991	.998	1.000	1.000	1.000	1.000	1.000	1.000	1.000	1.000	1.000	1.000	1.000	1.000
23	.358	.729	.907	.973	.993	.998	1.000	1.000	1.000	1.000	1.000	1.000	1.000	1.000	1.000	1.000	1.000	1.000	1.000
24	.723	.928	.983	.996	.999	1.000	1.000	1.000	1.000	1.000	1.000	1.000	1.000	1.000	1.000	1.000	1.000	1.000	1.000
25	1.000	1.000	1.000	1.000	1.000	1.000	1.000	1.000	1.000	1.000	1.000	1.000	1.000	1.000	1.000	1.000	1.000	1.000	1.000

d   Cumulative Probabilities for Values of p with d Defects   n = 26

d	.05	.10	.15	.20	.25	.30	.35	.40	.45	.50	.55	.60	.65	.70	.75	.80	.85	.90	.95
0	.000	.000	.000	.000	.000	.000	.000	.000	.000	.000	.000	.000	.000	.000	.001	.003	.015	.065	.264
1	.000	.000	.000	.000	.000	.000	.000	.000	.000	.000	.000	.000	.000	.001	.005	.023	.082	.251	.624
2	.000	.000	.000	.000	.000	.000	.000	.000	.000	.000	.000	.000	.001	.007	.026	.084	.230	.511	.861
3	.000	.000	.000	.000	.000	.000	.000	.000	.000	.000	.000	.002	.007	.026	.080	.207	.439	.741	.961
4	.000	.000	.000	.000	.000	.000	.000	.000	.000	.000	.001	.007	.024	.073	.184	.383	.650	.888	.991
5	.000	.000	.000	.000	.000	.000	.000	.000	.000	.001	.006	.021	.065	.163	.337	.577	.815	.960	.998
6	.000	.000	.000	.000	.000	.000	.000	.001	.005	.018	.056	.142	.297	.515	.747	.917	.988	1.000
7	.000	.000	.000	.000	.000	.000	.000	.001	.004	.014	.047	.122	.260	.460	.685	.869	.968	.997	1.000
8	.000	.000	.000	.000	.000	.000	.000	.002	.011	.038	.102	.226	.411	.627	.820	.941	.989	.999	1.000
9	.000	.000	.000	.000	.000	.000	.002	.008	.029	.084	.194	.364	.573	.770	.909	.977	.997	1.000	1.000
10	.000	.000	.000	.000	.000	.001	.005	.022	.067	.163	.320	.521	.722	.875	.960	.992	.999	1.000	1.000
11	.000	.000	.000	.000	.000	.003	.015	.052	.135	.279	.471	.674	.838	.940	.985	.998	1.000	1.000	1.000
12	.000	.000	.000	.000	.002	.009	.038	.108	.238	.423	.626	.801	.917	.974	.995	.999	1.000	1.000	1.000
13	.000	.000	.000	.001	.005	.026	.083	.199	.374	.577	.762	.892	.962	.991	.998	1.000	1.000	1.000	1.000
14	.000	.000	.000	.002	.015	.060	.162	.326	.529	.721	.865	.948	.985	.997	1.000	1.000	1.000	1.000	1.000
15	.000	.000	.001	.008	.040	.125	.278	.479	.680	.837	.933	.978	.995	.999	1.000	1.000	1.000	1.000	1.000
16	.000	.000	.003	.023	.091	.230	.427	.636	.806	.916	.971	.992	.998	1.000	1.000	1.000	1.000	1.000	1.000
17	.000	.001	.011	.059	.180	.373	.589	.774	.898	.962	.989	.998	1.000	1.000	1.000	1.000	1.000	1.000	1.000
18	.000	.003	.032	.131	.315	.540	.740	.878	.953	.986	.996	.999	1.000	1.000	1.000	1.000	1.000	1.000	1.000
19	.000	.012	.083	.253	.485	.703	.858	.944	.982	.995	.999	1.000	1.000	1.000	1.000	1.000	1.000	1.000	1.000
20	.002	.040	.185	.423	.663	.837	.935	.979	.994	.999	1.000	1.000	1.000	1.000	1.000	1.000	1.000	1.000	1.000
21	.009	.112	.350	.617	.816	.927	.976	.993	.999	1.000	1.000	1.000	1.000	1.000	1.000	1.000	1.000	1.000	1.000
22	.039	.259	.561	.793	.920	.974	.993	.998	1.000	1.000	1.000	1.000	1.000	1.000	1.000	1.000	1.000	1.000	1.000
23	.139	.489	.770	.916	.974	.993	.999	1.000	1.000	1.000	1.000	1.000	1.000	1.000	1.000	1.000	1.000	1.000	1.000
24	.376	.749	.918	.977	.995	.999	1.000	1.000	1.000	1.000	1.000	1.000	1.000	1.000	1.000	1.000	1.000	1.000	1.000
25	.736	.935	.985	.997	.999	1.000	1.000	1.000	1.000	1.000	1.000	1.000	1.000	1.000	1.000	1.000	1.000	1.000	1.000
26	1.000	1.000	1.000	1.000	1.000	1.000	1.000	1.000	1.000	1.000	1.000	1.000	1.000	1.000	1.000	1.000	1.000	1.000	1.000

d   Cumulative Probabilities for Values of p with d Defects   n = 27

d	.05	.10	.15	.20	.25	.30	.35	.40	.45	.50	.55	.60	.65	.70	.75	.80	.85	.90	.95
0	.000	.000	.000	.000	.000	.000	.000	.000	.000	.000	.000	.000	.000	.000	.000	.002	.012	.058	.250
1	.000	.000	.000	.000	.000	.000	.000	.000	.000	.000	.000	.000	.000	.001	.004	.019	.072	.233	.606
2	.000	.000	.000	.000	.000	.000	.000	.000	.000	.000	.000	.000	.001	.005	.021	.072	.207	.485	.850
3	.000	.000	.000	.000	.000	.000	.000	.000	.000	.000	.000	.001	.005	.020	.067	.182	.407	.718	.956
4	.000	.000	.000	.000	.000	.000	.000	.000	.000	.000	.001	.005	.018	.059	.158	.348	.619	.873	.990
5	.000	.000	.000	.000	.000	.000	.000	.000	.000	.001	.004	.015	.051	.136	.299	.539	.790	.953	.998
6	.000	.000	.000	.000	.000	.000	.000	.000	.001	.003	.013	.042	.115	.256	.471	.713	.901	.985	1.000
7	.000	.000	.000	.000	.000	.000	.000	.000	.002	.010	.034	.095	.218	.411	.643	.844	.960	.996	1.000
8	.000	.000	.000	.000	.000	.000	.000	.001	.007	.026	.077	.184	.358	.577	.786	.926	.986	.999	1.000
9	.000	.000	.000	.000	.000	.000	.001	.005	.019	.061	.153	.309	.516	.728	.887	.970	.996	1.000	1.000
10	.000	.000	.000	.000	.000	.000	.003	.013	.046	.124	.263	.458	.670	.843	.947	.989	.999	1.000	1.000
11	.000	.000	.000	.000	.000	.002	.009	.034	.098	.221	.403	.613	.798	.920	.978	.997	1.000	1.000	1.000
12	.000	.000	.000	.000	.001	.005	.023	.074	.181	.351	.556	.750	.889	.964	.992	.999	1.000	1.000	1.000
13	.000	.000	.000	.000	.002	.014	.054	.145	.300	.500	.700	.855	.946	.986	.998	1.000	1.000	1.000	1.000
14	.000	.000	.000	.001	.008	.036	.111	.250	.444	.649	.819	.926	.977	.995	.999	1.000	1.000	1.000	1.000
15	.000	.000	.000	.003	.022	.080	.202	.387	.597	.779	.902	.966	.991	.998	1.000	1.000	1.000	1.000	1.000
16	.000	.000	.001	.011	.053	.157	.330	.542	.737	.876	.954	.987	.997	1.000	1.000	1.000	1.000	1.000	1.000
17	.000	.000	.004	.030	.113	.272	.484	.691	.847	.939	.981	.995	.999	1.000	1.000	1.000	1.000	1.000	1.000
18	.000	.001	.014	.074	.214	.423	.642	.816	.923	.974	.993	.999	1.000	1.000	1.000	1.000	1.000	1.000	1.000
19	.000	.004	.040	.156	.357	.589	.782	.905	.966	.990	.998	1.000	1.000	1.000	1.000	1.000	1.000	1.000	1.000
20	.000	.015	.099	.287	.529	.744	.885	.958	.987	.997	.999	1.000	1.000	1.000	1.000	1.000	1.000	1.000	1.000
21	.002	.047	.210	.461	.701	.864	.949	.985	.996	.999	1.000	1.000	1.000	1.000	1.000	1.000	1.000	1.000	1.000
22	.010	.127	.381	.652	.842	.941	.982	.995	.999	1.000	1.000	1.000	1.000	1.000	1.000	1.000	1.000	1.000	1.000
23	.044	.282	.593	.818	.933	.980	.995	.999	1.000	1.000	1.000	1.000	1.000	1.000	1.000	1.000	1.000	1.000	1.000
24	.150	.515	.793	.928	.979	.995	.999	1.000	1.000	1.000	1.000	1.000	1.000	1.000	1.000	1.000	1.000	1.000	1.000
25	.394	.767	.928	.981	.996	.999	1.000	1.000	1.000	1.000	1.000	1.000	1.000	1.000	1.000	1.000	1.000	1.000	1.000
26	.750	.942	.988	.998	1.000	1.000	1.000	1.000	1.000	1.000	1.000	1.000	1.000	1.000	1.000	1.000	1.000	1.000	1.000
27	1.000	1.000	1.000	1.000	1.000	1.000	1.000	1.000	1.000	1.000	1.000	1.000	1.000	1.000	1.000	1.000	1.000	1.000	1.000

d   Cumulative Probabilities for Values of p with d Defects   n = 28

d	.05	.10	.15	.20	.25	.30	.35	.40	.45	.50	.55	.60	.65	.70	.75	.80	.85	.90	.95
0	.000	.000	.000	.000	.000	.000	.000	.000	.000	.000	.000	.000	.000	.000	.000	.002	.011	.052	.238
1	.000	.000	.000	.000	.000	.000	.000	.000	.000	.000	.000	.000	.000	.001	.003	.015	.063	.215	.588
2	.000	.000	.000	.000	.000	.000	.000	.000	.000	.000	.000	.000	.001	.004	.017	.061	.187	.459	.837
3	.000	.000	.000	.000	.000	.000	.000	.000	.000	.000	.000	.001	.004	.016	.055	.160	.377	.695	.951
4	.000	.000	.000	.000	.000	.000	.000	.000	.000	.000	.001	.003	.014	.047	.135	.315	.587	.858	.988
5	.000	.000	.000	.000	.000	.000	.000	.000	.000	.000	.003	.011	.039	.113	.264	.501	.765	.945	.998
6	.000	.000	.000	.000	.000	.000	.000	.000	.000	.002	.009	.031	.092	.220	.428	.678	.885	.982	1.000
7	.000	.000	.000	.000	.000	.000	.000	.000	.001	.006	.024	.074	.182	.365	.600	.818	.951	.995	1.000
8	.000	.000	.000	.000	.000	.000	.000	.001	.004	.018	.058	.148	.309	.528	.750	.910	.982	.999	1.000
9	.000	.000	.000	.000	.000	.000	.000	.003	.012	.044	.119	.259	.461	.682	.862	.961	.994	1.000	1.000
10	.000	.000	.000	.000	.000	.000	.002	.008	.031	.092	.213	.399	.616	.809	.932	.985	.998	1.000	1.000
11	.000	.000	.000	.000	.000	.001	.005	.022	.070	.172	.340	.551	.753	.897	.971	.995	1.000	1.000	1.000
12	.000	.000	.000	.000	.000	.003	.014	.050	.135	.286	.487	.695	.857	.951	.989	.999	1.000	1.000	1.000
13	.000	.000	.000	.000	.001	.008	.034	.102	.235	.425	.636	.813	.926	.979	.996	1.000	1.000	1.000	1.000
14	.000	.000	.000	.000	.004	.021	.074	.187	.364	.575	.765	.898	.966	.992	.999	1.000	1.000	1.000	1.000
15	.000	.000	.000	.001	.011	.049	.143	.305	.513	.714	.865	.950	.986	.997	1.000	1.000	1.000	1.000	1.000
16	.000	.000	.000	.005	.029	.103	.247	.449	.660	.828	.930	.978	.995	.999	1.000	1.000	1.000	1.000	1.000
17	.000	.000	.002	.015	.068	.191	.384	.601	.787	.908	.969	.992	.998	1.000	1.000	1.000	1.000	1.000	1.000
18	.000	.000	.006	.039	.138	.318	.539	.741	.881	.956	.988	.997	1.000	1.000	1.000	1.000	1.000	1.000	1.000
19	.000	.001	.018	.090	.250	.472	.691	.852	.942	.982	.996	.999	1.000	1.000	1.000	1.000	1.000	1.000	1.000
20	.000	.005	.049	.182	.400	.635	.818	.926	.976	.994	.999	1.000	1.000	1.000	1.000	1.000	1.000	1.000	1.000
21	.000	.018	.115	.322	.572	.780	.908	.969	.991	.998	1.000	1.000	1.000	1.000	1.000	1.000	1.000	1.000	1.000
22	.002	.055	.235	.499	.736	.887	.961	.989	.997	1.000	1.000	1.000	1.000	1.000	1.000	1.000	1.000	1.000	1.000
23	.012	.142	.413	.685	.865	.953	.986	.997	.999	1.000	1.000	1.000	1.000	1.000	1.000	1.000	1.000	1.000	1.000
24	.049	.305	.623	.840	.945	.984	.996	.999	1.000	1.000	1.000	1.000	1.000	1.000	1.000	1.000	1.000	1.000	1.000
25	.163	.541	.813	.939	.983	.996	.999	1.000	1.000	1.000	1.000	1.000	1.000	1.000	1.000	1.000	1.000	1.000	1.000
26	.412	.785	.937	.985	.997	.999	1.000	1.000	1.000	1.000	1.000	1.000	1.000	1.000	1.000	1.000	1.000	1.000	1.000
27	.762	.948	.989	.998	1.000	1.000	1.000	1.000	1.000	1.000	1.000	1.000	1.000	1.000	1.000	1.000	1.000	1.000	1.000
28	1.000	1.000	1.000	1.000	1.000	1.000	1.000	1.000	1.000	1.000	1.000	1.000	1.000	1.000	1.000	1.000	1.000	1.000	1.000

d Cumulative Probabilities for Values of p with d Defects   n = 29

d	.05	.10	.15	.20	.25	.30	.35	.40	.45	.50	.55	.60	.65	.70	.75	.80	.85	.90	.95
0	.000	.000	.000	.000	.000	.000	.000	.000	.000	.000	.000	.000	.000	.000	.000	.002	.009	.047	.226
1	.000	.000	.000	.000	.000	.000	.000	.000	.000	.000	.000	.000	.000	.000	.003	.013	.055	.199	.571
2	.000	.000	.000	.000	.000	.000	.000	.000	.000	.000	.000	.000	.001	.003	.013	.052	.168	.435	.825
3	.000	.000	.000	.000	.000	.000	.000	.000	.000	.000	.000	.000	.003	.012	.046	.140	.349	.671	.945
4	.000	.000	.000	.000	.000	.000	.000	.000	.000	.000	.000	.002	.010	.038	.115	.284	.555	.842	.986
5	.000	.000	.000	.000	.000	.000	.000	.000	.000	.000	.002	.008	.030	.093	.232	.463	.738	.936	.997
6	.000	.000	.000	.000	.000	.000	.000	.000	.000	.001	.006	.023	.074	.188	.387	.643	.867	.978	1.000
7	.000	.000	.000	.000	.000	.000	.000	.000	.001	.004	.017	.057	.151	.321	.557	.790	.941	.994	1.000
8	.000	.000	.000	.000	.000	.000	.000	.000	.003	.012	.043	.119	.265	.479	.713	.892	.978	.998	1.000
9	.000	.000	.000	.000	.000	.000	.000	.002	.008	.031	.091	.215	.408	.636	.834	.951	.993	1.000	1.000
10	.000	.000	.000	.000	.000	.000	.001	.005	.021	.068	.171	.343	.562	.771	.914	.980	.998	1.000	1.000
11	.000	.000	.000	.000	.000	.000	.003	.013	.049	.132	.283	.490	.705	.871	.961	.993	.999	1.000	1.000
12	.000	.000	.000	.000	.000	.001	.008	.033	.099	.229	.421	.637	.821	.935	.984	.998	1.000	1.000	1.000
13	.000	.000	.000	.000	.000	.004	.021	.071	.180	.356	.569	.766	.902	.971	.994	.999	1.000	1.000	1.000
14	.000	.000	.000	.000	.002	.012	.048	.136	.293	.500	.707	.864	.952	.988	.998	1.000	1.000	1.000	1.000
15	.000	.000	.000	.001	.006	.029	.098	.234	.431	.644	.820	.929	.979	.996	1.000	1.000	1.000	1.000	1.000
16	.000	.000	.000	.002	.016	.065	.179	.363	.579	.771	.901	.967	.992	.999	1.000	1.000	1.000	1.000	1.000
17	.000	.000	.001	.007	.039	.129	.295	.510	.717	.868	.951	.987	.997	1.000	1.000	1.000	1.000	1.000	1.000
18	.000	.000	.002	.020	.086	.229	.438	.657	.829	.932	.979	.995	.999	1.000	1.000	1.000	1.000	1.000	1.000
19	.000	.000	.007	.049	.166	.364	.592	.785	.909	.969	.992	.998	1.000	1.000	1.000	1.000	1.000	1.000	1.000
20	.000	.002	.022	.108	.287	.521	.735	.881	.957	.988	.997	1.000	1.000	1.000	1.000	1.000	1.000	1.000	1.000
21	.000	.006	.059	.210	.443	.679	.849	.943	.983	.996	.999	1.000	1.000	1.000	1.000	1.000	1.000	1.000	1.000
22	.000	.022	.133	.357	.613	.812	.926	.977	.994	.999	1.000	1.000	1.000	1.000	1.000	1.000	1.000	1.000	1.000
23	.003	.064	.262	.537	.768	.907	.970	.992	.998	1.000	1.000	1.000	1.000	1.000	1.000	1.000	1.000	1.000	1.000
24	.014	.158	.445	.716	.885	.962	.990	.998	1.000	1.000	1.000	1.000	1.000	1.000	1.000	1.000	1.000	1.000	1.000
25	.055	.329	.651	.860	.954	.988	.997	1.000	1.000	1.000	1.000	1.000	1.000	1.000	1.000	1.000	1.000	1.000	1.000
26	.175	.565	.832	.948	.987	.997	.999	1.000	1.000	1.000	1.000	1.000	1.000	1.000	1.000	1.000	1.000	1.000	1.000
27	.429	.801	.945	.987	.997	1.000	1.000	1.000	1.000	1.000	1.000	1.000	1.000	1.000	1.000	1.000	1.000	1.000	1.000
28	.774	.953	.991	.998	1.000	1.000	1.000	1.000	1.000	1.000	1.000	1.000	1.000	1.000	1.000	1.000	1.000	1.000	1.000
29	1.000	1.000	1.000	1.000	1.000	1.000	1.000	1.000	1.000	1.000	1.000	1.000	1.000	1.000	1.000	1.000	1.000	1.000	1.000

d Cumulative Probabilities for Values of p with d Defects

n = 30

d	.05	.10	.15	.20	.25	.30	.35	.40	.45	.50	.55	.60	.65	.70	.75	.80	.85	.90	.95
0	.000	.000	.000	.000	.000	.000	.000	.000	.000	.000	.000	.000	.000	.000	.000	.001	.008	.042	.215
1	.000	.000	.000	.000	.000	.000	.000	.000	.000	.000	.000	.000	.000	.000	.002	.011	.048	.184	.554
2	.000	.000	.000	.000	.000	.000	.000	.000	.000	.000	.000	.000	.000	.002	.011	.044	.151	.411	.812
3	.000	.000	.000	.000	.000	.000	.000	.000	.000	.000	.000	.000	.002	.009	.037	.123	.322	.647	.939
4	.000	.000	.000	.000	.000	.000	.000	.000	.000	.000	.000	.002	.008	.030	.098	.255	.524	.825	.984
5	.000	.000	.000	.000	.000	.000	.000	.000	.000	.000	.001	.006	.023	.077	.203	.428	.711	.927	.997
6	.000	.000	.000	.000	.000	.000	.000	.000	.000	.001	.004	.017	.059	.160	.348	.607	.847	.974	.999
7	.000	.000	.000	.000	.000	.000	.000	.000	.000	.003	.012	.044	.124	.281	.514	.761	.930	.992	1.000
8	.000	.000	.000	.000	.000	.000	.000	.000	.002	.008	.031	.094	.225	.432	.674	.871	.972	.998	1.000
9	.000	.000	.000	.000	.000	.000	.000	.001	.005	.021	.069	.176	.358	.589	.803	.939	.990	1.000	1.000
10	.000	.000	.000	.000	.000	.000	.000	.003	.014	.049	.135	.291	.508	.730	.894	.974	.997	1.000	1.000
11	.000	.000	.000	.000	.000	.000	.001	.008	.033	.100	.233	.431	.655	.841	.949	.991	.999	1.000	1.000
12	.000	.000	.000	.000	.000	.001	.005	.021	.071	.181	.359	.578	.780	.916	.978	.997	1.000	1.000	1.000
13	.000	.000	.000	.000	.000	.002	.012	.048	.136	.292	.502	.715	.874	.960	.992	.999	1.000	1.000	1.000
14	.000	.000	.000	.000	.001	.006	.030	.097	.231	.428	.645	.825	.935	.983	.997	1.000	1.000	1.000	1.000
15	.000	.000	.000	.000	.003	.017	.065	.175	.355	.572	.769	.903	.970	.994	.999	1.000	1.000	1.000	1.000
16	.000	.000	.000	.001	.008	.040	.126	.285	.498	.708	.864	.952	.988	.998	1.000	1.000	1.000	1.000	1.000
17	.000	.000	.000	.003	.022	.084	.220	.422	.641	.819	.929	.979	.995	.999	1.000	1.000	1.000	1.000	1.000
18	.000	.000	.001	.009	.051	.159	.345	.569	.767	.900	.967	.992	.999	1.000	1.000	1.000	1.000	1.000	1.000
19	.000	.000	.003	.026	.106	.270	.492	.709	.865	.951	.986	.997	1.000	1.000	1.000	1.000	1.000	1.000	1.000
20	.000	.000	.010	.061	.197	.411	.642	.824	.931	.979	.995	.999	1.000	1.000	1.000	1.000	1.000	1.000	1.000
21	.000	.002	.028	.129	.326	.568	.775	.906	.969	.992	.998	1.000	1.000	1.000	1.000	1.000	1.000	1.000	1.000
22	.000	.008	.070	.239	.486	.719	.876	.956	.988	.997	1.000	1.000	1.000	1.000	1.000	1.000	1.000	1.000	1.000
23	.001	.026	.153	.393	.652	.840	.941	.983	.996	.999	1.000	1.000	1.000	1.000	1.000	1.000	1.000	1.000	1.000
24	.003	.073	.289	.572	.797	.923	.977	.994	.999	1.000	1.000	1.000	1.000	1.000	1.000	1.000	1.000	1.000	1.000
25	.016	.175	.476	.745	.902	.970	.992	.998	1.000	1.000	1.000	1.000	1.000	1.000	1.000	1.000	1.000	1.000	1.000
26	.061	.353	.678	.877	.963	.991	.998	1.000	1.000	1.000	1.000	1.000	1.000	1.000	1.000	1.000	1.000	1.000	1.000
27	.188	.589	.849	.956	.989	.998	1.000	1.000	1.000	1.000	1.000	1.000	1.000	1.000	1.000	1.000	1.000	1.000	1.000
28	.446	.816	.952	.989	.998	1.000	1.000	1.000	1.000	1.000	1.000	1.000	1.000	1.000	1.000	1.000	1.000	1.000	1.000
29	.785	.958	.992	.999	1.000	1.000	1.000	1.000	1.000	1.000	1.000	1.000	1.000	1.000	1.000	1.000	1.000	1.000	1.000
30	1.000	1.000	1.000	1.000	1.000	1.000	1.000	1.000	1.000	1.000	1.000	1.000	1.000	1.000	1.000	1.000	1.000	1.000	1.000

d   Cumulative Probabilities for Values of p with d Defects   n = 31

d	.05	.10	.15	.20	.25	.30	.35	.40	.45	.50	.55	.60	.65	.70	.75	.80	.85	.90	.95
0	.000	.000	.000	.000	.000	.000	.000	.000	.000	.000	.000	.000	.000	.000	.000	.001	.006	.038	.204
1	.000	.000	.000	.000	.000	.000	.000	.000	.000	.000	.000	.000	.000	.000	.002	.009	.042	.170	.537
2	.000	.000	.000	.000	.000	.000	.000	.000	.000	.000	.000	.000	.000	.002	.008	.037	.136	.389	.799
3	.000	.000	.000	.000	.000	.000	.000	.000	.000	.000	.000	.000	.001	.007	.031	.107	.296	.624	.933
4	.000	.000	.000	.000	.000	.000	.000	.000	.000	.000	.000	.001	.006	.024	.083	.229	.494	.807	.982
5	.000	.000	.000	.000	.000	.000	.000	.000	.000	.000	.001	.004	.018	.063	.176	.393	.683	.917	.996
6	.000	.000	.000	.000	.000	.000	.000	.000	.000	.000	.003	.013	.046	.135	.312	.571	.827	.969	.999
7	.000	.000	.000	.000	.000	.000	.000	.000	.000	.002	.008	.033	.101	.245	.473	.730	.918	.990	1.000
8	.000	.000	.000	.000	.000	.000	.000	.000	.001	.005	.023	.074	.189	.386	.634	.849	.966	.997	1.000
9	.000	.000	.000	.000	.000	.000	.000	.000	.003	.015	.052	.143	.311	.542	.771	.925	.988	.999	1.000
10	.000	.000	.000	.000	.000	.000	.000	.002	.009	.035	.106	.245	.455	.688	.872	.967	.996	1.000	1.000
11	.000	.000	.000	.000	.000	.000	.001	.005	.023	.075	.189	.375	.603	.808	.936	.987	.999	1.000	1.000
12	.000	.000	.000	.000	.000	.000	.003	.013	.051	.141	.302	.520	.736	.893	.971	.996	1.000	1.000	1.000
13	.000	.000	.000	.000	.000	.001	.007	.032	.100	.237	.438	.660	.841	.947	.988	.999	1.000	1.000	1.000
14	.000	.000	.000	.000	.000	.003	.019	.068	.178	.360	.581	.781	.913	.976	.996	1.000	1.000	1.000	1.000
15	.000	.000	.000	.000	.001	.010	.042	.128	.287	.500	.713	.872	.958	.990	.999	1.000	1.000	1.000	1.000
16	.000	.000	.000	.000	.004	.024	.087	.219	.419	.640	.822	.932	.981	.997	1.000	1.000	1.000	1.000	1.000
17	.000	.000	.000	.001	.012	.053	.159	.340	.562	.763	.900	.968	.993	.999	1.000	1.000	1.000	1.000	1.000
18	.000	.000	.000	.004	.029	.107	.264	.480	.698	.859	.949	.987	.997	1.000	1.000	1.000	1.000	1.000	1.000
19	.000	.000	.001	.013	.064	.192	.397	.625	.811	.925	.977	.995	.999	1.000	1.000	1.000	1.000	1.000	1.000
20	.000	.000	.004	.033	.128	.312	.545	.755	.894	.965	.991	.998	1.000	1.000	1.000	1.000	1.000	1.000	1.000
21	.000	.001	.012	.075	.229	.458	.689	.857	.948	.985	.997	1.000	1.000	1.000	1.000	1.000	1.000	1.000	1.000
22	.000	.003	.034	.151	.366	.614	.811	.926	.977	.995	.999	1.000	1.000	1.000	1.000	1.000	1.000	1.000	1.000
23	.000	.010	.082	.270	.527	.755	.899	.967	.992	.998	1.000	1.000	1.000	1.000	1.000	1.000	1.000	1.000	1.000
24	.001	.031	.173	.429	.688	.865	.954	.987	.997	1.000	1.000	1.000	1.000	1.000	1.000	1.000	1.000	1.000	1.000
25	.004	.083	.317	.607	.824	.937	.982	.996	.999	1.000	1.000	1.000	1.000	1.000	1.000	1.000	1.000	1.000	1.000
26	.018	.193	.506	.771	.917	.976	.994	.999	1.000	1.000	1.000	1.000	1.000	1.000	1.000	1.000	1.000	1.000	1.000
27	.067	.376	.704	.893	.969	.993	.999	1.000	1.000	1.000	1.000	1.000	1.000	1.000	1.000	1.000	1.000	1.000	1.000
28	.201	.611	.864	.963	.992	.998	1.000	1.000	1.000	1.000	1.000	1.000	1.000	1.000	1.000	1.000	1.000	1.000	1.000
29	.463	.830	.958	.991	.998	1.000	1.000	1.000	1.000	1.000	1.000	1.000	1.000	1.000	1.000	1.000	1.000	1.000	1.000
30	.796	.962	.994	.999	1.000	1.000	1.000	1.000	1.000	1.000	1.000	1.000	1.000	1.000	1.000	1.000	1.000	1.000	1.000
31	1.000	1.000	1.000	1.000	1.000	1.000	1.000	1.000	1.000	1.000	1.000	1.000	1.000	1.000	1.000	1.000	1.000	1.000	1.000

d Cumulative Probabilities for Values of p with d Defects   n = 32

d	.05	.10	.15	.20	.25	.30	.35	.40	.45	.50	.55	.60	.65	.70	.75	.80	.85	.90	.95
0	.000	.000	.000	.000	.000	.000	.000	.000	.000	.000	.000	.000	.000	.000	.000	.001	.006	.034	.194
1	.000	.000	.000	.000	.000	.000	.000	.000	.000	.000	.000	.000	.000	.000	.001	.007	.037	.156	.520
2	.000	.000	.000	.000	.000	.000	.000	.000	.000	.000	.000	.000	.000	.001	.007	.032	.122	.367	.786
3	.000	.000	.000	.000	.000	.000	.000	.000	.000	.000	.000	.000	.001	.005	.025	.093	.272	.600	.926
4	.000	.000	.000	.000	.000	.000	.000	.000	.000	.000	.000	.001	.004	.019	.070	.204	.464	.789	.980
5	.000	.000	.000	.000	.000	.000	.000	.000	.000	.000	.000	.003	.013	.051	.153	.360	.654	.906	.995
6	.000	.000	.000	.000	.000	.000	.000	.000	.000	.000	.002	.009	.036	.113	.278	.535	.805	.964	.999
7	.000	.000	.000	.000	.000	.000	.000	.000	.000	.001	.006	.025	.082	.212	.432	.698	.904	.988	1.000
8	.000	.000	.000	.000	.000	.000	.000	.000	.001	.004	.016	.057	.158	.344	.594	.825	.959	.997	1.000
9	.000	.000	.000	.000	.000	.000	.000	.000	.002	.010	.039	.116	.268	.495	.737	.910	.984	.999	1.000
10	.000	.000	.000	.000	.000	.000	.000	.001	.006	.025	.082	.205	.405	.644	.846	.959	.995	1.000	1.000
11	.000	.000	.000	.000	.000	.000	.000	.003	.015	.055	.151	.323	.551	.772	.920	.983	.998	1.000	1.000
12	.000	.000	.000	.000	.000	.000	.001	.008	.035	.108	.251	.462	.690	.867	.962	.994	1.000	1.000	1.000
13	.000	.000	.000	.000	.000	.001	.004	.021	.073	.189	.377	.604	.804	.931	.984	.998	1.000	1.000	1.000
14	.000	.000	.000	.000	.000	.002	.011	.046	.135	.298	.517	.732	.888	.967	.994	.999	1.000	1.000	1.000
15	.000	.000	.000	.000	.001	.005	.027	.092	.227	.430	.654	.835	.942	.986	.998	1.000	1.000	1.000	1.000
16	.000	.000	.000	.000	.002	.014	.058	.165	.346	.570	.773	.908	.973	.995	.999	1.000	1.000	1.000	1.000

continued on following page

d Cumulative Probabilities for Values of p with d Defects n = 32

d	.05	.10	.15	.20	.25	.30	.35	.40	.45	.50	.55	.60	.65	.70	.75	.80	.85	.90	.95
17	.000	.000	.000	.001	.006	.033	.112	.268	.483	.702	.865	.954	.989	.998	1.000	1.000	1.000	1.000	1.000
18	.000	.000	.000	.002	.016	.069	.196	.396	.623	.811	.927	.979	.996	.999	1.000	1.000	1.000	1.000	1.000
19	.000	.000	.000	.006	.038	.133	.310	.538	.749	.892	.965	.992	.999	1.000	1.000	1.000	1.000	1.000	1.000
20	.000	.000	.002	.017	.080	.228	.449	.677	.849	.945	.985	.997	1.000	1.000	1.000	1.000	1.000	1.000	1.000
21	.000	.000	.005	.041	.154	.356	.595	.795	.918	.975	.994	.999	1.000	1.000	1.000	1.000	1.000	1.000	1.000
22	.000	.001	.016	.090	.263	.505	.732	.884	.961	.990	.998	1.000	1.000	1.000	1.000	1.000	1.000	1.000	1.000
23	.000	.003	.041	.175	.406	.656	.842	.943	.984	.996	.999	1.000	1.000	1.000	1.000	1.000	1.000	1.000	1.000
24	.000	.012	.096	.302	.568	.788	.918	.975	.994	.999	1.000	1.000	1.000	1.000	1.000	1.000	1.000	1.000	1.000
25	.001	.036	.195	.465	.722	.887	.964	.991	.998	1.000	1.000	1.000	1.000	1.000	1.000	1.000	1.000	1.000	1.000
26	.005	.094	.346	.640	.847	.949	.987	.997	1.000	1.000	1.000	1.000	1.000	1.000	1.000	1.000	1.000	1.000	1.000
27	.020	.211	.536	.796	.930	.981	.996	.999	1.000	1.000	1.000	1.000	1.000	1.000	1.000	1.000	1.000	1.000	1.000
28	.074	.400	.728	.907	.975	.995	.999	1.000	1.000	1.000	1.000	1.000	1.000	1.000	1.000	1.000	1.000	1.000	1.000
29	.214	.633	.878	.968	.993	.999	1.000	1.000	1.000	1.000	1.000	1.000	1.000	1.000	1.000	1.000	1.000	1.000	1.000
30	.480	.844	.963	.993	.999	1.000	1.000	1.000	1.000	1.000	1.000	1.000	1.000	1.000	1.000	1.000	1.000	1.000	1.000
31	.806	.966	.994	.999	1.000	1.000	1.000	1.000	1.000	1.000	1.000	1.000	1.000	1.000	1.000	1.000	1.000	1.000	1.000
32	1.000	1.000	1.000	1.000	1.000	1.000	1.000	1.000	1.000	1.000	1.000	1.000	1.000	1.000	1.000	1.000	1.000	1.000	1.000

d Cumulative Probabilities for Values of p with d Defects   n = 33

d	.05	.10	.15	.20	.25	.30	.35	.40	.45	.50	.55	.60	.65	.70	.75	.80	.85	.90	.95
0	.000	.000	.000	.000	.000	.000	.000	.000	.000	.000	.000	.000	.000	.000	.000	.001	.005	.031	.184
1	.000	.000	.000	.000	.000	.000	.000	.000	.000	.000	.000	.000	.000	.000	.001	.006	.032	.144	.504
2	.000	.000	.000	.000	.000	.000	.000	.000	.000	.000	.000	.000	.000	.001	.005	.027	.109	.346	.773
3	.000	.000	.000	.000	.000	.000	.000	.000	.000	.000	.000	.000	.001	.004	.021	.081	.250	.577	.919
4	.000	.000	.000	.000	.000	.000	.000	.000	.000	.000	.000	.000	.003	.015	.059	.182	.436	.770	.977
5	.000	.000	.000	.000	.000	.000	.000	.000	.000	.000	.000	.002	.010	.041	.132	.329	.626	.894	.995
6	.000	.000	.000	.000	.000	.000	.000	.000	.000	.000	.001	.007	.028	.094	.247	.500	.783	.958	.999
7	.000	.000	.000	.000	.000	.000	.000	.000	.000	.001	.004	.019	.066	.182	.394	.666	.889	.986	1.000
8	.000	.000	.000	.000	.000	.000	.000	.000	.000	.002	.012	.044	.132	.304	.553	.800	.951	.996	1.000
9	.000	.000	.000	.000	.000	.000	.000	.000	.001	.007	.029	.092	.230	.450	.701	.893	.981	.999	1.000
10	.000	.000	.000	.000	.000	.000	.000	.001	.004	.018	.062	.169	.357	.599	.819	.949	.993	1.000	1.000
11	.000	.000	.000	.000	.000	.000	.000	.002	.010	.040	.120	.276	.500	.733	.901	.978	.998	1.000	1.000
12	.000	.000	.000	.000	.000	.000	.001	.005	.024	.081	.206	.406	.641	.839	.952	.992	.999	1.000	1.000
13	.000	.000	.000	.000	.000	.000	.002	.013	.052	.148	.320	.547	.764	.912	.979	.997	1.000	1.000	1.000
14	.000	.000	.000	.000	.000	.001	.007	.031	.101	.243	.454	.681	.859	.956	.992	.999	1.000	1.000	1.000
15	.000	.000	.000	.000	.000	.003	.017	.065	.177	.364	.592	.794	.923	.980	.997	1.000	1.000	1.000	1.000
16	.000	.000	.000	.000	.001	.008	.038	.121	.281	.500	.719	.879	.962	.992	.999	1.000	1.000	1.000	1.000

continued on following page

d Cumulative Probabilities for Values of p with d Defects   n = 33

d	.05	.10	.15	.20	.25	.30	.35	.40	.45	.50	.55	.60	.65	.70	.75	.80	.85	.90	.95
17	.000	.000	.000	.000	.003	.020	.077	.206	.408	.636	.823	.935	.983	.997	1.000	1.000	1.000	1.000	1.000
18	.000	.000	.000	.001	.008	.044	.141	.319	.546	.757	.899	.969	.993	.999	1.000	1.000	1.000	1.000	1.000
19	.000	.000	.000	.003	.021	.088	.236	.453	.680	.852	.948	.987	.998	1.000	1.000	1.000	1.000	1.000	1.000
20	.000	.000	.001	.008	.048	.161	.359	.594	.794	.919	.976	.995	.999	1.000	1.000	1.000	1.000	1.000	1.000
21	.000	.000	.002	.022	.099	.267	.500	.724	.880	.960	.990	.998	1.000	1.000	1.000	1.000	1.000	1.000	1.000
22	.000	.000	.007	.051	.181	.401	.643	.831	.938	.982	.996	.999	1.000	1.000	1.000	1.000	1.000	1.000	1.000
23	.000	.001	.019	.107	.299	.550	.770	.908	.971	.993	.999	1.000	1.000	1.000	1.000	1.000	1.000	1.000	1.000
24	.000	.004	.049	.200	.447	.696	868	.956	.988	.998	1.000	1.000	1.000	1.000	1.000	1.000	1.000	1.000	1.000
25	.000	.014	.111	.334	.606	.818	.934	.981	.996	.999	1.000	1.000	1.000	1.000	1.000	1.000	1.000	1.000	1.000
26	.001	.042	.217	.500	.753	.906	.972	.993	.999	1.000	1.000	1.000	1.000	1.000	1.000	1.000	1.000	1.000	1.000
27	.005	.106	.374	.671	.868	.959	.990	.998	1.000	1.000	1.000	1.000	1.000	1.000	1.000	1.000	1.000	1.000	1.000
28	.023	.230	.564	.818	.941	.985	.997	1.000	1.000	1.000	1.000	1.000	1.000	1.000	1.000	1.000	1.000	1.000	1.000
29	.081	.423	.750	.919	.979	.996	.999	1.000	1.000	1.000	1.000	1.000	1.000	1.000	1.000	1.000	1.000	1.000	1.000
30	.227	.654	.891	.973	.995	.999	1.000	1.000	1.000	1.000	1.000	1.000	1.000	1.000	1.000	1.000	1.000	1.000	1.000
31	.496	.856	.968	.994	.999	1.000	1.000	1.000	1.000	1.000	1.000	1.000	1.000	1.000	1.000	1.000	1.000	1.000	1.000
32	.816	.969	.995	.999	1.000	1.000	1.000	1.000	1.000	1.000	1.000	1.000	1.000	1.000	1.000	1.000	1.000	1.000	1.000
33	1.000	1.000	1.000	1.000	1.000	1.000	1.000	1.000	1.000	1.000	1.000	1.000	1.000	1.000	1.000	1.000	1.000	1.000	1.000

d Cumulative Probabilities for Values of p with d Defects   n = 34

d	.05	.10	.15	.20	.25	.30	.35	.40	.45	.50	.55	.60	.65	.70	.75	.80	.85	.90	.95
0	.000	.000	.000	.000	.000	.000	.000	.000	.000	.000	.000	.000	.000	.000	.000	.001	.004	.028	.175
1	.000	.000	.000	.000	.000	.000	.000	.000	.000	.000	.000	.000	.000	.000	.001	.005	.028	.133	.488
2	.000	.000	.000	.000	.000	.000	.000	.000	.000	.000	.000	.000	.000	.001	.004	.023	.097	.326	.759
3	.000	.000	.000	.000	.000	.000	.000	.000	.000	.000	.000	.000	.000	.003	.017	.070	.228	.554	.912
4	.000	.000	.000	.000	.000	.000	.000	.000	.000	.000	.000	.000	.002	.012	.049	.162	.408	.750	.974
5	.000	.000	.000	.000	.000	.000	.000	.000	.000	.000	.000	.001	.008	.033	.114	.300	.597	.881	.994
6	.000	.000	.000	.000	.000	.000	.000	.000	.000	.000	.001	.005	.022	.079	.218	.466	.759	.952	.999
7	.000	.000	.000	.000	.000	.000	.000	.000	.000	.000	.003	.014	.053	.156	.357	.633	.873	.983	1.000
8	.000	.000	.000	.000	.000	.000	.000	.000	.000	.001	.008	.034	.109	.268	.513	.773	.941	.995	1.000
9	.000	.000	.000	.000	.000	.000	.000	.000	.001	.005	.021	.073	.196	.406	.664	.875	.976	.999	1.000
10	.000	.000	.000	.000	.000	.000	.000	.000	.002	.012	.047	.138	.313	.554	.789	.938	.991	1.000	1.000
11	.000	.000	.000	.000	.000	.000	.000	.001	.006	.029	.094	.233	.450	.693	.881	.973	.997	1.000	1.000
12	.000	.000	.000	.000	.000	.000	.000	.003	.016	.061	.167	.354	.592	.807	.939	.989	.999	1.000	1.000
13	.000	.000	.000	.000	.000	.000	.001	.008	.037	.115	.269	.491	.721	.890	.972	.996	1.000	1.000	1.000
14	.000	.000	.000	.000·	.000	.000	.004	.020	.074	.196	.394	.627	.826	.943	.988	.999	1.000	1.000	1.000
15	.000	.000	.000	.000	.000	.001	.010	.044	.135	.304	.530	.749	.901	.973	.996	1.000	1.000	1.000	1.000
16	.000	.000	.000	.000	.000	.004	.024	.087	.224	.432	.662	.845	.949	.989	.999	1.000	1.000	1.000	1.000
17	.000	.000	.000	.000	.001	.011	.051	.155	.338	.568	.776	.913	.976	.996	1.000	1.000	1.000	1.000	1.000

continued on following page

d   Cumulative Probabilities for Values of p with d Defects   n = 34

d	.05	.10	.15	.20	.25	.30	.35	.40	.45	.50	.55	.60	.65	.70	.75	.80	.85	.90	.95
18	.000	.000	.000	.000	.004	.027	.099	.251	.470	.696	.865	.956	.990	.999	1.000	1.000	1.000	1.000	1.000
19	.000	.000	.000	.001	.012	.057	.174	.373	.606	.804	.926	.980	.996	1.000	1.000	1.000	1.000	1.000	1.000
20	.000	.000	.000	.004	.028	.110	.279	.509	.731	.885	.963	.992	.999	1.000	1.000	1.000	1.000	1.000	1.000
21	.000	.000	.001	.011	.061	.193	.408	.646	.833	.939	.984	.997	1.000	1.000	1.000	1.000	1.000	1.000	1.000
22	.000	.000	.003	.027	.119	.307	.550	.767	.906	.971	.994	.999	1.000	1.000	1.000	1.000	1.000	1.000	1.000
23	.000	.000	.009	.062	.211	.446	.687	.862	.953	.988	.998	1.000	1.000	1.000	1.000	1.000	1.000	1.000	1.000
24	.000	.001	.024	.125	.336	.594	.804	.927	.979	.995	.999	1.000	1.000	1.000	1.000	1.000	1.000	1.000	1.000
25	.000	.005	.059	.227	.487	.732	.891	.966	.992	.999	1.000	1.000	1.000	1.000	1.000	1.000	1.000	1.000	1.000
26	.000	.017	.127	.367	.643	.844	.947	.986	.997	1.000	1.000	1.000	1.000	1.000	1.000	1.000	1.000	1.000	1.000
27	.001	.048	.241	.534	.782	.921	.978	.995	.999	1.000	1.000	1.000	1.000	1.000	1.000	1.000	1.000	1.000	1.000
28	.006	.119	.403	.700	.886	.967	.992	.999	1.000	1.000	1.000	1.000	1.000	1.000	1.000	1.000	1.000	1.000	1.000
29	.026	.250	.592	.838	.951	.988	.998	1.000	1.000	1.000	1.000	1.000	1.000	1.000	1.000	1.000	1.000	1.000	1.000
30	.088	.446	.772	.930	.983	.997	1.000	1.000	1.000	1.000	1.000	1.000	1.000	1.000	1.000	1.000	1.000	1.000	1.000
31	.241	.674	.903	.977	.996	.999	1.000	1.000	1.000	1.000	1.000	1.000	1.000	1.000	1.000	1.000	1.000	1.000	1.000
32	.512	.867	.972	.995	.999	1.000	1.000	1.000	1.000	1.000	1.000	1.000	1.000	1.000	1.000	1.000	1.000	1.000	1.000
33	.825	.972	.996	.999	1.000	1.000	1.000	1.000	1.000	1.000	1.000	1.000	1.000	1.000	1.000	1.000	1.000	1.000	1.000
34	1.000	1.000	1.000	1.000	1.000	1.000	1.000	1.000	1.000	1.000	1.000	1.000	1.000	1.000	1.000	1.000	1.000	1.000	1.000

d   Cumulative Probabilities for Values of p with d Defects   n = 35

d	.05	.10	.15	.20	.25	.30	.35	.40	.45	.50	.55	.60	.65	.70	.75	.80	.85	.90	.95
0	.000	.000	.000	.000	.000	.000	.000	.000	.000	.000	.000	.000	.000	.000	.000	.000	.003	.025	.166
1	.000	.000	.000	.000	.000	.000	.000	.000	.000	.000	.000	.000	.000	.000	.001	.004	.024	.122	.472
2	.000	.000	.000	.000	.000	.000	.000	.000	.000	.000	.000	.000	.000	.000	.003	.019	.087	.306	.746
3	.000	.000	.000	.000	.000	.000	.000	.000	.000	.000	.000	.000	.000	.002	.014	.061	.209	.531	.904
4	.000	.000	.000	.000	.000	.000	.000	.000	.000	.000	.000	.000	.002	.009	.041	.143	.381	.731	.971
5	.000	.000	.000	.000	.000	.000	.000	.000	.000	.000	.000	.001	.006	.027	.098	.272	.569	.868	.993
6	.000	.000	.000	.000	.000	.000	.000	.000	.000	.000	.001	.003	.017	.065	.192	.433	.735	.945	.998
7	.000	.000	.000	.000	.000	.000	.000	.000	.000	.000	.002	.010	.042	.133	.322	.599	.856	.980	1.000
8	.000	.000	.000	.000	.000	.000	.000	.000	.000	.001	.006	.026	.089	.234	.474	.745	.931	.994	1.000
9	.000	.000	.000	.000	.000	.000	.000	.000	.000	.003	.015	.058	.165	.365	.626	.854	.971	.998	1.000
10	.000	.000	.000	.000	.000	.000	.000	.000	.001	.008	.035	.112	.272	.510	.758	.925	.989	1.000	1.000
11	.000	.000	.000	.000	.000	.000	.000	.001	.004	.020	.073	.195	.402	.652	.858	.966	.996	1.000	1.000
12	.000	.000	.000	.000	.000	.000	.000	.002	.011	.045	.134	.306	.542	.773	.924	.986	.999	1.000	1.000
13	.000	.000	.000	.000	.000	.000	.001	.005	.026	.088	.223	.436	.676	.865	.964	.995	1.000	1.000	1.000
14	.000	.000	.000	.000	.000	.000	.002	.013	.054	.155	.338	.573	.789	.927	.984	.998	1.000	1.000	1.000
15	.000	.000	.000	.000	.000	.001	.006	.030	.102	.250	.469	.700	.874	.964	.994	.999	1.000	1.000	1.000
16	.000	.000	.000	.000	.000	.002	.015	.062	.175	.368	.602	.807	.932	.984	.998	1.000	1.000	1.000	1.000
17	.000	.000	.000	.000	.001	.006	.034	.114	.275	.500	.725	.886	.966	.994	.999	1.000	1.000	1.000	1.000

continued on following page

d Cumulative Probabilities for Values of p with d Defects   n = 35

d	.05	.10	.15	.20	.25	.30	.35	.40	.45	.50	.55	.60	.65	.70	.75	.80	.85	.90	.95
18	.000	.000	.000	.000	.002	.016	.068	.193	.398	.632	.825	.938	.985	.998	1.000	1.000	1.000	1.000	1.000
19	.000	.000	.000	.001	.006	.036	.126	.300	.531	.750	.898	.970	.994	.999	1.000	1.000	1.000	1.000	1.000
20	.000	.000	.000	.002	.016	.073	.211	.427	.662	.845	.946	.987	.998	1.000	1.000	1.000	1.000	1.000	1.000
21	.000	.000	.000	.005	.036	.135	.324	.564	.777	.912	.974	.995	.999	1.000	1.000	1.000	1.000	1.000	1.000
22	.000	.000	.001	.014	.076	.227	.458	.694	.866	.955	.989	.998	1.000	1.000	1.000	1.000	1.000	1.000	1.000
23	.000	.000	.004	.034	.142	.348	.598	.805	.927	.980	.996	.999	1.000	1.000	1.000	1.000	1.000	1.000	1.000
24	.000	.000	.011	.075	.242	.490	.728	.888	.965	.992	.999	1.000	1.000	1.000	1.000	1.000	1.000	1.000	1.000
25	.000	.002	.029	.146	.374	.635	.835	.942	.985	.997	1.000	1.000	1.000	1.000	1.000	1.000	1.000	1.000	1.000
26	.000	.006	.069	.255	.526	.766	.911	.974	.994	.999	1.000	1.000	1.000	1.000	1.000	1.000	1.000	1.000	1.000
27	.000	.020	.144	.401	.678	.867	.958	.990	.998	1.000	1.000	1.000	1.000	1.000	1.000	1.000	1.000	1.000	1.000
28	.002	.055	.265	.567	.808	.935	.983	.997	.999	1.000	1.000	1.000	1.000	1.000	1.000	1.000	1.000	1.000	1.000
29	.007	.132	.431	.728	.902	.973	.994	.999	1.000	1.000	1.000	1.000	1.000	1.000	1.000	1.000	1.000	1.000	1.000
30	.029	.269	.619	.857	.959	.991	.998	1.000	1.000	1.000	1.000	1.000	1.000	1.000	1.000	1.000	1.000	1.000	1.000
31	.096	.469	.791	.939	.986	.998	1.000	1.000	1.000	1.000	1.000	1.000	1.000	1.000	1.000	1.000	1.000	1.000	1.000
32	.254	.694	.913	.981	.997	1.000	1.000	1.000	1.000	1.000	1.000	1.000	1.000	1.000	1.000	1.000	1.000	1.000	1.000
33	.528	.878	.976	.996	.999	1.000	1.000	1.000	1.000	1.000	1.000	1.000	1.000	1.000	1.000	1.000	1.000	1.000	1.000
34	.834	.975	.997	1.000	1.000	1.000	1.000	1.000	1.000	1.000	1.000	1.000	1.000	1.000	1.000	1.000	1.000	1.000	1.000
35	1.000	1.000	1.000	1.000	1.000	1.000	1.000	1.000	1.000	1.000	1.000	1.000	1.000	1.000	1.000	1.000	1.000	1.000	1.000

d Cumulative Probabilities for Values of p with d Defects   n = 36

d	.05	.10	.15	.20	.25	.30	.35	.40	.45	.50	.55	.60	.65	.70	.75	.80	.85	.90	.95
0	.000	.000	.000	.000	.000	.000	.000	.000	.000	.000	.000	.000	.000	.000	.000	.000	.003	.023	.158
1	.000	.000	.000	.000	.000	.000	.000	.000	.000	.000	.000	.000	.000	.000	.000	.003	.021	.113	.457
2	.000	.000	.000	.000	.000	.000	.000	.000	.000	.000	.000	.000	.000	.000	.003	.016	.078	.288	.732
3	.000	.000	.000	.000	.000	.000	.000	.000	.000	.000	.000	.000	.000	.002	.011	.052	.191	.509	.896
4	.000	.000	.000	.000	.000	.000	.000	.000	.000	.000	.000	.000	.001	.007	.034	.127	.355	.711	.968
5	.000	.000	.000	.000	.000	.000	.000	.000	.000	.000	.000	.001	.004	.022	.083	.246	.541	.855	.992
6	.000	.000	.000	.000	.000	.000	.000	.000	.000	.000	.000	.002	.013	.054	.168	.401	.710	.937	.998
7	.000	.000	.000	.000	.000	.000	.000	.000	.000	.000	.001	.007	.033	.112	.290	.566	.838	.976	1.000
8	.000	.000	.000	.000	.000	.000	.000	.000	.000	.001	.004	.020	.073	.204	.436	.716	.920	.992	1.000
9	.000	.000	.000	.000	.000	.000	.000	.000	.000	.002	.011	.045	.138	.325	.588	.832	.965	.998	1.000
10	.000	.000	.000	.000	.000	.000	.000	.000	.001	.006	.026	.090	.234	.466	.725	.911	.986	.999	1.000
11	.000	.000	.000	.000	.000	.000	.000	.000	.003	.014	.056	.162	.356	.609	.833	.958	.995	1.000	1.000
12	.000	.000	.000	.000	.000	.000	.000	.001	.007	.033	.107	.262	.493	.737	.908	.982	.999	1.000	1.000
13	.000	.000	.000	.000	.000	.000	.000	.003	.018	.066	.183	.384	.629	.837	.954	.993	1.000	1.000	1.000
14	.000	.000	.000	.000	.000	.000	.001	.008	.038	.121	.286	.518	.750	.908	.979	.998	1.000	1.000	1.000
15	.000	.000	.000	.000	.000	.000	.004	.020	.075	.203	.410	.649	.845	.953	.991	.999	1.000	1.000	1.000
16	.000	.000	.000	.000	.000	.001	.009	.043	.135	.309	.542	.764	.912	.978	.997	1.000	1.000	1.000	1.000
17	.000	.000	.000	.000	.000	.004	.022	.083	.220	.434	.670	.854	.954	.991	.999	1.000	1.000	1.000	1.000
18	.000	.000	.000	.000	.001	.009	.046	.146	.330	.566	.780	.917	.978	.996	1.000	1.000	1.000	1.000	1.000

continued on following page

d Cumulative Probabilities for Values of p with d Defects n = 36

d	.05	.10	.15	.20	.25	.30	.35	.40	.45	.50	.55	.60	.65	.70	.75	.80	.85	.90	.95
19	.000	.000	.000	.000	.003	.022	.088	.236	.458	.691	.865	.957	.991	.999	1.000	1.000	1.000	1.000	1.000
20	.000	.000	.000	.001	.009	.047	.155	.351	.590	.797	.925	.980	.996	1.000	1.000	1.000	1.000	1.000	1.000
21	.000	.000	.000	.002	.021	.092	.250	.482	.714	.879	.962	.992	.999	1.000	1.000	1.000	1.000	1.000	1.000
22	.000	.000	.000	.007	.046	.163	.371	.616	.817	.934	.982	.997	1.000	1.000	1.000	1.000	1.000	1.000	1.000
23	.000	.000	.001	.018	.092	.263	.507	.738	.893	.967	.993	.999	1.000	1.000	1.000	1.000	1.000	1.000	1.000
24	.000	.000	.005	.042	.167	.391	.644	.838	.944	.986	.997	1.000	1.000	1.000	1.000	1.000	1.000	1.000	1.000
25	.000	.001	.014	.089	.275	.534	.766	.910	.974	.994	.999	1.000	1.000	1.000	1.000	1.000	1.000	1.000	1.000
26	.000	.002	.035	.168	.412	.675	.862	.955	.989	.998	1.000	1.000	1.000	1.000	1.000	1.000	1.000	1.000	1.000
27	.000	.008	.080	.284	.564	.796	.927	.980	.996	.999	1.000	1.000	1.000	1.000	1.000	1.000	1.000	1.000	1.000
28	.000	.024	.162	.434	.710	.888	.967	.993	.999	1.000	1.000	1.000	1.000	1.000	1.000	1.000	1.000	1.000	1.000
29	.002	.063	.290	.599	.832	.946	.987	.998	1.000	1.000	1.000	1.000	1.000	1.000	1.000	1.000	1.000	1.000	1.000
30	.008	.145	.459	.754	.917	.978	.996	.999	1.000	1.000	1.000	1.000	1.000	1.000	1.000	1.000	1.000	1.000	1.000
31	.032	.289	.645	.873	.966	.993	.999	1.000	1.000	1.000	1.000	1.000	1.000	1.000	1.000	1.000	1.000	1.000	1.000
32	.104	.491	.809	.948	.989	.998	1.000	1.000	1.000	1.000	1.000	1.000	1.000	1.000	1.000	1.000	1.000	1.000	1.000
33	.268	.712	.922	.984	.997	1.000	1.000	1.000	1.000	1.000	1.000	1.000	1.000	1.000	1.000	1.000	1.000	1.000	1.000
34	.543	.887	.979	.997	1.000	1.000	1.000	1.000	1.000	1.000	1.000	1.000	1.000	1.000	1.000	1.000	1.000	1.000	1.000
35	.842	.977	.997	1.000	1.000	1.000	1.000	1.000	1.000	1.000	1.000	1.000	1.000	1.000	1.000	1.000	1.000	1.000	1.000
36	1.000	1.000	1.000	1.000	1.000	1.000	1.000	1.000	1.000	1.000	1.000	1.000	1.000	1.000	1.000	1.000	1.000	1.000	1.000

d Cumulative Probabilities for Values of p with d Defects   n = 37

d	.05	.10	.15	.20	.25	.30	.35	.40	.45	.50	.55	.60	.65	.70	.75	.80	.85	.90	.95
0	.000	.000	.000	.000	.000	.000	.000	.000	.000	.000	.000	.000	.000	.000	.000	.000	.002	.020	.150
1	.000	.000	.000	.000	.000	.000	.000	.000	.000	.000	.000	.000	.000	.000	.000	.003	.018	.104	.442
2	.000	.000	.000	.000	.000	.000	.000	.000	.000	.000	.000	.000	.000	.000	.002	.013	.069	.270	.718
3	.000	.000	.000	.000	.000	.000	.000	.000	.000	.000	.000	.000	.000	.001	.009	.045	.174	.486	.888
4	.000	.000	.000	.000	.000	.000	.000	.000	.000	.000	.000	.000	.001	.006	.028	.112	.330	.691	.964
5	.000	.000	.000	.000	.000	.000	.000	.000	.000	.000	.000	.000	.003	.017	.071	.222	.513	.840	.990
6	.000	.000	.000	.000	.000	.000	.000	.000	.000	.000	.000	.002	.010	.044	.147	.370	.685	.929	.998
7	.000	.000	.000	.000	.000	.000	.000	.000	.000	.000	.001	.005	.026	.095	.259	.533	.819	.973	1.000
8	.000	.000	.000	.000	.000	.000	.000	.000	.000	.000	.003	.015	.059	.176	.400	.686	.908	.991	1.000
9	.000	.000	.000	.000	.000	.000	.000	.000	.000	.001	.008	.035	.115	.289	.550	.809	.958	.997	1.000
10	.000	.000	.000	.000	.000	.000	.000	.000	.001	.004	.019	.072	.201	.424	.691	.895	.983	.999	1.000
11	.000	.000	.000	.000	.000	.000	.000	.000	.002	.010	.043	.133	.314	.566	.806	.948	.994	1.000	1.000
12	.000	.000	.000	.000	.000	.000	.000	.001	.005	.024	.084	.222	.445	.698	.889	.977	.998	1.000	1.000
13	.000	.000	.000	.000	.000	.000	.000	.002	.012	.049	.149	.335	.582	.807	.942	.991	.999	1.000	1.000
14	.000	.000	.000	.000	.000	.000	.001	.005	.027	.094	.240	.464	.707	.887	.973	.997	1.000	1.000	1.000
15	.000	.000	.000	.000	.000	.000	.002	.013	.055	.162	.354	.597	.811	.940	.988	.999	1.000	1.000	1.000
16	.000	.000	.000	.000	.000	.001	.006	.029	.102	.256	.482	.718	.888	.971	.995	1.000	1.000	1.000	1.000
17	.000	.000	.000	.000	.000	.002	.014	.059	.173	.371	.612	.818	.939	.987	.998	1.000	1.000	1.000	1.000
18	.000	.000	.000	.000	.001	.005	.030	.108	.270	.500	.730	.892	.970	.995	.999	1.000	1.000	1.000	1.000

continued on following page

d Cumulative Probabilities for Values of p with d Defects

n = 37

d	.05	.10	.15	.20	.25	.30	.35	.40	.45	.50	.55	.60	.65	.70	.75	.80	.85	.90	.95
19	.000	.000	.000	.000	.002	.013	.061	.182	.388	.629	.827	.941	.986	.998	1.000	1.000	1.000	1.000	1.000
20	.000	.000	.000	.000	.005	.029	.112	.282	.518	.744	.898	.971	.994	.999	1.000	1.000	1.000	1.000	1.000
21	.000	.000	.000	.001	.012	.060	.189	.403	.646	.838	.945	.987	.998	1.000	1.000	1.000	1.000	1.000	1.000
22	.000	.000	.000	.003	.027	.113	.293	.536	.760	.906	.973	.995	.999	1.000	1.000	1.000	1.000	1.000	1.000
23	.000	.000	.001	.009	.058	.193	.418	.665	.851	.951	.988	.998	1.000	1.000	1.000	1.000	1.000	1.000	1.000
24	.000	.000	.002	.023	.111	.302	.555	.778	.916	.976	.995	.999	1.000	1.000	1.000	1.000	1.000	1.000	1.000
25	.000	.000	.006	.052	.194	.434	.686	.867	.957	.990	.998	1.000	1.000	1.000	1.000	1.000	1.000	1.000	1.000
26	.000	.001	.017	.105	.309	.576	.799	.928	.981	.996	.999	1.000	1.000	1.000	1.000	1.000	1.000	1.000	1.000
27	.000	.003	.042	.191	.450	.711	.885	.965	.992	.999	1.000	1.000	1.000	1.000	1.000	1.000	1.000	1.000	1.000
28	.000	.009	.092	.314	.600	.824	.941	.985	.997	1.000	1.000	1.000	1.000	1.000	1.000	1.000	1.000	1.000	1.000
29	.000	.027	.181	.467	.741	.905	.974	.995	.999	1.000	1.000	1.000	1.000	1.000	1.000	1.000	1.000	1.000	1.000
30	.002	.071	.315	.630	.853	.956	.990	.998	1.000	1.000	1.000	1.000	1.000	1.000	1.000	1.000	1.000	1.000	1.000
31	.010	.160	.487	.778	.929	.983	.997	1.000	1.000	1.000	1.000	1.000	1.000	1.000	1.000	1.000	1.000	1.000	1.000
32	.036	.309	.670	.888	.972	.994	.999	1.000	1.000	1.000	1.000	1.000	1.000	1.000	1.000	1.000	1.000	1.000	1.000
33	.112	.514	.826	.955	.991	.999	1.000	1.000	1.000	1.000	1.000	1.000	1.000	1.000	1.000	1.000	1.000	1.000	1.000
34	.282	.730	.931	.987	.998	1.000	1.000	1.000	1.000	1.000	1.000	1.000	1.000	1.000	1.000	1.000	1.000	1.000	1.000
35	.558	.896	.982	.997	1.000	1.000	1.000	1.000	1.000	1.000	1.000	1.000	1.000	1.000	1.000	1.000	1.000	1.000	1.000
36	.850	.980	.998	1.000	1.000	1.000	1.000	1.000	1.000	1.000	1.000	1.000	1.000	1.000	1.000	1.000	1.000	1.000	1.000
37	1.000	1.000	1.000	1.000	1.000	1.000	1.000	1.000	1.000	1.000	1.000	1.000	1.000	1.000	1.000	1.000	1.000	1.000	1.000

214 Assessing Child Survival Programs

d Cumulative Probabilities for Values of p with d Defects　　　　n = 38

d	.05	.10	.15	.20	.25	.30	.35	.40	.45	.50	.55	.60	.65	.70	.75	.80	.85	.90	.95
0	.000	.000	.000	.000	.000	.000	.000	.000	.000	.000	.000	.000	.000	.000	.000	.000	.002	.018	.142
1	.000	.000	.000	.000	.000	.000	.000	.000	.000	.000	.000	.000	.000	.000	.000	.002	.016	.095	.427
2	.000	.000	.000	.000	.000	.000	.000	.000	.000	.000	.000	.000	.000	.000	.002	.011	.062	.254	.704
3	.000	.000	.000	.000	.000	.000	.000	.000	.000	.000	.000	.000	.000	.001	.007	.039	.158	.465	.880
4	.000	.000	.000	.000	.000	.000	.000	.000	.000	.000	.000	.000	.001	.004	.024	.099	.307	.670	.960
5	.000	.000	.000	.000	.000	.000	.000	.000	.000	.000	.000	.000	.002	.014	.060	.200	.485	.825	.989
6	.000	.000	.000	.000	.000	.000	.000	.000	.000	.000	.000	.001	.008	.036	.128	.340	.659	.920	.997
7	.000	.000	.000	.000	.000	.000	.000	.000	.000	.000	.001	.004	.020	.079	.231	.500	.799	.968	1.000
8	.000	.000	.000	.000	.000	.000	.000	.000	.000	.000	.002	.011	.047	.152	.365	.655	.894	.989	1.000
9	.000	.000	.000	.000	.000	.000	.000	.000	.000	.001	.006	.027	.096	.255	.513	.784	.951	.997	1.000
10	.000	.000	.000	.000	.000	.000	.000	.000	.000	.003	.014	.057	.171	.384	.656	.878	.979	.999	1.000
11	.000	.000	.000	.000	.000	.000	.000	.000	.001	.007	.032	.109	.274	.524	.777	.938	.992	1.000	1.000
12	.000	.000	.000	.000	.000	.000	.000	.000	.003	.017	.065	.186	.399	.659	.868	.971	.997	1.000	1.000
13	.000	.000	.000	.000	.000	.000	.000	.001	.008	.036	.120	.290	.534	.774	.929	.988	.999	1.000	1.000
14	.000	.000	.000	.000	.000	.000	.000	.003	.019	.072	.199	.413	.663	.863	.965	.995	1.000	1.000	1.000
15	.000	.000	.000	.000	.000	.000	.001	.008	.039	.128	.303	.544	.775	.924	.984	.998	1.000	1.000	1.000
16	.000	.000	.000	.000	.000	.000	.003	.019	.076	.209	.425	.670	.861	.961	.994	1.000	1.000	1.000	1.000
17	.000	.000	.000	.000	.000	.001	.008	.041	.134	.314	.554	.778	.921	.982	.998	1.000	1.000	1.000	1.000
18	.000	.000	.000	.000	.000	.003	.019	.078	.217	.436	.677	.862	.959	.992	.999	1.000	1.000	1.000	1.000
19	.000	.000	.000	.000	.001	.008	.041	.138	.323	.564	.783	.922	.981	.997	1.000	1.000	1.000	1.000	1.000

continued on following page

d Cumulative Probabilities for Values of p with d Defects   n = 38

	.05	.10	.15	.20	.25	.30	.35	.40	.45	.50	.55	.60	.65	.70	.75	.80	.85	.90	.95
20	.000	.000	.000	.000	.002	.018	.079	.222	.446	.686	.866	.959	.992	.999	1.000	1.000	1.000	1.000	1.000
21	.000	.000	.000	.000	.006	.039	.139	.330	.575	.791	.924	.981	.997	1.000	1.000	1.000	1.000	1.000	1.000
22	.000	.000	.000	.002	.016	.076	.225	.456	.697	.872	.961	.992	.999	1.000	1.000	1.000	1.000	1.000	1.000
23	.000	.000	.000	.005	.035	.137	.337	.587	.801	.928	.981	.997	1.000	1.000	1.000	1.000	1.000	1.000	1.000
24	.000	.000	.001	.012	.071	.226	.466	.710	.880	.964	.992	.999	1.000	1.000	1.000	1.000	1.000	1.000	1.000
25	.000	.000	.003	.029	.132	.341	.601	.814	.935	.983	.997	1.000	1.000	1.000	1.000	1.000	1.000	1.000	1.000
26	.000	.000	.008	.062	.223	.476	.726	.891	.968	.993	.999	1.000	1.000	1.000	1.000	1.000	1.000	1.000	1.000
27	.000	.001	.021	.122	.344	.616	.829	.943	.986	.997	1.000	1.000	1.000	1.000	1.000	1.000	1.000	1.000	1.000
28	.000	.003	.049	.216	.487	.745	.904	.973	.994	.999	1.000	1.000	1.000	1.000	1.000	1.000	1.000	1.000	1.000
29	.000	.011	.106	.345	.635	.848	.953	.989	.998	1.000	1.000	1.000	1.000	1.000	1.000	1.000	1.000	1.000	1.000
30	.000	.032	.201	.500	.769	.921	.980	.996	.999	1.000	1.000	1.000	1.000	1.000	1.000	1.000	1.000	1.000	1.000
31	.003	.080	.341	.660	.872	.964	.992	.999	1.000	1.000	1.000	1.000	1.000	1.000	1.000	1.000	1.000	1.000	1.000
32	.011	.175	.515	.800	.940	.986	.998	1.000	1.000	1.000	1.000	1.000	1.000	1.000	1.000	1.000	1.000	1.000	1.000
33	.040	.330	.693	.901	.976	.996	.999	1.000	1.000	1.000	1.000	1.000	1.000	1.000	1.000	1.000	1.000	1.000	1.000
34	.120	.535	.842	.961	.993	.999	1.000	1.000	1.000	1.000	1.000	1.000	1.000	1.000	1.000	1.000	1.000	1.000	1.000
35	.296	.746	.938	.989	.998	1.000	1.000	1.000	1.000	1.000	1.000	1.000	1.000	1.000	1.000	1.000	1.000	1.000	1.000
36	.573	.905	.984	.998	1.000	1.000	1.000	1.000	1.000	1.000	1.000	1.000	1.000	1.000	1.000	1.000	1.000	1.000	1.000
37	.858	.982	.998	1.000	1.000	1.000	1.000	1.000	1.000	1.000	1.000	1.000	1.000	1.000	1.000	1.000	1.000	1.000	1.000
38	1.000	1.000	1.000	1.000	1.000	1.000	1.000	1.000	1.000	1.000	1.000	1.000	1.000	1.000	1.000	1.000	1.000	1.000	1.000

d Cumulative Probabilities for Values of p with d Defects n = 39

d	.05	.10	.15	.20	.25	.30	.35	.40	.45	.50	.55	.60	.65	.70	.75	.80	.85	.90	.95
0	.000	.000	.000	.000	.000	.000	.000	.000	.000	.000	.000	.000	.000	.000	.000	.000	.002	.016	.135
1	.000	.000	.000	.000	.000	.000	.000	.000	.000	.000	.000	.000	.000	.000	.000	.002	.014	.088	.413
2	.000	.000	.000	.000	.000	.000	.000	.000	.000	.000	.000	.000	.000	.000	.001	.009	.055	.238	.691
3	.000	.000	.000	.000	.000	.000	.000	.000	.000	.000	.000	.000	.000	.001	.006	.033	.143	.444	.871
4	.000	.000	.000	.000	.000	.000	.000	.000	.000	.000	.000	.000	.000	.003	.019	.087	.284	.650	.956
5	.000	.000	.000	.000	.000	.000	.000	.000	.000	.000	.000	.000	.002	.011	.051	.180	.459	.810	.988
6	.000	.000	.000	.000	.000	.000	.000	.000	.000	.000	.000	.001	.006	.029	.111	.312	.633	.911	.997
7	.000	.000	.000	.000	.000	.000	.000	.000	.000	.000	.000	.003	.016	.066	.206	.468	.778	.963	.999
8	.000	.000	.000	.000	.000	.000	.000	.000	.000	.000	.001	.008	.038	.130	.331	.624	.880	.987	1.000
9	.000	.000	.000	.000	.000	.000	.000	.000	.000	.001	.004	.020	.079	.224	.476	.759	.942	.996	1.000
10	.000	.000	.000	.000	.000	.000	.000	.000	.000	.002	.010	.045	.145	.345	.620	.859	.975	.999	1.000
11	.000	.000	.000	.000	.000	.000	.000	.000	.001	.005	.024	.088	.238	.482	.747	.926	.990	1.000	1.000
12	.000	.000	.000	.000	.000	.000	.000	.000	.002	.012	.050	.155	.355	.618	.846	.965	.997	1.000	1.000
13	.000	.000	.000	.000	.000	.000	.000	.001	.005	.027	.095	.248	.487	.740	.914	.985	.999	1.000	1.000
14	.000	.000	.000	.000	.000	.000	.000	.002	.013	.054	.163	.363	.618	.836	.956	.994	1.000	1.000	1.000
15	.000	.000	.000	.000	.000	.000	.001	.005	.028	.100	.256	.491	.736	.906	.980	.998	1.000	1.000	1.000
16	.000	.000	.000	.000	.000	.000	.002	.013	.056	.168	.370	.619	.831	.950	.991	.999	1.000	1.000	1.000
17	.000	.000	.000	.000	.000	.001	.005	.028	.102	.261	.496	.735	.900	.976	.997	1.000	1.000	1.000	1.000
18	.000	.000	.000	.000	.000	.002	.012	.056	.171	.375	.622	.829	.946	.989	.999	1.000	1.000	1.000	1.000
19	.000	.000	.000	.000	.000	.004	.027	.102	.264	.500	.736	.898	.973	.996	1.000	1.000	1.000	1.000	1.000
20	.000	.000	.000	.000	.001	.011	.054	.171	.378	.625	.829	.944	.988	.998	1.000	1.000	1.000	1.000	1.000

continued on following page

d Cumulative Probabilities for Values of p with d Defects n = 39

d	.05	.10	.15	.20	.25	.30	.35	.40	.45	.50	.55	.60	.65	.70	.75	.80	.85	.90	.95
21	.000	.000	.000	.000	.003	.024	.100	.265	.504	.739	.898	.972	.995	.999	1.000	1.000	1.000	1.000	1.000
22	.000	.000	.000	.001	.009	.050	.169	.381	.630	.832	.944	.987	.998	1.000	1.000	1.000	1.000	1.000	1.000
23	.000	.000	.000	.002	.020	.094	.264	.509	.744	.900	.972	.995	.999	1.000	1.000	1.000	1.000	1.000	1.000
24	.000	.000	.000	.006	.044	.164	.382	.637	.837	.946	.987	.998	1.000	1.000	1.000	1.000	1.000	1.000	1.000
25	.000	.000	.001	.015	.086	.260	.513	.752	.905	.973	.995	.999	1.000	1.000	1.000	1.000	1.000	1.000	1.000
26	.000	.000	.003	.035	.154	.382	.645	.845	.950	.988	.998	1.000	1.000	1.000	1.000	1.000	1.000	1.000	1.000
27	.000	.000	.010	.074	.253	.518	.762	.912	.976	.995	.999	1.000	1.000	1.000	1.000	1.000	1.000	1.000	1.000
28	.000	.001	.025	.141	.380	.655	.855	.955	.990	.998	1.000	1.000	1.000	1.000	1.000	1.000	1.000	1.000	1.000
29	.000	.004	.058	.241	.524	.776	.921	.980	.996	.999	1.000	1.000	1.000	1.000	1.000	1.000	1.000	1.000	1.000
30	.000	.013	.120	.376	.669	.870	.962	.992	.999	1.000	1.000	1.000	1.000	1.000	1.000	1.000	1.000	1.000	1.000
31	.001	.037	.222	.532	.794	.934	.984	.997	1.000	1.000	1.000	1.000	1.000	1.000	1.000	1.000	1.000	1.000	1.000
32	.003	.089	.367	.688	.889	.971	.994	.999	1.000	1.000	1.000	1.000	1.000	1.000	1.000	1.000	1.000	1.000	1.000
33	.012	.190	.541	.820	.949	.989	.998	1.000	1.000	1.000	1.000	1.000	1.000	1.000	1.000	1.000	1.000	1.000	1.000
34	.044	.350	.716	.913	.981	.997	1.000	1.000	1.000	1.000	1.000	1.000	1.000	1.000	1.000	1.000	1.000	1.000	1.000
35	.129	.556	.857	.967	.994	.999	1.000	1.000	1.000	1.000	1.000	1.000	1.000	1.000	1.000	1.000	1.000	1.000	1.000
36	.309	.762	.945	.991	.999	1.000	1.000	1.000	1.000	1.000	1.000	1.000	1.000	1.000	1.000	1.000	1.000	1.000	1.000
37	.587	.912	.986	.998	1.000	1.000	1.000	1.000	1.000	1.000	1.000	1.000	1.000	1.000	1.000	1.000	1.000	1.000	1.000
38	.865	.984	.998	1.000	1.000	1.000	1.000	1.000	1.000	1.000	1.000	1.000	1.000	1.000	1.000	1.000	1.000	1.000	1.000
39	1.000	1.000	1.000	1.000	1.000	1.000	1.000	1.000	1.000	1.000	1.000	1.000	1.000	1.000	1.000	1.000	1.000	1.000	1.000

d Cumulative Probabilities for Values of p with d Defects n = 40

d	.05	.10	.15	.20	.25	.30	.35	.40	.45	.50	.55	.60	.65	.70	.75	.80	.85	.90	.95
0	.000	.000	.000	.000	.000	.000	.000	.000	.000	.000	.000	.000	.000	.000	.000	.000	.002	.015	.129
1	.000	.000	.000	.000	.000	.000	.000	.000	.000	.000	.000	.000	.000	.000	.000	.001	.012	.080	.399
2	.000	.000	.000	.000	.000	.000	.000	.000	.000	.000	.000	.000	.000	.000	.001	.008	.049	.223	.677
3	.000	.000	.000	.000	.000	.000	.000	.000	.000	.000	.000	.000	.000	.001	.005	.028	.130	.423	.862
4	.000	.000	.000	.000	.000	.000	.000	.000	.000	.000	.000	.000	.000	.003	.016	.076	.263	.629	.952
5	.000	.000	.000	.000	.000	.000	.000	.000	.000	.000	.000	.000	.001	.009	.043	.161	.433	.794	.986
6	.000	.000	.000	.000	.000	.000	.000	.000	.000	.000	.000	.001	.004	.024	.096	.286	.607	.900	.997
7	.000	.000	.000	.000	.000	.000	.000	.000	.000	.000	.000	.002	.012	.055	.182	.437	.756	.958	.999
8	.000	.000	.000	.000	.000	.000	.000	.000	.000	.000	.001	.006	.030	.111	.300	.593	.865	.985	1.000
9	.000	.000	.000	.000	.000	.000	.000	.000	.000	.000	.003	.016	.064	.196	.440	.732	.933	.995	1.000
10	.000	.000	.000	.000	.000	.000	.000	.000	.000	.001	.007	.035	.121	.309	.584	.839	.970	.999	1.000
11	.000	.000	.000	.000	.000	.000	.000	.000	.000	.003	.018	.071	.205	.441	.715	.912	.988	1.000	1.000
12	.000	.000	.000	.000	.000	.000	.000	.000	.001	.008	.039	.129	.314	.577	.821	.957	.996	1.000	1.000
13	.000	.000	.000	.000	.000	.000	.000	.000	.003	.019	.075	.211	.441	.703	.897	.981	.999	1.000	1.000
14	.000	.000	.000	.000	.000	.000	.000	.001	.009	.040	.133	.317	.572	.807	.946	.992	1.000	1.000	1.000
15	.000	.000	.000	.000	.000	.000	.000	.003	.020	.077	.214	.440	.695	.885	.974	.997	1.000	1.000	1.000
16	.000	.000	.000	.000	.000	.000	.001	.008	.041	.134	.319	.568	.798	.937	.988	.999	1.000	1.000	1.000
17	.000	.000	.000	.000	.000	.000	.003	.019	.077	.215	.439	.689	.876	.968	.995	1.000	1.000	1.000	1.000
18	.000	.000	.000	.000	.000	.001	.008	.039	.133	.318	.565	.791	.930	.985	.998	1.000	1.000	1.000	1.000
19	.000	.000	.000	.000	.000	.002	.017	.074	.213	.437	.684	.870	.964	.994	.999	1.000	1.000	1.000	1.000
20	.000	.000	.000	.000	.001	.006	.036	.130	.316	.563	.787	.926	.983	.998	1.000	1.000	1.000	1.000	1.000

continued on following page

d Cumulative Probabilities for Values of p with d Defects   n = 40

d	.05	.10	.15	.20	.25	.30	.35	.40	.45	.50	.55	.60	.65	.70	.75	.80	.85	.90	.95
21	.000	.000	.000	.000	.002	.015	.070	.209	.435	.682	.867	.961	.992	.999	1.000	1.000	1.000	1.000	1.000
22	.000	.000	.000	.000	.005	.032	.124	.311	.561	.785	.923	.981	.997	1.000	1.000	1.000	1.000	1.000	1.000
23	.000	.000	.000	.001	.012	.063	.202	.432	.681	.866	.959	.992	.999	1.000	1.000	1.000	1.000	1.000	1.000
24	.000	.000	.000	.003	.026	.115	.305	.560	.786	.923	.980	.997	1.000	1.000	1.000	1.000	1.000	1.000	1.000
25	.000	.000	.000	.008	.054	.193	.428	.683	.867	.960	.991	.999	1.000	1.000	1.000	1.000	1.000	1.000	1.000
26	.000	.000	.001	.019	.103	.297	.559	.789	.925	.981	.997	1.000	1.000	1.000	1.000	1.000	1.000	1.000	1.000
27	.000	.000	.004	.043	.179	.423	.686	.871	.961	.992	.999	1.000	1.000	1.000	1.000	1.000	1.000	1.000	1.000
28	.000	.000	.012	.088	.285	.559	.795	.929	.982	.997	1.000	1.000	1.000	1.000	1.000	1.000	1.000	1.000	1.000
29	.000	.001	.030	.161	.416	.691	.879	.965	.993	.999	1.000	1.000	1.000	1.000	1.000	1.000	1.000	1.000	1.000
30	.000	.005	.067	.268	.560	.804	.936	.984	.997	1.000	1.000	1.000	1.000	1.000	1.000	1.000	1.000	1.000	1.000
31	.000	.015	.135	.407	.700	.889	.970	.994	.999	1.000	1.000	1.000	1.000	1.000	1.000	1.000	1.000	1.000	1.000
32	.001	.042	.244	.563	.818	.945	.988	.998	1.000	1.000	1.000	1.000	1.000	1.000	1.000	1.000	1.000	1.000	1.000
33	.003	.100	.393	.714	.904	.976	.996	.999	1.000	1.000	1.000	1.000	1.000	1.000	1.000	1.000	1.000	1.000	1.000
34	.014	.206	.567	.839	.957	.991	.999	1.000	1.000	1.000	1.000	1.000	1.000	1.000	1.000	1.000	1.000	1.000	1.000
35	.048	.371	.737	.924	.984	.997	1.000	1.000	1.000	1.000	1.000	1.000	1.000	1.000	1.000	1.000	1.000	1.000	1.000
36	.138	.577	.870	.972	.995	.999	1.000	1.000	1.000	1.000	1.000	1.000	1.000	1.000	1.000	1.000	1.000	1.000	1.000
37	.323	.777	.951	.992	.999	1.000	1.000	1.000	1.000	1.000	1.000	1.000	1.000	1.000	1.000	1.000	1.000	1.000	1.000
38	.601	.920	.988	.999	1.000	1.000	1.000	1.000	1.000	1.000	1.000	1.000	1.000	1.000	1.000	1.000	1.000	1.000	1.000
39	.871	.985	.998	1.000	1.000	1.000	1.000	1.000	1.000	1.000	1.000	1.000	1.000	1.000	1.000	1.000	1.000	1.000	1.000
40	1.000	1.000	1.000	1.000	1.000	1.000	1.000	1.000	1.000	1.000	1.000	1.000	1.000	1.000	1.000	1.000	1.000	1.000	1.000

d   Cumulative Probabilities for Values of p with d Defects   n = 41

d	.05	.10	.15	.20	.25	.30	.35	.40	.45	.50	.55	.60	.65	.70	.75	.80	.85	.90	.95
0	.000	.000	.000	.000	.000	.000	.000	.000	.000	.000	.000	.000	.000	.000	.000	.000	.001	.013	.122
1	.000	.000	.000	.000	.000	.000	.000	.000	.000	.000	.000	.000	.000	.000	.000	.001	.011	.074	.386
2	.000	.000	.000	.000	.000	.000	.000	.000	.000	.000	.000	.000	.000	.000	.001	.007	.043	.209	.663
3	.000	.000	.000	.000	.000	.000	.000	.000	.000	.000	.000	.000	.000	.000	.004	.024	.118	.403	.853
4	.000	.000	.000	.000	.000	.000	.000	.000	.000	.000	.000	.000	.000	.002	.013	.066	.243	.608	.947
5	.000	.000	.000	.000	.000	.000	.000	.000	.000	.000	.000	.000	.001	.007	.036	.144	.407	.777	.984
6	.000	.000	.000	.000	.000	.000	.000	.000	.000	.000	.000	.000	.003	.019	.083	.261	.581	.890	.996
7	.000	.000	.000	.000	.000	.000	.000	.000	.000	.000	.000	.001	.010	.046	.161	.407	.734	.952	.999
8	.000	.000	.000	.000	.000	.000	.000	.000	.000	.000	.001	.004	.024	.094	.270	.562	.848	.982	1.000
9	.000	.000	.000	.000	.000	.000	.000	.000	.000	.000	.002	.012	.052	.170	.405	.704	.923	.994	1.000
10	.000	.000	.000	.000	.000	.000	.000	.000	.000	.001	.005	.027	.102	.275	.548	.818	.964	.998	1.000
11	.000	.000	.000	.000	.000	.000	.000	.000	.000	.002	.013	.057	.176	.401	.682	.898	.985	1.000	1.000
12	.000	.000	.000	.000	.000	.000	.000	.000	.001	.006	.029	.105	.276	.536	.794	.948	.995	1.000	1.000
13	.000	.000	.000	.000	.000	.000	.000	.000	.002	.014	.059	.178	.397	.665	.878	.976	.998	1.000	1.000
14	.000	.000	.000	.000	.000	.000	.000	.001	.006	.030	.107	.275	.526	.776	.933	.990	.999	1.000	1.000
15	.000	.000	.000	.000	.000	.000	.000	.002	.014	.059	.177	.391	.652	.862	.967	.996	1.000	1.000	1.000
16	.000	.000	.000	.000	.000	.000	.001	.005	.029	.106	.272	.517	.762	.921	.985	.999	1.000	1.000	1.000
17	.000	.000	.000	.000	.000	.000	.002	.013	.057	.174	.385	.640	.849	.959	.994	1.000	1.000	1.000	1.000
18	.000	.000	.000	.000	.000	.000	.005	.027	.102	.266	.508	.750	.911	.980	.998	1.000	1.000	1.000	1.000
19	.000	.000	.000	.000	.000	.001	.011	.053	.169	.378	.631	.839	.952	.991	.999	1.000	1.000	1.000	1.000
20	.000	.000	.000	.000	.000	.004	.024	.097	.259	.500	.741	.903	.976	.996	1.000	1.000	1.000	1.000	1.000
21	.000	.000	.000	.000	.001	.009	.048	.161	.369	.622	.831	.947	.989	.999	1.000	1.000	1.000	1.000	1.000

continued on following page

d Cumulative Probabilities for Values of p with d Defects   n = 41

d	.05	.10	.15	.20	.25	.30	.35	.40	.45	.50	.55	.60	.65	.70	.75	.80	.85	.90	.95
22	.000	.000	.000	.000	.002	.020	.089	.250	.492	.734	.898	.973	.995	1.000	1.000	1.000	1.000	1.000	1.000
23	.000	.000	.000	.000	.006	.041	.151	.360	.615	.826	.943	.987	.998	1.000	1.000	1.000	1.000	1.000	1.000
24	.000	.000	.000	.001	.015	.079	.238	.483	.728	.894	.971	.995	.999	1.000	1.000	1.000	1.000	1.000	1.000
25	.000	.000	.000	.004	.033	.138	.348	.609	.823	.941	.986	.998	1.000	1.000	1.000	1.000	1.000	1.000	1.000
26	.000	.000	.001	.010	.067	.224	.474	.725	.893	.970	.994	.999	1.000	1.000	1.000	1.000	1.000	1.000	1.000
27	.000	.000	.002	.024	.122	.335	.603	.822	.941	.986	.998	1.000	1.000	1.000	1.000	1.000	1.000	1.000	1.000
28	.000	.000	.005	.052	.206	.464	.724	.895	.971	.994	.999	1.000	1.000	1.000	1.000	1.000	1.000	1.000	1.000
29	.000	.000	.015	.102	.318	.599	.824	.943	.987	.998	1.000	1.000	1.000	1.000	1.000	1.000	1.000	1.000	1.000
30	.000	.002	.036	.182	.452	.725	.898	.973	.995	.999	1.000	1.000	1.000	1.000	1.000	1.000	1.000	1.000	1.000
31	.000	.006	.077	.296	.595	.830	.948	.988	.998	1.000	1.000	1.000	1.000	1.000	1.000	1.000	1.000	1.000	1.000
32	.000	.018	.152	.438	.730	.906	.976	.996	.999	1.000	1.000	1.000	1.000	1.000	1.000	1.000	1.000	1.000	1.000
33	.001	.048	.266	.593	.839	.954	.990	.999	1.000	1.000	1.000	1.000	1.000	1.000	1.000	1.000	1.000	1.000	1.000
34	.004	.110	.419	.739	.917	.981	.997	1.000	1.000	1.000	1.000	1.000	1.000	1.000	1.000	1.000	1.000	1.000	1.000
35	.016	.223	.593	.856	.964	.993	.999	1.000	1.000	1.000	1.000	1.000	1.000	1.000	1.000	1.000	1.000	1.000	1.000
36	.053	.392	.757	.934	.987	.998	1.000	1.000	1.000	1.000	1.000	1.000	1.000	1.000	1.000	1.000	1.000	1.000	1.000
37	.147	.597	.882	.976	.996	1.000	1.000	1.000	1.000	1.000	1.000	1.000	1.000	1.000	1.000	1.000	1.000	1.000	1.000
38	.337	.791	.957	.993	.999	1.000	1.000	1.000	1.000	1.000	1.000	1.000	1.000	1.000	1.000	1.000	1.000	1.000	1.000
39	.614	.926	.989	.999	1.000	1.000	1.000	1.000	1.000	1.000	1.000	1.000	1.000	1.000	1.000	1.000	1.000	1.000	1.000
40	.878	.987	.999	1.000	1.000	1.000	1.000	1.000	1.000	1.000	1.000	1.000	1.000	1.000	1.000	1.000	1.000	1.000	1.000
41	1.000	1.000	1.000	1.000	1.000	1.000	1.000	1.000	1.000	1.000	1.000	1.000	1.000	1.000	1.000	1.000	1.000	1.000	1.000

d Cumulative Probabilities for Values of p with d Defects   n = 42

	.05	.10	.15	.20	.25	.30	.35	.40	.45	.50	.55	.60	.65	.70	.75	.80	.85	.90	.95
0	.000	.000	.000	.000	.000	.000	.000	.000	.000	.000	.000	.000	.000	.000	.000	.000	.001	.012	.116
1	.000	.000	.000	.000	.000	.000	.000	.000	.000	.000	.000	.000	.000	.000	.000	.001	.009	.068	.372
2	.000	.000	.000	.000	.000	.000	.000	.000	.000	.000	.000	.000	.000	.000	.001	.006	.038	.195	.649
3	.000	.000	.000	.000	.000	.000	.000	.000	.000	.000	.000	.000	.000	.000	.003	.021	.107	.384	.843
4	.000	.000	.000	.000	.000	.000	.000	.000	.000	.000	.000	.000	.000	.002	.011	.058	.225	.588	.943
5	.000	.000	.000	.000	.000	.000	.000	.000	.000	.000	.000	.000	.001	.005	.031	.129	.383	.760	.983
6	.000	.000	.000	.000	.000	.000	.000	.000	.000	.000	.000	.000	.002	.015	.071	.238	.555	.879	.996
7	.000	.000	.000	.000	.000	.000	.000	.000	.000	.000	.000	.001	.007	.038	.141	.378	.711	.946	.999
8	.000	.000	.000	.000	.000	.000	.000	.000	.000	.000	.000	.003	.019	.080	.243	.531	.831	.979	1.000
9	.000	.000	.000	.000	.000	.000	.000	.000	.000	.000	.001	.009	.043	.148	.371	.676	.911	.993	1.000
10	.000	.000	.000	.000	.000	.000	.000	.000	.000	.000	.004	.021	.084	.244	.512	.795	.958	.998	1.000
11	.000	.000	.000	.000	.000	.000	.000	.000	.000	.001	.010	.045	.150	.363	.649	.882	.982	.999	1.000
12	.000	.000	.000	.000	.000	.000	.000	.000	.000	.004	.022	.086	.241	.496	.766	.938	.993	1.000	1.000
13	.000	.000	.000	.000	.000	.000	.000	.000	.001	.010	.045	.149	.354	.627	.857	.970	.998	1.000	1.000
14	.000	.000	.000	.000	.000	.000	.000	.000	.004	.022	.085	.236	.481	.743	.919	.987	.999	1.000	1.000
15	.000	.000	.000	.000	.000	.000	.000	.001	.009	.044	.146	.345	.608	.836	.958	.995	1.000	1.000	1.000
16	.000	.000	.000	.000	.000	.000	.000	.003	.021	.082	.229	.467	.723	.903	.980	.998	1.000	1.000	1.000
17	.000	.000	.000	.000	.000	.000	.001	.008	.042	.140	.334	.591	.818	.947	.991	.999	1.000	1.000	1.000
18	.000	.000	.000	.000	.000	.000	.003	.018	.077	.220	.453	.706	.889	.974	.997	1.000	1.000	1.000	1.000
19	.000	.000	.000	.000	.000	.001	.007	.038	.132	.322	.576	.803	.938	.988	.999	1.000	1.000	1.000	1.000
20	.000	.000	.000	.000	.000	.002	.015	.071	.210	.439	.691	.878	.968	.995	1.000	1.000	1.000	1.000	1.000
21	.000	.000	.000	.000	.000	.005	.032	.122	.309	.561	.790	.929	.985	.998	1.000	1.000	1.000	1.000	1.000

continued on following page

d Cumulative Probabilities for Values of p with d Defects   n = 42

	.05	.10	.15	.20	.25	.30	.35	.40	.45	.50	.55	.60	.65	.70	.75	.80	.85	.90	.95
22	.000	.000	.000	.000	.001	.012	.062	.197	.424	.678	.868	.962	.993	.999	1.000	1.000	1.000	1.000	1.000
23	.000	.000	.000	.000	.003	.026	.111	.294	.547	.780	.923	.982	.997	1.000	1.000	1.000	1.000	1.000	1.000
24	.000	.000	.000	.001	.009	.053	.182	.409	.666	.860	.958	.992	.999	1.000	1.000	1.000	1.000	1.000	1.000
25	.000	.000	.000	.002	.020	.097	.277	.533	.771	.918	.979	.997	1.000	1.000	1.000	1.000	1.000	1.000	1.000
26	.000	.000	.000	.005	.042	.164	.392	.655	.854	.956	.991	.999	1.000	1.000	1.000	1.000	1.000	1.000	1.000
27	.000	.000	.001	.013	.081	.257	.519	.764	.915	.978	.996	1.000	1.000	1.000	1.000	1.000	1.000	1.000	1.000
28	.000	.000	.002	.030	.143	.373	.646	.851	.955	.990	.999	1.000	1.000	1.000	1.000	1.000	1.000	1.000	1.000
29	.000	.000	.007	.062	.234	.504	.759	.914	.978	.996	1.000	1.000	1.000	1.000	1.000	1.000	1.000	1.000	1.000
30	.000	.001	.018	.118	.351	.637	.850	.955	.990	.999	1.000	1.000	1.000	1.000	1.000	1.000	1.000	1.000	1.000
31	.000	.002	.042	.205	.488	.756	.916	.979	.996	1.000	1.000	1.000	1.000	1.000	1.000	1.000	1.000	1.000	1.000
32	.000	.007	.089	.324	.629	.852	.957	.991	.999	1.000	1.000	1.000	1.000	1.000	1.000	1.000	1.000	1.000	1.000
33	.000	.021	.169	.469	.757	.920	.981	.997	1.000	1.000	1.000	1.000	1.000	1.000	1.000	1.000	1.000	1.000	1.000
34	.001	.054	.289	.622	.859	.962	.993	.999	1.000	1.000	1.000	1.000	1.000	1.000	1.000	1.000	1.000	1.000	1.000
35	.004	.121	.445	.762	.929	.985	.998	1.000	1.000	1.000	1.000	1.000	1.000	1.000	1.000	1.000	1.000	1.000	1.000
36	.017	.240	.617	.871	.969	.995	.999	1.000	1.000	1.000	1.000	1.000	1.000	1.000	1.000	1.000	1.000	1.000	1.000
37	.057	.412	.775	.942	.989	.998	1.000	1.000	1.000	1.000	1.000	1.000	1.000	1.000	1.000	1.000	1.000	1.000	1.000
38	.157	.616	.893	.979	.997	1.000	1.000	1.000	1.000	1.000	1.000	1.000	1.000	1.000	1.000	1.000	1.000	1.000	1.000
39	.351	.805	.962	.994	.999	1.000	1.000	1.000	1.000	1.000	1.000	1.000	1.000	1.000	1.000	1.000	1.000	1.000	1.000
40	.628	.932	.991	.999	1.000	1.000	1.000	1.000	1.000	1.000	1.000	1.000	1.000	1.000	1.000	1.000	1.000	1.000	1.000
41	.884	.988	.999	1.000	1.000	1.000	1.000	1.000	1.000	1.000	1.000	1.000	1.000	1.000	1.000	1.000	1.000	1.000	1.000
42	1.000	1.000	1.000	1.000	1.000	1.000	1.000	1.000	1.000	1.000	1.000	1.000	1.000	1.000	1.000	1.000	1.000	1.000	1.000

d Cumulative Probabilities for Values of p with d Defects   n = 43

d	.05	.10	.15	.20	.25	.30	.35	.40	.45	.50	.55	.60	.65	.70	.75	.80	.85	.90	.95
0	.000	.000	.000	.000	.000	.000	.000	.000	.000	.000	.000	.000	.000	.000	.000	.000	.001	.011	.110
1	.000	.000	.000	.000	.000	.000	.000	.000	.000	.000	.000	.000	.000	.000	.000	.001	.008	.062	.360
2	.000	.000	.000	.000	.000	.000	.000	.000	.000	.000	.000	.000	.000	.000	.000	.005	.034	.182	.635
3	.000	.000	.000	.000	.000	.000	.000	.000	.000	.000	.000	.000	.000	.000	.002	.018	.096	.365	.833
4	.000	.000	.000	.000	.000	.000	.000	.000	.000	.000	.000	.000	.000	.001	.009	.051	.207	.567	.938
5	.000	.000	.000	.000	.000	.000	.000	.000	.000	.000	.000	.000	.001	.004	.026	.115	.359	.743	.981
6	.000	.000	.000	.000	.000	.000	.000	.000	.000	.000	.000	.000	.002	.012	.061	.216	.529	.867	.995
7	.000	.000	.000	.000	.000	.000	.000	.000	.000	.000	.000	.001	.006	.031	.124	.350	.687	.939	.999
8	.000	.000	.000	.000	.000	.000	.000	.000	.000	.000	.000	.002	.015	.067	.217	.500	.813	.976	1.000
9	.000	.000	.000	.000	.000	.000	.000	.000	.000	.000	.001	.007	.034	.127	.339	.647	.899	.991	1.000
10	.000	.000	.000	.000	.000	.000	.000	.000	.000	.000	.003	.016	.070	.215	.477	.771	.951	.997	1.000
11	.000	.000	.000	.000	.000	.000	.000	.000	.000	.001	.007	.035	.127	.327	.615	.864	.979	.999	1.000
12	.000	.000	.000	.000	.000	.000	.000	.000	.000	.003	.016	.070	.209	.456	.737	.927	.992	1.000	1.000
13	.000	.000	.000	.000	.000	.000	.000	.000	.001	.007	.035	.124	.315	.587	.834	.964	.997	1.000	1.000
14	.000	.000	.000	.000	.000	.000	.000	.000	.002	.016	.067	.201	.437	.708	.904	.984	.999	1.000	1.000
15	.000	.000	.000	.000	.000	.000	.000	.001	.006	.033	.118	.301	.563	.808	.949	.993	1.000	1.000	1.000
16	.000	.000	.000	.000	.000	.000	.000	.002	.014	.063	.192	.418	.683	.883	.975	.997	1.000	1.000	1.000
17	.000	.000	.000	.000	.000	.000	.001	.005	.030	.111	.287	.541	.785	.934	.989	.999	1.000	1.000	1.000
18	.000	.000	.000	.000	.000	.000	.002	.012	.058	.180	.399	.660	.864	.966	.995	1.000	1.000	1.000	1.000
19	.000	.000	.000	.000	.000	.000	.004	.026	.102	.271	.520	.764	.921	.984	.998	1.000	1.000	1.000	1.000
20	.000	.000	.000	.000	.000	.001	.010	.051	.167	.380	.639	.848	.957	.993	.999	1.000	1.000	1.000	1.000
21	.000	.000	.000	.000	.000	.003	.021	.091	.254	.500	.746	.909	.979	.997	1.000	1.000	1.000	1.000	1.000

continued on following page

d   Cumulative Probabilities for Values of p with d Defects   n = 43

d	.05	.10	.15	.20	.25	.30	.35	.40	.45	.50	.55	.60	.65	.70	.75	.80	.85	.90	.95
22	.000	.000	.000	.000	.001	.007	.043	.152	.361	.620	.833	.949*	.990	.999	1.000	1.000	1.000	1.000	1.000
23	.000	.000	.000	.000	.002	.016	.079	.236	.480	.729	.898	.974	.996	1.000	1.000	1.000	1.000	1.000	1.000
24	.000	.000	.000	.000	.005	.034	.136	.340	.601	.820	.942	.988	.998	1.000	1.000	1.000	1.000	1.000	1.000
25	.000	.000	.000	.001	.011	.066	.215	.459	.713	.889	.970	.995	.999	1.000	1.000	1.000	1.000	1.000	1.000
26	.000	.000	.000	.003	.025	.117	.317	.582	.808	.937	.986	.998	1.000	1.000	1.000	1.000	1.000	1.000	1.000
27	.000	.000	.000	.007	.051	.192	.437	.699	.882	.967	.994	.999	1.000	1.000	1.000	1.000	1.000	1.000	1.000
28	.000	.000	.001	.016	.096	.292	.563	.799	.933	.984	.998	1.000	1.000	1.000	1.000	1.000	1.000	1.000	1.000
29	.000	.000	.003	.036	.166	.413	.685	.876	.965	.993	.999	1.000	1.000	1.000	1.000	1.000	1.000	1.000	1.000
30	.000	.000	.008	.073	.263	.544	.791	.930	.984	.997	1.000	1.000	1.000	1.000	1.000	1.000	1.000	1.000	1.000
31	.000	.001	.021	.136	.385	.673	.873	.965	.993	.999	1.000	1.000	1.000	1.000	1.000	1.000	1.000	1.000	1.000
32	.000	.003	.049	.229	.523	.785	.930	.984	.997	1.000	1.000	1.000	1.000	1.000	1.000	1.000	1.000	1.000	1.000
33	.000	.009	.101	.353	.661	.873	.966	.993	.999	1.000	1.000	1.000	1.000	1.000	1.000	1.000	1.000	1.000	1.000
34	.000	.024	.187	.500	.783	.933	.985	.998*	1.000	1.000	1.000	1.000	1.000	1.000	1.000	1.000	1.000	1.000	1.000
35	.001	.061	.313	.650	.876	.969	.994	.999	1.000	1.000	1.000	1.000	1.000	1.000	1.000	1.000	1.000	1.000	1.000
36	.005	.133	.471	.784	.939	.988	.998	1.000	1.000	1.000	1.000	1.000	1.000	1.000	1.000	1.000	1.000	1.000	1.000
37	.019	.257	.641	.885	.974	.996	.999	1.000	1.000	1.000	1.000	1.000	1.000	1.000	1.000	1.000	1.000	1.000	1.000
38	.062	.433	.793	.949	.991	.999	1.000	1.000	1.000	1.000	1.000	1.000	1.000	1.000	1.000	1.000	1.000	1.000	1.000
39	.167	.635	.904	.982	.998	1.000	1.000	1.000	1.000	1.000	1.000	1.000	1.000	1.000	1.000	1.000	1.000	1.000	1.000
40	.365	.818	.966	.995	1.000	1.000	1.000	1.000	1.000	1.000	1.000	1.000	1.000	1.000	1.000	1.000	1.000	1.000	1.000
41	.640	.938	.992	.999	1.000	1.000	1.000	1.000	1.000	1.000	1.000	1.000	1.000	1.000	1.000	1.000	1.000	1.000	1.000
42	.890	.989	.999	1.000	1.000	1.000	1.000	1.000	1.000	1.000	1.000	1.000	1.000	1.000	1.000	1.000	1.000	1.000	1.000
43	1.000	1.000	1.000	1.000	1.000	1.000	1.000	1.000	1.000	1.000	1.000	1.000	1.000	1.000	1.000	1.000	1.000	1.000	1.000

d Cumulative Probabilities for Values of p with d Defects   n = 44

d	.05	.10	.15	.20	.25	.30	.35	.40	.45	.50	.55	.60	.65	.70	.75	.80	.85	.90	.95
0	.000	.000	.000	.000	.000	.000	.000	.000	.000	.000	.000	.000	.000	.000	.000	.000	.001	.010	.105
1	.000	.000	.000	.000	.000	.000	.000	.000	.000	.000	.000	.000	.000	.000	.000	.001	.007	.057	.347
2	.000	.000	.000	.000	.000	.000	.000	.000	.000	.000	.000	.000	.000	.000	.000	.004	.030	.170	.621
3	.000	.000	.000	.000	.000	.000	.000	.000	.000	.000	.000	.000	.000	.000	.002	.015	.087	.347	.823
4	.000	.000	.000	.000	.000	.000	.000	.000	.000	.000	.000	.000	.000	.001	.007	.044	.190	.547	.933
5	.000	.000	.000	.000	.000	.000	.000	.000	.000	.000	.000	.000	.000	.003	.021	.102	.336	.726	.978
6	.000	.000	.000	.000	.000	.000	.000	.000	.000	.000	.000	.000	.001	.010	.052	.196	.503	.854	.994
7	.000	.000	.000	.000	.000	.000	.000	.000	.000	.000	.000	.001	.004	.026	.108	.323	.663	.932	.999
8	.000	.000	.000	.000	.000	.000	.000	.000	.000	.000	.000	.002	.012	.056	.194	.470	.794	.972	1.000
9	.000	.000	.000	.000	.000	.000	.000	.000	.000	.000	.001	.005	.027	.109	.309	.617	.886	.990	1.000
10	.000	.000	.000	.000	.000	.000	.000	.000	.000	.000	.002	.012	.057	.189	.442	.746	.943	.997	1.000
11	.000	.000	.000	.000	.000	.000	.000	.000	.000	.001	.005	.028	.107	.294	.580	.846	.974	.999	1.000
12	.000	.000	.000	.000	.000	.000	.000	.000	.000	.002	.012	.056	.180	.417	.706	.914	.990	1.000	1.000
13	.000	.000	.000	.000	.000	.000	.000	.000	.001	.005	.027	.102	.278	.548	.810	.956	.996	1.000	1.000
14	.000	.000	.000	.000	.000	.000	.000	.000	.002	.011	.053	.170	.394	.672	.886	.980	.999	1.000	1.000
15	.000	.000	.000	.000	.000	.000	.000	.000	.004	.024	.095	.261	.519	.778	.937	.991	1.000	1.000	1.000
16	.000	.000	.000	.000	.000	.000	.000	.001	.010	.048	.159	.371	.641	.861	.968	.997	1.000	1.000	1.000
17	.000	.000	.000	.000	.000	.000	.000	.003	.021	.087	.244	.492	.749	.919	.985	.999	1.000	1.000	1.000
18	.000	.000	.000	.000	.000	.000	.001	.008	.042	.146	.349	.613	.837	.956	.994	1.000	1.000	1.000	1.000
19	.000	.000	.000	.000	.000	.000	.003	.018	.078	.226	.466	.723	.901	.978	.997	1.000	1.000	1.000	1.000
20	.000	.000	.000	.000	.000	.001	.006	.036	.131	.326	.586	.814	.944	.990	.999	1.000	1.000	1.000	1.000
21	.000	.000	.000	.000	.000	.002	.014	.067	.206	.440	.698	.884	.971	.996	1.000	1.000	1.000	1.000	1.000
22	.000	.000	.000	.000	.000	.004	.029	.116	.302	.560	.794	.933	.986	.998	1.000	1.000	1.000	1.000	1.000

continued on following page

d Cumulative Probabilities for Values of p with d Defects

n = 44

d	.05	.10	.15	.20	.25	.30	.35	.40	.45	.50	.55	.60	.65	.70	.75	.80	.85	.90	.95
23	.000	.000	.000	.000	.001	.010	.056	.186	.414	.674	.869	.964	.994	.999	1.000	1.000	1.000	1.000	1.000
24	.000	.000	.000	.000	.003	.022	.099	.277	.534	.774	.922	.982	.997	1.000	1.000	1.000	1.000	1.000	1.000
25	.000	.000	.000	.000	.006	.044	.163	.387	.651	.854	.958	.992	.999	1.000	1.000	1.000	1.000	1.000	1.000
26	.000	.000	.000	.001	.015	.081	.251	.508	.756	.913	.979	.997	1.000	1.000	1.000	1.000	1.000	1.000	1.000
27	.000	.000	.000	.003	.032	.139	.359	.629	.841	.952	.990	.999	1.000	1.000	1.000	1.000	1.000	1.000	1.000
28	.000	.000	.000	.009	.063	.222	.481	.739	.905	.976	.996	1.000	1.000	1.000	1.000	1.000	1.000	1.000	1.000
29	.000	.000	.001	.020	.114	.328	.606	.830	.947	.989	.998	1.000	1.000	1.000	1.000	1.000	1.000	1.000	1.000
30	.000	.000	.004	.044	.190	.452	.722	.898	.973	.995	.999	1.000	1.000	1.000	1.000	1.000	1.000	1.000	1.000
31	.000	.000	.010	.086	.294	.583	.820	.944	.988	.998	1.000	1.000	1.000	1.000	1.000	1.000	1.000	1.000	1.000
32	.000	.001	.026	.154	.420	.706	.893	.972	.995	.999	1.000	1.000	1.000	1.000	1.000	1.000	1.000	1.000	1.000
33	.000	.003	.057	.254	.558	.811	.943	.988	.998	1.000	1.000	1.000	1.000	1.000	1.000	1.000	1.000	1.000	1.000
34	.000	.010	.114	.383	.691	.891	.973	.995	.999	1.000	1.000	1.000	1.000	1.000	1.000	1.000	1.000	1.000	1.000
35	.000	.028	.206	.530	.806	.944	.988	.998	1.000	1.000	1.000	1.000	1.000	1.000	1.000	1.000	1.000	1.000	1.000
36	.001	.068	.337	.677	.892	.974	.996	.999	1.000	1.000	1.000	1.000	1.000	1.000	1.000	1.000	1.000	1.000	1.000
37	.006	.146	.497	.804	.948	.990	.999	1.000	1.000	1.000	1.000	1.000	1.000	1.000	1.000	1.000	1.000	1.000	1.000
38	.022	.274	.664	.898	.979	.997	1.000	1.000	1.000	1.000	1.000	1.000	1.000	1.000	1.000	1.000	1.000	1.000	1.000
39	.067	.453	.810	.956	.993	.999	1.000	1.000	1.000	1.000	1.000	1.000	1.000	1.000	1.000	1.000	1.000	1.000	1.000
40	.177	.653	.913	.985	.998	1.000	1.000	1.000	1.000	1.000	1.000	1.000	1.000	1.000	1.000	1.000	1.000	1.000	1.000
41	.379	.830	.970	.996	1.000	1.000	1.000	1.000	1.000	1.000	1.000	1.000	1.000	1.000	1.000	1.000	1.000	1.000	1.000
42	.653	.943	.993	.999	1.000	1.000	1.000	1.000	1.000	1.000	1.000	1.000	1.000	1.000	1.000	1.000	1.000	1.000	1.000
43	.895	.990	.999	1.000	1.000	1.000	1.000	1.000	1.000	1.000	1.000	1.000	1.000	1.000	1.000	1.000	1.000	1.000	1.000
44	1.000	1.000	1.000	1.000	1.000	1.000	1.000	1.000	1.000	1.000	1.000	1.000	1.000	1.000	1.000	1.000	1.000	1.000	1.000

d Cumulative Probabilities for Values of p with d Defects   n = 45

d	.05	.10	.15	.20	.25	.30	.35	.40	.45	.50	.55	.60	.65	.70	.75	.80	.85	.90	.95
0	.000	.000	.000	.000	.000	.000	.000	.000	.000	.000	.000	.000	.000	.000	.000	.000	.001	.009	.099
1	.000	.000	.000	.000	.000	.000	.000	.000	.000	.000	.000	.000	.000	.000	.000	.001	.006	.052	.335
2	.000	.000	.000	.000	.000	.000	.000	.000	.000	.000	.000	.000	.000	.000	.000	.003	.027	.159	.608
3	.000	.000	.000	.000	.000	.000	.000	.000	.000	.000	.000	.000	.000	.000	.002	.013	.078	.329	.813
4	.000	.000	.000	.000	.000	.000	.000	.000	.000	.000	.000	.000	.000	.001	.006	.038	.175	.527	.927
5	.000	.000	.000	.000	.000	.000	.000	.000	.000	.000	.000	.000	.000	.003	.018	.090	.314	.708	.976
6	.000	.000	.000	.000	.000	.000	.000	.000	.000	.000	.000	.000	.001	.008	.045	.177	.478	.841	.993
7	.000	.000	.000	.000	.000	.000	.000	.000	.000	.000	.000	.000	.003	.021	.094	.297	.639	.924	.998
8	.000	.000	.000	.000	.000	.000	.000	.000	.000	.000	.000	.001	.009	.047	.173	.441	.775	.968	1.000
9	.000	.000	.000	.000	.000	.000	.000	.000	.000	.000	.000	.004	.022	.093	.280	.588	.873	.988	1.000
10	.000	.000	.000	.000	.000	.000	.000	.000	.000	.000	.001	.009	.047	.165	.409	.720	.935	.996	1.000
11	.000	.000	.000	.000	.000	.000	.000	.000	.000	.000	.004	.022	.090	.262	.546	.826	.970	.999	1.000
12	.000	.000	.000	.000	.000	.000	.000	.000	.000	.001	.009	.045	.155	.380	.675	.901	.987	1.000	1.000
13	.000	.000	.000	.000	.000	.000	.000	.000	.000	.003	.020	.084	.244	.509	.784	.948	.995	1.000	1.000
14	.000	.000	.000	.000	.000	.000	.000	.000	.001	.008	.041	.143	.353	.635	.867	.975	.998	1.000	1.000
15	.000	.000	.000	.000	.000	.000	.000	.000	.003	.018	.076	.225	.475	.746	.925	.989	.999	1.000	1.000
16	.000	.000	.000	.000	.000	.000	.000	.001	.007	.036	.130	.327	.598	.836	.961	.996	1.000	1.000	1.000
17	.000	.000	.000	.000	.000	.000	.000	.002	.015	.068	.206	.444	.711	.901	.981	.998	1.000	1.000	1.000
18	.000	.000	.000	.000	.000	.000	.001	.005	.031	.116	.302	.564	.806	.945	.992	.999	1.000	1.000	1.000
19	.000	.000	.000	.000	.000	.000	.001	.012	.058	.186	.413	.679	.879	.972	.997	1.000	1.000	1.000	1.000
20	.000	.000	.000	.000	.000	.000	.004	.025	.102	.276	.532	.778	.929	.986	.999	1.000	1.000	1.000	1.000
21	.000	.000	.000	.000	.000	.001	.009	.048	.165	.383	.647	.856	.962	.994	1.000	1.000	1.000	1.000	1.000
22	.000	.000	.000	.000	.000	.002	.019	.086	.249	.500	.751	.914	.981	.998	1.000	1.000	1.000	1.000	1.000

continued on following page

d Cumulative Probabilities for Values of p with d Defects   n = 45

d	.05	.10	.15	.20	.25	.30	.35	.40	.45	.50	.55	.60	.65	.70	.75	.80	.85	.90	.95
23	.000	.000	.000	.000	.000	.006	.038	.144	.353	.617	.835	.952	.991	.999	1.000	1.000	1.000	1.000	1.000
24	.000	.000	.000	.000	.001	.014	.071	.222	.468	.724	.898	.975	.996	1.000	1.000	1.000	1.000	1.000	1.000
25	.000	.000	.000	.000	.003	.028	.121	.321	.587	.814	.942	.988	.999	1.000	1.000	1.000	1.000	1.000	1.000
26	.000	.000	.000	.001	.008	.055	.194	.436	.698	.884	.969	.995	.999	1.000	1.000	1.000	1.000	1.000	1.000
27	.000	.000	.000	.002	.019	.099	.289	.556	.794	.932	.985	.998	1.000	1.000	1.000	1.000	1.000	1.000	1.000
28	.000	.000	.000	.004	.039	.164	.402	.673	.870	.964	.993	.999	1.000	1.000	1.000	1.000	1.000	1.000	1.000
29	.000	.000	.001	.011	.075	.254	.525	.775	.924	.982	.997	1.000	1.000	1.000	1.000	1.000	1.000	1.000	1.000
30	.000	.000	.002	.025	.133	.365	.647	.857	.959	.992	.999	1.000	1.000	1.000	1.000	1.000	1.000	1.000	1.000
31	.000	.000	.005	.052	.216	.491	.756	.916	.980	.997	1.000	1.000	1.000	1.000	1.000	1.000	1.000	1.000	1.000
32	.000	.000	.013	.099	.325	.620	.845	.955	.991	.999	1.000	1.000	1.000	1.000	1.000	1.000	1.000	1.000	1.000
33	.000	.001	.030	.174	.454	.738	.910	.978	.996	1.000	1.000	1.000	1.000	1.000	1.000	1.000	1.000	1.000	1.000
34	.000	.004	.065	.280	.591	.835	.953	.991	.999	1.000	1.000	1.000	1.000	1.000	1.000	1.000	1.000	1.000	1.000
35	.000	.012	.127	.412	.720	.907	.978	.996	1.000	1.000	1.000	1.000	1.000	1.000	1.000	1.000	1.000	1.000	1.000
36	.000	.032	.225	.559	.827	.953	.991	.999	1.000	1.000	1.000	1.000	1.000	1.000	1.000	1.000	1.000	1.000	1.000
37	.002	.076	.361	.703	.906	.979	.997	1.000	1.000	1.000	1.000	1.000	1.000	1.000	1.000	1.000	1.000	1.000	1.000
38	.007	.159	.522	.823	.955	.992	.999	1.000	1.000	1.000	1.000	1.000	1.000	1.000	1.000	1.000	1.000	1.000	1.000
39	.024	.292	.686	.910	.982	.997	1.000	1.000	1.000	1.000	1.000	1.000	1.000	1.000	1.000	1.000	1.000	1.000	1.000
40	.073	.473	.825	.962	.994	.999	1.000	1.000	1.000	1.000	1.000	1.000	1.000	1.000	1.000	1.000	1.000	1.000	1.000
41	.187	.671	.922	.987	.998	1.000	1.000	1.000	1.000	1.000	1.000	1.000	1.000	1.000	1.000	1.000	1.000	1.000	1.000
42	.392	.841	.973	.997	1.000	1.000	1.000	1.000	1.000	1.000	1.000	1.000	1.000	1.000	1.000	1.000	1.000	1.000	1.000
43	.665	.948	.994	.999	1.000	1.000	1.000	1.000	1.000	1.000	1.000	1.000	1.000	1.000	1.000	1.000	1.000	1.000	1.000
44	.901	.991	.999	1.000	1.000	1.000	1.000	1.000	1.000	1.000	1.000	1.000	1.000	1.000	1.000	1.000	1.000	1.000	1.000
45	1.000	1.000	1.000	1.000	1.000	1.000	1.000	1.000	1.000	1.000	1.000	1.000	1.000	1.000	1.000	1.000	1.000	1.000	1.000

d Cumulative Probabilities for Values of p with d Defects   n = 46

d	.05	.10	.15	.20	.25	.30	.35	.40	.45	.50	.55	.60	.65	.70	.75	.80	.85	.90	.95
0	.000	.000	.000	.000	.000	.000	.000	.000	.000	.000	.000	.000	.000	.000	.000	.000	.001	.008	.094
1	.000	.000	.000	.000	.000	.000	.000	.000	.000	.000	.000	.000	.000	.000	.000	.000	.005	.048	.323
2	.000	.000	.000	.000	.000	.000	.000	.000	.000	.000	.000	.000	.000	.000	.000	.003	.023	.148	.594
3	.000	.000	.000	.000	.000	.000	.000	.000	.000	.000	.000	.000	.000	.000	.001	.011	.071	.312	.803
4	.000	.000	.000	.000	.000	.000	.000	.000	.000	.000	.000	.000	.000	.001	.005	.033	.160	.507	.921
5	.000	.000	.000	.000	.000	.000	.000	.000	.000	.000	.000	.000	.000	.002	.015	.080	.293	.690	.974
6	.000	.000	.000	.000	.000	.000	.000	.000	.000	.000	.000	.000	.001	.006	.038	.159	.454	.828	.992
7	.000	.000	.000	.000	.000	.000	.000	.000	.000	.000	.000	.000	.003	.017	.082	.273	.615	.916	.998
8	.000	.000	.000	.000	.000	.000	.000	.000	.000	.000	.000	.001	.007	.039	.153	.412	.754	.964	1.000
9	.000	.000	.000	.000	.000	.000	.000	.000	.000	.000	.000	.003	.017	.079	.253	.559	.858	.986	1.000
10	.000	.000	.000	.000	.000	.000	.000	.000	.000	.000	.001	.007	.038	.143	.377	.694	.926	.995	1.000
11	.000	.000	.000	.000	.000	.000	.000	.000	.000	.000	.003	.017	.075	.233	.511	.805	.965	.998	1.000
12	.000	.000	.000	.000	.000	.000	.000	.000	.000	.001	.007	.035	.132	.345	.643	.886	.985	1.000	1.000
13	.000	.000	.000	.000	.000	.000	.000	.000	.000	.002	.015	.068	.213	.470	.757	.938	.994	1.000	1.000
14	.000	.000	.000	.000	.000	.000	.000	.000	.001	.006	.032	.119	.315	.597	.847	.970	.998	1.000	1.000
15	.000	.000	.000	.000	.000	.000	.000	.000	.002	.013	.060	.192	.433	.713	.910	.986	.999	1.000	1.000
16	.000	.000	.000	.000	.000	.000	.000	.000	.005	.027	.106	.286	.555	.809	.952	.994	1.000	1.000	1.000
17	.000	.000	.000	.000	.000	.000	.000	.001	.010	.052	.172	.397	.672	.882	.976	.998	1.000	1.000	1.000
18	.000	.000	.000	.000	.000	.000	.000	.003	.022	.092	.258	.516	.773	.932	.989	.999	1.000	1.000	1.000
19	.000	.000	.000	.000	.000	.000	.001	.008	.043	.151	.363	.633	.853	.964	.995	1.000	1.000	1.000	1.000
20	.000	.000	.000	.000	.000	.000	.002	.017	.078	.231	.478	.738	.911	.982	.998	1.000	1.000	1.000	1.000
21	.000	.000	.000	.000	.000	.000	.006	.034	.130	.329	.595	.825	.950	.992	.999	1.000	1.000	1.000	1.000
22	.000	.000	.000	.000	.000	.001	.012	.064	.203	.441	.704	.891	.974	.997	1.000	1.000	1.000	1.000	1.000
23	.000	.000	.000	.000	.000	.003	.026	.109	.296	.559	.797	.936	.988	.999	1.000	1.000	1.000	1.000	1.000

continued on following page

d Cumulative Probabilities for Values of p with d Defects   n = 46

	.05	.10	.15	.20	.25	.30	.35	.40	.45	.50	.55	.60	.65	.70	.75	.80	.85	.90	.95
24	.000	.000	.000	.000	.001	.008	.050	.175	.405	.671	.870	.966	.994	1.000	1.000	1.000	1.000	1.000	1.000
25	.000	.000	.000	.000	.002	.018	.089	.262	.522	.769	.922	.983	.998	1.000	1.000	1.000	1.000	1.000	1.000
26	.000	.000	.000	.000	.005	.036	.147	.367	.637	.849	.957	.992	.999	1.000	1.000	1.000	1.000	1.000	1.000
27	.000	.000	.000	.001	.011	.068	.227	.484	.742	.908	.978	.997	1.000	1.000	1.000	1.000	1.000	1.000	1.000
28	.000	.000	.000	.002	.024	.118	.328	.603	.828	.948	.990	.999	1.000	1.000	1.000	1.000	1.000	1.000	1.000
29	.000	.000	.000	.006	.048	.191	.445	.714	.894	.973	.995	1.000	1.000	1.000	1.000	1.000	1.000	1.000	1.000
30	.000	.000	.001	.014	.090	.287	.567	.808	.940	.987	.998	1.000	1.000	1.000	1.000	1.000	1.000	1.000	1.000
31	.000	.000	.002	.030	.153	.403	.685	.881	.968	.994	.999	1.000	1.000	1.000	1.000	1.000	1.000	1.000	1.000
32	.000	.000	.006	.062	.243	.530	.787	.932	.985	.998	1.000	1.000	1.000	1.000	1.000	1.000	1.000	1.000	1.000
33	.000	.000	.015	.114	.357	.655	.868	.965	.993	.999	1.000	1.000	1.000	1.000	1.000	1.000	1.000	1.000	1.000
34	.000	.002	.035	.195	.489	.767	.925	.983	.997	1.000	1.000	1.000	1.000	1.000	1.000	1.000	1.000	1.000	1.000
35	.000	.005	.074	.306	.623	.857	.962	.993	.999	1.000	1.000	1.000	1.000	1.000	1.000	1.000	1.000	1.000	1.000
36	.000	.014	.142	.441	.747	.921	.983	.997	1.000	1.000	1.000	1.000	1.000	1.000	1.000	1.000	1.000	1.000	1.000
37	.000	.036	.246	.588	.847	.961	.993	.999	1.000	1.000	1.000	1.000	1.000	1.000	1.000	1.000	1.000	1.000	1.000
38	.002	.084	.385	.727	.918	.983	.997	1.000	1.000	1.000	1.000	1.000	1.000	1.000	1.000	1.000	1.000	1.000	1.000
39	.008	.172	.546	.841	.962	.994	.999	1.000	1.000	1.000	1.000	1.000	1.000	1.000	1.000	1.000	1.000	1.000	1.000
40	.026	.310	.707	.920	.985	.998	1.000	1.000	1.000	1.000	1.000	1.000	1.000	1.000	1.000	1.000	1.000	1.000	1.000
41	.079	.493	.840	.967	.995	.999	1.000	1.000	1.000	1.000	1.000	1.000	1.000	1.000	1.000	1.000	1.000	1.000	1.000
42	.197	.688	.929	.989	.999	1.000	1.000	1.000	1.000	1.000	1.000	1.000	1.000	1.000	1.000	1.000	1.000	1.000	1.000
43	.406	.852	.977	.997	1.000	1.000	1.000	1.000	1.000	1.000	1.000	1.000	1.000	1.000	1.000	1.000	1.000	1.000	1.000
44	.677	.952	.995	1.000	1.000	1.000	1.000	1.000	1.000	1.000	1.000	1.000	1.000	1.000	1.000	1.000	1.000	1.000	1.000
45	.906	.992	.999	1.000	1.000	1.000	1.000	1.000	1.000	1.000	1.000	1.000	1.000	1.000	1.000	1.000	1.000	1.000	1.000
46	1.000	1.000	1.000	1.000	1.000	1.000	1.000	1.000	1.000	1.000	1.000	1.000	1.000	1.000	1.000	1.000	1.000	1.000	1.000

d   Cumulative Probabilities for Values of p with d Defects

n = 47

	.05	.10	.15	.20	.25	.30	.35	.40	.45	.50	.55	.60	.65	.70	.75	.80	.85	.90	.95
0	.000	.000	.000	.000	.000	.000	.000	.000	.000	.000	.000	.000	.000	.000	.000	.000	.000	.007	.090
1	.000	.000	.000	.000	.000	.000	.000	.000	.000	.000	.000	.000	.000	.000	.000	.000	.004	.044	.312
2	.000	.000	.000	.000	.000	.000	.000	.000	.000	.000	.000	.000	.000	.000	.000	.002	.021	.138	.580
3	.000	.000	.000	.000	.000	.000	.000	.000	.000	.000	.000	.000	.000	.000	.001	.009	.064	.296	.793
4	.000	.000	.000	.000	.000	.000	.000	.000	.000	.000	.000	.000	.000	.000	.004	.029	.147	.488	.915
5	.000	.000	.000	.000	.000	.000	.000	.000	.000	.000	.000	.000	.000	.002	.012	.070	.273	.671	.971
6	.000	.000	.000	.000	.000	.000	.000	.000	.000	.000	.000	.000	.001	.005	.032	.144	.430	.814	.992
7	.000	.000	.000	.000	.000	.000	.000	.000	.000	.000	.000	.000	.002	.014	.071	.251	.591	.907	.998
8	.000	.000	.000	.000	.000	.000	.000	.000	.000	.000	.000	.001	.005	.033	.135	.384	.733	.959	1.000
9	.000	.000	.000	.000	.000	.000	.000	.000	.000	.000	.000	.002	.014	.067	.228	.529	.842	.984	1.000
10	.000	.000	.000	.000	.000	.000	.000	.000	.000	.000	.001	.005	.031	.124	.346	.667	.915	.994	1.000
11	.000	.000	.000	.000	.000	.000	.000	.000	.000	.000	.002	.013	.062	.206	.478	.783	.959	.998	1.000
12	.000	.000	.000	.000	.000	.000	.000	.000	.000	.001	.005	.028	.112	.311	.610	.869	.982	.999	1.000
13	.000	.000	.000	.000	.000	.000	.000	.000	.000	.002	.011	.055	.184	.433	.728	.928	.993	1.000	1.000
14	.000	.000	.000	.000	.000	.000	.000	.000	.000	.004	.024	.099	.279	.559	.824	.963	.997	1.000	1.000
15	.000	.000	.000	.000	.000	.000	.000	.000	.001	.009	.047	.163	.391	.678	.894	.983	.999	1.000	1.000
16	.000	.000	.000	.000	.000	.000	.000	.000	.003	.020	.085	.249	.512	.780	.941	.993	1.000	1.000	1.000
17	.000	.000	.000	.000	.000	.000	.000	.001	.007	.039	.142	.353	.631	.860	.970	.997	1.000	1.000	1.000
18	.000	.000	.000	.000	.000	.000	.000	.002	.016	.072	.219	.468	.737	.917	.986	.999	1.000	1.000	1.000
19	.000	.000	.000	.000	.000	.000	.001	.005	.032	.121	.316	.586	.825	.954	.994	1.000	1.000	1.000	1.000
20	.000	.000	.000	.000	.000	.000	.001	.012	.059	.191	.426	.696	.891	.977	.997	1.000	1.000	1.000	1.000
21	.000	.000	.000	.000	.000	.000	.003	.024	.101	.280	.543	.790	.937	.989	.999	1.000	1.000	1.000	1.000
22	.000	.000	.000	.000	.000	.001	.008	.046	.163	.385	.655	.864	.966	.995	1.000	1.000	1.000	1.000	1.000
23	.000	.000	.000	.000	.000	.002	.017	.082	.245	.500	.755	.918	.983	.998	1.000	1.000	1.000	1.000	1.000

continued on following page

d   Cumulative Probabilities for Values of p with d Defects   n = 47

d	.05	.10	.15	.20	.25	.30	.35	.40	.45	.50	.55	.60	.65	.70	.75	.80	.85	.90	.95
24	.000	.000	.000	.000	.000	.005	.034	.136	.345	.615	.837	.954	.992	.999	1.000	1.000	1.000	1.000	1.000
25	.000	.000	.000	.000	.001	.011	.063	.210	.457	.720	.899	.976	.997	1.000	1.000	1.000	1.000	1.000	1.000
26	.000	.000	.000	.000	.003	.023	.109	.304	.574	.809	.941	.988	.999	1.000	1.000	1.000	1.000	1.000	1.000
27	.000	.000	.000	.000	.006	.046	.175	.414	.684	.879	.968	.995	.999	1.000	1.000	1.000	1.000	1.000	1.000
28	.000	.000	.000	.001	.014	.083	.263	.532	.781	.928	.984	.998	1.000	1.000	1.000	1.000	1.000	1.000	1.000
29	.000	.000	.000	.003	.030	.140	.369	.647	.858	.961	.993	.999	1.000	1.000	1.000	1.000	1.000	1.000	1.000
30	.000	.000	.000	.007	.059	.220	.488	.751	.915	.980	.997	1.000	1.000	1.000	1.000	1.000	1.000	1.000	1.000
31	.000	.000	.001	.017	.106	.322	.609	.837	.953	.991	.999	1.000	1.000	1.000	1.000	1.000	1.000	1.000	1.000
32	.000	.000	.003	.037	.176	.441	.721	.901	.976	.996	1.000	1.000	1.000	1.000	1.000	1.000	1.000	1.000	1.000
33	.000	.000	.007	.072	.272	.567	.816	.945	.989	.998	1.000	1.000	1.000	1.000	1.000	1.000	1.000	1.000	1.000
34	.000	.001	.018	.131	.390	.689	.888	.972	.995	.999	1.000	1.000	1.000	1.000	1.000	1.000	1.000	1.000	1.000
35	.000	.002	.041	.217	.522	.794	.938	.987	.998	1.000	1.000	1.000	1.000	1.000	1.000	1.000	1.000	1.000	1.000
36	.000	.006	.085	.333	.654	.876	.969	.995	.999	1.000	1.000	1.000	1.000	1.000	1.000	1.000	1.000	1.000	1.000
37	.000	.016	.158	.471	.772	.933	.986	.998	1.000	1.000	1.000	1.000	1.000	1.000	1.000	1.000	1.000	1.000	1.000
38	.000	.041	.267	.616	.865	.967	.995	.999	1.000	1.000	1.000	1.000	1.000	1.000	1.000	1.000	1.000	1.000	1.000
39	.002	.093	.409	.749	.929	.986	.998	1.000	1.000	1.000	1.000	1.000	1.000	1.000	1.000	1.000	1.000	1.000	1.000
40	.008	.186	.570	.856	.968	.995	.999	1.000	1.000	1.000	1.000	1.000	1.000	1.000	1.000	1.000	1.000	1.000	1.000
41	.029	.329	.727	.930	.988	.998	1.000	1.000	1.000	1.000	1.000	1.000	1.000	1.000	1.000	1.000	1.000	1.000	1.000
42	.085	.512	.853	.971	.996	1.000	1.000	1.000	1.000	1.000	1.000	1.000	1.000	1.000	1.000	1.000	1.000	1.000	1.000
43	.207	.704	.936	.991	.999	1.000	1.000	1.000	1.000	1.000	1.000	1.000	1.000	1.000	1.000	1.000	1.000	1.000	1.000
44	.420	.862	.979	.998	1.000	1.000	1.000	1.000	1.000	1.000	1.000	1.000	1.000	1.000	1.000	1.000	1.000	1.000	1.000
45	.688	.956	.996	1.000	1.000	1.000	1.000	1.000	1.000	1.000	1.000	1.000	1.000	1.000	1.000	1.000	1.000	1.000	1.000
46	.910	.993	1.000	1.000	1.000	1.000	1.000	1.000	1.000	1.000	1.000	1.000	1.000	1.000	1.000	1.000	1.000	1.000	1.000
47	1.000	1.000	1.000	1.000	1.000	1.000	1.000	1.000	1.000	1.000	1.000	1.000	1.000	1.000	1.000	1.000	1.000	1.000	1.000

d Cumulative Probabilities for Values of p with d Defects   n = 48

	.05	.10	.15	.20	.25	.30	.35	.40	.45	.50	.55	.60	.65	.70	.75	.80	.85	.90	.95
0	.000	.000	.000	.000	.000	.000	.000	.000	.000	.000	.000	.000	.000	.000	.000	.000	.000	.006	.085
1	.000	.000	.000	.000	.000	.000	.000	.000	.000	.000	.000	.000	.000	.000	.000	.000	.004	.040	.301
2	.000	.000	.000	.000	.000	.000	.000	.000	.000	.000	.000	.000	.000	.000	.000	.002	.018	.129	.567
3	.000	.000	.000	.000	.000	.000	.000	.000	.000	.000	.000	.000	.000	.000	.001	.008	.057	.280	.782
4	.000	.000	.000	.000	.000	.000	.000	.000	.000	.000	.000	.000	.000	.000	.003	.025	.134	.469	.909
5	.000	.000	.000	.000	.000	.000	.000	.000	.000	.000	.000	.000	.000	.001	.010	.062	.254	.653	.968
6	.000	.000	.000	.000	.000	.000	.000	.000	.000	.000	.000	.000	.000	.004	.027	.129	.406	.800	.991
7	.000	.000	.000	.000	.000	.000	.000	.000	.000	.000	.000	.000	.001	.011	.061	.229	.567	.898	.998
8	.000	.000	.000	.000	.000	.000	.000	.000	.000	.000	.000	.000	.004	.027	.119	.358	.712	.954	.999
9	.000	.000	.000	.000	.000	.000	.000	.000	.000	.000	.000	.001	.011	.057	.205	.500	.826	.981	1.000
10	.000	.000	.000	.000	.000	.000	.000	.000	.000	.000	.000	.004	.025	.107	.316	.639	.904	.993	1.000
11	.000	.000	.000	.000	.000	.000	.000	.000	.000	.000	.001	.010	.051	.181	.445	.759	.952	.998	1.000
12	.000	.000	.000	.000	.000	.000	.000	.000	.000	.000	.003	.022	.094	.280	.577	.852	.978	.999	1.000
13	.000	.000	.000	.000	.000	.000	.000	.000	.000	.001	.008	.044	.159	.396	.699	.916	.991	1.000	1.000
14	.000	.000	.000	.000	.000	.000	.000	.000	.000	.003	.018	.081	.246	.521	.800	.956	.997	1.000	1.000
15	.000	.000	.000	.000	.000	.000	.000	.000	.001	.007	.037	.137	.352	.642	.877	.979	.999	1.000	1.000
16	.000	.000	.000	.000	.000	.000	.000	.000	.002	.015	.068	.214	.470	.749	.930	.991	1.000	1.000	1.000
17	.000	.000	.000	.000	.000	.000	.000	.001	.005	.030	.117	.311	.589	.836	.963	.996	1.000	1.000	1.000
18	.000	.000	.000	.000	.000	.000	.000	.001	.011	.056	.185	.422	.700	.900	.982	.999	1.000	1.000	1.000
19	.000	.000	.000	.000	.000	.000	.000	.003	.023	.097	.272	.539	.794	.943	.992	.999	1.000	1.000	1.000
20	.000	.000	.000	.000	.000	.000	.001	.008	.044	.156	.377	.652	.868	.970	.996	1.000	1.000	1.000	1.000
21	.000	.000	.000	.000	.000	.000	.002	.017	.078	.235	.490	.753	.921	.985	.999	1.000	1.000	1.000	1.000
22	.000	.000	.000	.000	.000	.000	.005	.033	.129	.333	.605	.835	.956	.993	1.000	1.000	1.000	1.000	1.000
23	.000	.000	.000	.000	.000	.001	.011	.060	.200	.443	.710	.897	.977	.997	1.000	1.000	1.000	1.000	1.000
24	.000	.000	.000	.000	.000	.003	.023	.103	.290	.557	.800	.940	.989	.999	1.000	1.000	1.000	1.000	1.000

continued on following page

d Cumulative Probabilities for Values of p with d Defects   n = 48

d	.05	.10	.15	.20	.25	.30	.35	.40	.45	.50	.55	.60	.65	.70	.75	.80	.85	.90	.95
25	.000	.000	.000	.000	.000	.007	.044	.165	.395	.667	.871	.967	.995	1.000	1.000	1.000	1.000	1.000	1.000
26	.000	.000	.000	.000	.001	.015	.079	.247	.510	.765	.922	.983	.998	1.000	1.000	1.000	1.000	1.000	1.000
27	.000	.000	.000	.000	.004	.030	.132	.348	.623	.844	.956	.992	.999	1.000	1.000	1.000	1.000	1.000	1.000
28	.000	.000	.000	.001	.008	.057	.206	.461	.728	.903	.977	.997	1.000	1.000	1.000	1.000	1.000	1.000	1.000
29	.000	.000	.000	.001	.018	.100	.300	.578	.815	.944	.989	.999	1.000	1.000	1.000	1.000	1.000	1.000	1.000
30	.000	.000	.000	.004	.037	.164	.411	.689	.883	.970	.995	.999	1.000	1.000	1.000	1.000	1.000	1.000	1.000
31	.000	.000	.000	.009	.070	.251	.530	.786	.932	.985	.998	1.000	1.000	1.000	1.000	1.000	1.000	1.000	1.000
32	.000	.000	.001	.021	.123	.358	.648	.863	.963	.993	.999	1.000	1.000	1.000	1.000	1.000	1.000	1.000	1.000
33	.000	.000	.003	.044	.200	.479	.754	.919	.982	.997	1.000	1.000	1.000	1.000	1.000	1.000	1.000	1.000	1.000
34	.000	.000	.009	.084	.301	.604	.841	.956	.992	.999	1.000	1.000	1.000	1.000	1.000	1.000	1.000	1.000	1.000
35	.000	.001	.022	.148	.423	.720	.906	.978	.997	1.000	1.000	1.000	1.000	1.000	1.000	1.000	1.000	1.000	1.000
36	.000	.002	.048	.241	.555	.819	.949	.990	.999	1.000	1.000	1.000	1.000	1.000	1.000	1.000	1.000	1.000	1.000
37	.000	.007	.096	.361	.684	.893	.975	.996	1.000	1.000	1.000	1.000	1.000	1.000	1.000	1.000	1.000	1.000	1.000
38	.000	.019	.174	.500	.795	.943	.989	.999	1.000	1.000	1.000	1.000	1.000	1.000	1.000	1.000	1.000	1.000	1.000
39	.001	.046	.288	.642	.881	.973	.996	1.000	1.000	1.000	1.000	1.000	1.000	1.000	1.000	1.000	1.000	1.000	1.000
40	.002	.102	.433	.771	.939	.989	.999	1.000	1.000	1.000	1.000	1.000	1.000	1.000	1.000	1.000	1.000	1.000	1.000
41	.009	.200	.594	.871	.973	.996	1.000	1.000	1.000	1.000	1.000	1.000	1.000	1.000	1.000	1.000	1.000	1.000	1.000
42	.032	.347	.746	.938	.990	.999	1.000	1.000	1.000	1.000	1.000	1.000	1.000	1.000	1.000	1.000	1.000	1.000	1.000
43	.091	.531	.866	.975	.997	1.000	1.000	1.000	1.000	1.000	1.000	1.000	1.000	1.000	1.000	1.000	1.000	1.000	1.000
44	.218	.720	.943	.992	.999	1.000	1.000	1.000	1.000	1.000	1.000	1.000	1.000	1.000	1.000	1.000	1.000	1.000	1.000
45	.433	.871	.982	.998	1.000	1.000	1.000	1.000	1.000	1.000	1.000	1.000	1.000	1.000	1.000	1.000	1.000	1.000	1.000
46	.699	.960	.996	1.000	1.000	1.000	1.000	1.000	1.000	1.000	1.000	1.000	1.000	1.000	1.000	1.000	1.000	1.000	1.000
47	.915	.994	1.000	1.000	1.000	1.000	1.000	1.000	1.000	1.000	1.000	1.000	1.000	1.000	1.000	1.000	1.000	1.000	1.000
48	1.000	1.000	1.000	1.000	1.000	1.000	1.000	1.000	1.000	1.000	1.000	1.000	1.000	1.000	1.000	1.000	1.000	1.000	1.000

d Cumulative Probabilities for Values of p with d Defects   n = 49

d	.05	.10	.15	.20	.25	.30	.35	.40	.45	.50	.55	.60	.65	.70	.75	.80	.85	.90	.95
0	.000	.000	.000	.000	.000	.000	.000	.000	.000	.000	.000	.000	.000	.000	.000	.000	.000	.006	.081
1	.000	.000	.000	.000	.000	.000	.000	.000	.000	.000	.000	.000	.000	.000	.000	.000	.003	.037	.290
2	.000	.000	.000	.000	.000	.000	.000	.000	.000	.000	.000	.000	.000	.000	.000	.002	.016	.120	.554
3	.000	.000	.000	.000	.000	.000	.000	.000	.000	.000	.000	.000	.000	.000	.001	.007	.051	.265	.771
4	.000	.000	.000	.000	.000	.000	.000	.000	.000	.000	.000	.000	.000	.000	.003	.021	.123	.450	.903
5	.000	.000	.000	.000	.000	.000	.000	.000	.000	.000	.000	.000	.000	.001	.009	.055	.236	.635	.965
6	.000	.000	.000	.000	.000	.000	.000	.000	.000	.000	.000	.000	.000	.003	.023	.116	.383	.785	.989
7	.000	.000	.000	.000	.000	.000	.000	.000	.000	.000	.000	.000	.001	.009	.053	.209	.543	.888	.997
8	.000	.000	.000	.000	.000	.000	.000	.000	.000	.000	.000	.000	.003	.022	.105	.332	.690	.948	.999
9	.000	.000	.000	.000	.000	.000	.000	.000	.000	.000	.000	.001	.009	.048	.183	.472	.809	.978	1.000
10	.000	.000	.000	.000	.000	.000	.000	.000	.000	.000	.000	.003	.020	.092	.288	.612	.893	.992	1.000
11	.000	.000	.000	.000	.000	.000	.000	.000	.000	.000	.001	.008	.042	.159	.413	.735	.945	.997	1.000
12	.000	.000	.000	.000	.000	.000	.000	.000	.000	.000	.002	.017	.079	.250	.544	.834	.974	.999	1.000
13	.000	.000	.000	.000	.000	.000	.000	.000	.000	.001	.006	.035	.136	.361	.668	.903	.989	1.000	1.000
14	.000	.000	.000	.000	.000	.000	.000	.000	.000	.002	.014	.066	.215	.484	.775	.948	.996	1.000	1.000
15	.000	.000	.000	.000	.000	.000	.000	.000	.000	.005	.029	.115	.315	.606	.858	.974	.998	1.000	1.000
16	.000	.000	.000	.000	.000	.000	.000	.000	.001	.011	.054	.184	.429	.717	.916	.988	.999	1.000	1.000
17	.000	.000	.000	.000	.000	.000	.000	.000	.003	.022	.095	.272	.548	.810	.954	.995	1.000	1.000	1.000
18	.000	.000	.000	.000	.000	.000	.000	.001	.008	.043	.154	.378	.661	.881	.977	.998	1.000	1.000	1.000
19	.000	.000	.000	.000	.000	.000	.000	.002	.016	.076	.233	.492	.761	.930	.989	.999	1.000	1.000	1.000
20	.000	.000	.000	.000	.000	.000	.000	.005	.032	.126	.330	.607	.842	.962	.995	1.000	1.000	1.000	1.000
21	.000	.000	.000	.000	.000	.000	.001	.011	.059	.196	.439	.712	.902	.981	.998	1.000	1.000	1.000	1.000
22	.000	.000	.000	.000	.000	.000	.003	.023	.101	.284	.553	.802	.943	.991	.999	1.000	1.000	1.000	1.000
23	.000	.000	.000	.000	.000	.001	.007	.044	.161	.388	.663	.872	.969	.996	1.000	1.000	1.000	1.000	1.000
24	.000	.000	.000	.000	.000	.002	.015	.078	.240	.500	.760	.922	.985	.998	1.000	1.000	1.000	1.000	1.000

continued on following page

d   Cumulative Probabilities for Values of p with d Defects   n = 49

d	.05	.10	.15	.20	.25	.30	.35	.40	.45	.50	.55	.60	.65	.70	.75	.80	.85	.90	.95
25	.000	.000	.000	.000	.000	.004	.031	.128	.337	.612	.839	.956	.993	.999	1.000	1.000	1.000	1.000	1.000
26	.000	.000	.000	.000	.001	.009	.057	.198	.447	.716	.899	.977	.997	1.000	1.000	1.000	1.000	1.000	1.000
27	.000	.000	.000	.000	.002	.019	.098	.288	.561	.804	.941	.989	.999	1.000	1.000	1.000	1.000	1.000	1.000
28	.000	.000	.000	.000	.005	.038	.158	.393	.670	.874	.968	.995	1.000	1.000	1.000	1.000	1.000	1.000	1.000
29	.000	.000	.000	.001	.011	.070	.239	.508	.767	.924	.984	.998	1.000	1.000	1.000	1.000	1.000	1.000	1.000
30	.000	.000	.000	.002	.023	.119	.339	.622	.846	.957	.992	.999	1.000	1.000	1.000	1.000	1.000	1.000	1.000
31	.000	.000	.000	.005	.046	.190	.452	.728	.905	.978	.997	1.000	1.000	1.000	1.000	1.000	1.000	1.000	1.000
32	.000	.000	.001	.012	.084	.283	.571	.816	.946	.989	.999	1.000	1.000	1.000	1.000	1.000	1.000	1.000	1.000
33	.000	.000	.002	.026	.142	.394	.685	.885	.971	.995	1.000	1.000	1.000	1.000	1.000	1.000	1.000	1.000	1.000
34	.000	.000	.004	.052	.225	.516	.785	.934	.986	.998	1.000	1.000	1.000	1.000	1.000	1.000	1.000	1.000	1.000
35	.000	.000	.011	.097	.332	.639	.864	.965	.994	.999	1.000	1.000	1.000	1.000	1.000	1.000	1.000	1.000	1.000
36	.000	.001	.026	.166	.456	.750	.921	.983	.998	1.000	1.000	1.000	1.000	1.000	1.000	1.000	1.000	1.000	1.000
37	.000	.003	.055	.265	.587	.841	.958	.992	.999	1.000	1.000	1.000	1.000	1.000	1.000	1.000	1.000	1.000	1.000
38	.000	.008	.107	.388	.712	.908	.980	.997	1.000	1.000	1.000	1.000	1.000	1.000	1.000	1.000	1.000	1.000	1.000
39	.000	.022	.191	.528	.817	.952	.991	.999	1.000	1.000	1.000	1.000	1.000	1.000	1.000	1.000	1.000	1.000	1.000
40	.001	.052	.310	.668	.895	.978	.997	1.000	1.000	1.000	1.000	1.000	1.000	1.000	1.000	1.000	1.000	1.000	1.000
41	.003	.112	.457	.791	.947	.991	.999	1.000	1.000	1.000	1.000	1.000	1.000	1.000	1.000	1.000	1.000	1.000	1.000
42	.011	.215	.617	.884	.977	.997	1.000	1.000	1.000	1.000	1.000	1.000	1.000	1.000	1.000	1.000	1.000	1.000	1.000
43	.035	.365	.764	.945	.991	.999	1.000	1.000	1.000	1.000	1.000	1.000	1.000	1.000	1.000	1.000	1.000	1.000	1.000
44	.097	.550	.877	.979	.997	1.000	1.000	1.000	1.000	1.000	1.000	1.000	1.000	1.000	1.000	1.000	1.000	1.000	1.000
45	.229	.735	.949	.993	.999	1.000	1.000	1.000	1.000	1.000	1.000	1.000	1.000	1.000	1.000	1.000	1.000	1.000	1.000
46	.446	.880	.984	.998	1.000	1.000	1.000	1.000	1.000	1.000	1.000	1.000	1.000	1.000	1.000	1.000	1.000	1.000	1.000
47	.710	.963	.997	1.000	1.000	1.000	1.000	1.000	1.000	1.000	1.000	1.000	1.000	1.000	1.000	1.000	1.000	1.000	1.000
48	.919	.994	1.000	1.000	1.000	1.000	1.000	1.000	1.000	1.000	1.000	1.000	1.000	1.000	1.000	1.000	1.000	1.000	1.000
49	1.000	1.000	1.000	1.000	1.000	1.000	1.000	1.000	1.000	1.000	1.000	1.000	1.000	1.000	1.000	1.000	1.000	1.000	1.000

d Cumulative Probabilities for Values of p with d Defects n = 50

d	.05	.10	.15	.20	.25	.30	.35	.40	.45	.50	.55	.60	.65	.70	.75	.80	.85	.90	.95
0	.000	.000	.000	.000	.000	.000	.000	.000	.000	.000	.000	.000	.000	.000	.000	.000	.000	.005	.077
1	.000	.000	.000	.000	.000	.000	.000	.000	.000	.000	.000	.000	.000	.000	.000	.000	.003	.034	.279
2	.000	.000	.000	.000	.000	.000	.000	.000	.000	.000	.000	.000	.000	.000	.000	.001	.014	.112	.541
3	.000	.000	.000	.000	.000	.000	.000	.000	.000	.000	.000	.000	.000	.000	.000	.006	.046	.250	.760
4	.000	.000	.000	.000	.000	.000	.000	.000	.000	.000	.000	.000	.000	.000	.002	.018	.112	.431	.896
5	.000	.000	.000	.000	.000	.000	.000	.000	.000	.000	.000	.000	.000	.001	.007	.048	.219	.616	.962
6	.000	.000	.000	.000	.000	.000	.000	.000	.000	.000	.000	.000	.000	.002	.019	.103	.361	.770	.988
7	.000	.000	.000	.000	.000	.000	.000	.000	.000	.000	.000	.000	.001	.007	.045	.190	.519	.878	.997
8	.000	.000	.000	.000	.000	.000	.000	.000	.000	.000	.000	.000	.002	.018	.092	.307	.668	.942	.999
9	.000	.000	.000	.000	.000	.000	.000	.000	.000	.000	.000	.001	.007	.040	.164	.444	.791	.975	1.000
10	.000	.000	.000	.000	.000	.000	.000	.000	.000	.000	.000	.002	.016	.079	.262	.584	.880	.991	1.000
11	.000	.000	.000	.000	.000	.000	.000	.000	.000	.000	.001	.006	.034	.139	.382	.711	.937	.997	1.000
12	.000	.000	.000	.000	.000	.000	.000	.000	.000	.000	.002	.013	.066	.223	.511	.814	.970	.999	1.000
13	.000	.000	.000	.000	.000	.000	.000	.000	.000	.000	.004	.028	.116	.328	.637	.889	.987	1.000	1.000
14	.000	.000	.000	.000	.000	.000	.000	.000	.000	.001	.010	.054	.188	.447	.748	.939	.995	1.000	1.000
15	.000	.000	.000	.000	.000	.000	.000	.000	.000	.003	.022	.096	.280	.569	.837	.969	.998	1.000	1.000
16	.000	.000	.000	.000	.000	.000	.000	.000	.001	.008	.043	.156	.389	.684	.902	.986	.999	1.000	1.000
17	.000	.000	.000	.000	.000	.000	.000	.000	.002	.016	.077	.237	.506	.782	.945	.994	1.000	1.000	1.000
18	.000	.000	.000	.000	.000	.000	.000	.001	.005	.032	.127	.336	.622	.859	.971	.997	1.000	1.000	1.000
19	.000	.000	.000	.000	.000	.000	.000	.001	.012	.059	.197	.446	.726	.915	.986	.999	1.000	1.000	1.000
20	.000	.000	.000	.000	.000	.000	.000	.003	.024	.101	.286	.561	.814	.952	.994	1.000	1.000	1.000	1.000
21	.000	.000	.000	.000	.000	.000	.001	.008	.044	.161	.390	.670	.881	.975	.997	1.000	1.000	1.000	1.000
22	.000	.000	.000	.000	.000	.000	.002	.016	.078	.240	.502	.766	.929	.988	.999	1.000	1.000	1.000	1.000
23	.000	.000	.000	.000	.000	.000	.005	.031	.128	.336	.613	.844	.960	.994	1.000	1.000	1.000	1.000	1.000
24	.000	.000	.000	.000	.000	.001	.010	.057	.197	.444	.716	.902	.979	.998	1.000	1.000	1.000	1.000	1.000
25	.000	.000	.000	.000	.000	.002	.021	.098	.284	.556	.803	.943	.990	.999	1.000	1.000	1.000	1.000	1.000

continued on following page

d Cumulative Probabilities for Values of p with d Defects   n = 50

d	.05	.10	.15	.20	.25	.30	.35	.40	.45	.50	.55	.60	.65	.70	.75	.80	.85	.90	.95
26	.000	.000	.000	.000	.000	.006	.040	.156	.387	.664	.872	.969	.995	1.000	1.000	1.000	1.000	1.000	1.000
27	.000	.000	.000	.000	.001	.012	.071	.234	.498	.760	.922	.984	.998	1.000	1.000	1.000	1.000	1.000	1.000
28	.000	.000	.000	.000	.003	.025	.119	.330	.610	.839	.956	.992	.999	1.000	1.000	1.000	1.000	1.000	1.000
29	.000	.000	.000	.000	.006	.048	.186	.439	.714	.899	.976	.997	1.000	1.000	1.000	1.000	1.000	1.000	1.000
30	.000	.000	.000	.001	.014	.085	.274	.554	.803	.941	.988	.999	1.000	1.000	1.000	1.000	1.000	1.000	1.000
31	.000	.000	.000	.003	.029	.141	.378	.664	.873	.968	.995	.999	1.000	1.000	1.000	1.000	1.000	1.000	1.000
32	.000	.000	.000	.006	.055	.218	.494	.763	.923	.984	.998	1.000	1.000	1.000	1.000	1.000	1.000	1.000	1.000
33	.000	.000	.001	.014	.098	.316	.611	.844	.957	.992	.999	1.000	1.000	1.000	1.000	1.000	1.000	1.000	1.000
34	.000	.000	.002	.031	.163	.431	.720	.904	.978	.997	1.000	1.000	1.000	1.000	1.000	1.000	1.000	1.000	1.000
35	.000	.000	.005	.061	.252	.553	.812	.946	.990	.999	1.000	1.000	1.000	1.000	1.000	1.000	1.000	1.000	1.000
36	.000	.000	.013	.111	.363	.672	.884	.972	.996	1.000	1.000	1.000	1.000	1.000	1.000	1.000	1.000	1.000	1.000
37	.000	.001	.030	.186	.489	.777	.934	.987	.998	1.000	1.000	1.000	1.000	1.000	1.000	1.000	1.000	1.000	1.000
38	.000	.003	.063	.289	.618	.861	.966	.994	.999	1.000	1.000	1.000	1.000	1.000	1.000	1.000	1.000	1.000	1.000
39	.000	.009	.120	.416	.738	.921	.984	.998	1.000	1.000	1.000	1.000	1.000	1.000	1.000	1.000	1.000	1.000	1.000
40	.000	.025	.209	.556	.836	.960	.993	.999	1.000	1.000	1.000	1.000	1.000	1.000	1.000	1.000	1.000	1.000	1.000
41	.001	.058	.332	.693	.908	.982	.998	1.000	1.000	1.000	1.000	1.000	1.000	1.000	1.000	1.000	1.000	1.000	1.000
42	.003	.122	.481	.810	.955	.993	.999	1.000	1.000	1.000	1.000	1.000	1.000	1.000	1.000	1.000	1.000	1.000	1.000
43	.012	.230	.639	.897	.981	.998	1.000	1.000	1.000	1.000	1.000	1.000	1.000	1.000	1.000	1.000	1.000	1.000	1.000
44	.038	.384	.781	.952	.993	.999	1.000	1.000	1.000	1.000	1.000	1.000	1.000	1.000	1.000	1.000	1.000	1.000	1.000
45	.104	.569	.888	.982	.998	1.000	1.000	1.000	1.000	1.000	1.000	1.000	1.000	1.000	1.000	1.000	1.000	1.000	1.000
46	.240	.750	.954	.994	1.000	1.000	1.000	1.000	1.000	1.000	1.000	1.000	1.000	1.000	1.000	1.000	1.000	1.000	1.000
47	.459	.888	.986	.999	1.000	1.000	1.000	1.000	1.000	1.000	1.000	1.000	1.000	1.000	1.000	1.000	1.000	1.000	1.000
48	.721	.966	.997	1.000	1.000	1.000	1.000	1.000	1.000	1.000	1.000	1.000	1.000	1.000	1.000	1.000	1.000	1.000	1.000
49	.923	.995	1.000	1.000	1.000	1.000	1.000	1.000	1.000	1.000	1.000	1.000	1.000	1.000	1.000	1.000	1.000	1.000	1.000
50	1.000	1.000	1.000	1.000	1.000	1.000	1.000	1.000	1.000	1.000	1.000	1.000	1.000	1.000	1.000	1.000	1.000	1.000	1.000

References

Ashby, Eric. 1956. *An Introduction to Cybernetics.* New York: John Wiley and Sons.

Barrios, Juan Ignacio. 1988. Data from the Commission on Information, Ministry of Health, San José, Costa Rica.

Berggren, W. L., D.C. Ewbank, and G.G. Berggren. 1981. "Reduction of Mortality in Rural Haiti Through a Primary Health Care Program." *New England Journal of Medicine,* 304:1324-1330.

Campbell, Donald T. 1969. "Reforms as Experiments." *The American Psychologist,* 24(4):409-428.

Campbell, Donald T. 1984. "Can We Be Scientific in Applied Social Science?" *Evaluation Studies: Review Annual,* vol. 9, edited by R.F. Conner, D.G. Altman and C. Jackson. Beverly Hills, CA: Sage Publications.

Campbell, Donald T. and Julian C. Stanley. 1966. *Experimental and Quasi Experimental Designs for Research.* Chicago: Rand McNally. (First edition published in 1963.)

Carter, N.M. and J.B. Cullen. 1984. "A Comparison of Centralization/Decentralization of Decision-Making Concepts." *Journal of Management,* 10: 267.

Casley, Dennis J. and Krishna Kumar. 1987. *Project Monitoring and Evaluation in Agriculture.* Baltimore, MD: Johns Hopkins University Press.

Casley, Dennis J. and Denis A. Lury. 1982. *Monitoring and Evaluation of Agricultural and Rural Development Projects.* Baltimore, MD: Johns Hopkins University Press.

Clignet, Remi and Carroll Long. 1975. "Notes on the Research Designs to be Used in the Evaluation of Bank Projects Involving Shelter Components." *Urban and Regional Economics.* Washington, DC: World Bank.

Commission on Information for Costa Rica. 1988. Personal Communication. Ministry of Health. San José, Costa Rica.

Cook, Thomas and Donald T. Campbell. 1979. *Quasi-Experimentation: Design and Analysis Issues for Field Settings.* Chicago: Rand McNally.

Dodge, H.F. and H.G. Romig. 1959. *Sampling Inspection Tables: Single and Double Sampling.* New York: John Wiley and Sons.

Duncan, A.J. 1965. *Quality Control and Industrial Statistics.* Richard D. Irwing. Homewood, Illinois.

Edmunds, S. and S. Paul. 1984. "Training guide for the implementation of development projects." International Association of Schools and Institutes of Administration, Working Group IV. August.

Ferrero, Carlos and S. Boada-Martinez. 1985. "Transparencias Sobre Evaluación del Programma de Salud Rural de Costa Rica." PAHO.

Ghana Health Assessment Project Team. 1981. "A quantitative method of assessing the health impact of different diseases in less developed countries." *International Journal of Epidemiology,* 10:78-80.

Gonzalez-Vega, C. 1985. "Health Improvements in Costa Rica: The Socio-Economic Background." Paper delivered at the Rockefeller Conference. Bellagio, Italy.

Hage, Jerald. 1980. *Theories of Organizations: Form, Processes, and Transformations.* New York: John Wiley and Sons.

Henderson, R.H. and T. Sundaresan. 1982. "Cluster Sampling to Assess Immunization Coverage: A Review of Experience with a Simplified Sampling Method." *Bulletin of the World Health Organization,* 60:253-260.

Herrera, M. Guillermo. 1983. Personal Communication. Harvard School of Public Health. Boston, MA.

Herrera, M.G., J.O. Mora, N. Christiansen, N. Ortiz, J. Clement, L. Vouri, B. Paredes, M. Wagner and D. Waber. 1980a. "Effects of Nutritional Supplementation and Early Education on Physical and Cognitive Development." *Life-Span Developmental Psychology, Intervention.* New York: Academic Press, Inc.

Herrera, M.G., J.O. Mora, B. Paredes and M. Wagner. 1980b. "Maternal Weight/ Height and the Effects of Food Supplementation During Pregnancy and Lactation." *Maternal Nutrition During Pregnancy and Lactation.* Vienna: Huber.

Kaplan, Abraham. 1963. *The Conduct of Inquiry: Methodology for Behavioral Science.* New York: Harper and Row.

Keare, Douglas and Scott Parris. 1982. "Evaluation of Shelter Programs for the Urban Poor: Principal Findings." World Bank Staff Working Paper 547. Washington, D.C.: World Bank.

La Nación. August 1978. Buenos Aires, Argentina.

Lawrence, Paul R. and Jay W. Lorsch. 1967. "Differentiation and integration in complex organizations." *Administrative Sciences Quarterly,* 12(June):235-247.

Lemeshow, Stanley and George Stroh, Jr. 1986. "Sampling Techniques for Evaluating Health Parameters in Developing Countries." Washington, DC: National Research Council.

Lemeshow, Stanley and George Stroh, Jr.. 1989. "Quality Assurance Sampling for Evaluating Health Parameters in Developing Countries." *Survey Methodology,* 15:71-81.

Lemeshow, S., A. Tserkovnyi, J.L. Tulloch, J.E. Dowd, S.K. Lwanga, and J. Keja. 1985. "A Computer Simulation of the EPI Survey Strategy." *International Journal of Epidemiology,* 14(3):473-481.

MacMahon, Brian and Thomas F. Pugh. 1970. *Epidemiology: Principles and Methods.* Boston: Little, Brown and Co.

Mangelsdorf, Karen Ruffing. 1988. "Administrative decentralization and development: Some conflicting evidence from Ecuador." *International Review of Administrative Sciences,* 54:67-88.

Mansfield, R. and K. Alam. 1985. "Decentralization, management development and organizational performance in a developing country." *Productivity Review,* 14(3):33.

March, James G. and Herbert Simon. 1958. *Organizations*. New York: John Wiley and Sons.

Miller, C.M. and R.G. Knapp. 1979. "Item Inspection Control." Chapter 11 in *Evaluating Quality of Care: Analytic Procedures-Monitoring Techniques*. Rockville, MD: Aspen.

Mora, J.O., A. Amenzquita, L. Castro, N. Christiansen, J. Clement, F. Cobos, H.D. Cremer, S. Dragastin, M. Elias, M.G. Herrera, N. Ortiz, F. Pardo, B. Paredes, C. Ramos, R. Riley, H. Rodriguez, L. Vouri, M. Wagner and F.J. Stare. 1974. "Nutrition, Health and Social Factors Related to Intellectual Performance." *World Rev. Nutr. Diet.*, 19:205.

Mora, J.O., L. Navarro, J. Clement, M. Wagner, B. Paredes and G.H. Herrera. 1978a. "The Effect of Nutritional Supplementation on Calorie and Protein Intake of Pregnant Women." *Nutritional Reports International*, 17:217.

Mora, J.O., M. Wagner, J. Suescun, N. Christiansen, J. Clement, and G.H. Herrera. 1978b. "Nutritional Supplementation and the Outcome of Pregnancy: III. Perinatal and Neonatal Mortality." *Nutritional Reports International*, 18:167.

Mora, J.O., B. Paredes, M. Wagner, L. Navarro, L. Vuori, J. Suescun, N. Christiansen, J. Clement, and G.H. Herrera. 1979. "Nutritional Supplementation and the Outcome of Pregnancy: I. Birth Weight." *American Journal of Clinical Nutrition*, 32:455-462.

Pan American Health Organization. 1988. Panamerican Conference, June-July. Washington, DC.

Pennings, Johannes. 1973. "Measures of Organizational Structure: A Methodological Note." *American Journal of Sociology*, 79(November):686-704.

Price, James L. 1972. *Handbook of Organizational Management*. Lexington, MA: Heath.

Reinke, W.A. 1988. "Industrial Sampling Plans: Prospects for Public Health Applications." Occasional Paper No. 2. Institute for International Programs, The Johns Hopkins University School of Hygiene and Public Health.

Rondinelli, Dennis A., et al. 1984. *Decentralization In Developing Countries: A Review of Recent Experience*. World Bank Staff Working Paper No. 481. Washington, DC: World Bank, pp. 10-22.

Rosero, L., C. Grimaldo, C. Raabe. 1990. "Monitoring a primary health care programme with lot quality assurance sampling." *Health Policy and Planning* 5(1):30-39.

Sáenz, L. 1985. *Salud sin Riqueza: El Caso de Costa Rica*. MOH: Costa Rica.

Shepard, Donald S., Laye Sanoh and Emmou Coffi. 1986. "Cost Effectiveness of the Expanded Programme on Immunization in the Ivory Coast: A Preliminary Assessment. *Social Science and Medicine*, 22 (3):369-377.

Smith, B. 1979. "The Measurement of Decentralization." *International Review of Administrative Sciences* 45(3):215.

Steinbruner, John D. 1974. *The Cybernetic Theory of Decision: New Dimensions of Political Analysis*. Princeton, NJ: Princeton University Press.

Stroh, George. Undated, c. 1985. "Rationale for the Development and Trial of Q.C. Sampling Designs in Program Evaluation." (Obtained from the files of Donald Shepard.)

Thompson, James. 1967. *Organizations in Action*. New York: McGraw Hill.

UN, Development Administration Division. 1982. *Some Major Issues in Public Administration for Development*, SICA second series, No. 2. Austin: University of Texas Press.

Valadez, Joseph J. 1985a. "Quantitative and Qualitative Methods for Monitoring and Evaluation." Pan American Health Organization, HSS-I.

Valadez, Joseph J. 1985b. "Weighted Group Judgement for Qualitative Evaluation and Decision Making." Washington, DC. Pan American Health Organization (WHO). HSS-SNIS-28.

Valadez, Joseph J. 1990. Memo to Dr. James Heiby, Office of Health, Bureau of Science and Technology, Agency for International Development.

Valadez, Joseph J. with Esmee Bellalta. 1984. "MACUL: The Influences of Tasks on the Development of Social and Physical Spaces." *Human Organization*, 43:146-154.

Valadez, Joseph J. and Paul Ulrich. 1989. "Can Sampling of the Costa Rican Health Archives Provide the Same Data as More Costly Household Surveys?" Harvard Institute for International Development Report. PRICOR Project.

Valadez, Joseph J., William Vargas Vargas, and Lori DiPrete. 1990. "Supervision of Primary Health Care in Costa Rica: Time Well Spent?" *Health Policy and Planning*, 5(2).

Valadez, Joseph J., William Vargas Vargas, Ajiuio Rivera, and Rosa Zoila. 1988. "Diagnosis of the Measles Vaccination Subsystem of the Costa Rican Primary Health Care System: Understanding Low Vaccination Coverage and Low Quality Service Delivery." Harvard Institute for International Development Report. PRICOR Project.

Valadez, Joseph J. and Leisa Weld. 1991. "Maternal Recall Error of Child Vaccination Status in a Developing Nation." *American Journal of Public Health*, December.

van Putten, J.G.. 1978. "Changes in two-thirds of the world: Who wants to be part of them?" *Public Management*, December:12.

Villegas, Hugo. 1978. "Costa Rica: Recursos Humanos y Participación de la Comunidad en los Servícios de Salud en el Médio Rural," Buletín de la Oficina Sanitária Panamericana, 84(1).

Webb, Eugene, et al. 1966. *Unobtrusive Measures*. Chicago: Rand McNally.

Weber, Max. 1947. *The Theory of Social and Economic Organization*. New York: Oxford University Press.

World Health Organization. Undated. Expanded Programme on Immunization. *Training for Mid-Level Managers: Evaluate Vaccination Coverage*.

Index

A

age distribution   47, 49, 116
Agency for International Development   22
alpha   86-7, 98, 119, 145, 156
attrition   55, 156
attrition or mortality   45, 55

B

BCG   111, 117, 121, 122
beta   7-8, 98, 119, 145, 156
binomial   70-8, 133, 177
binomial distribution   78, 80-1, 177

C

centralized   94, 145, 147, 160, 162, 169, 170
child survival programs   5, 50, 61, 95, 97, 177
classification error   72, 84-6, 89, 91, 134-5, 145
cluster sampling   68, 69, 70, 170, 171
cold chain   13-14, 40, 129, 130-1, 134, 136-9, 163, 166
compensatory equalization   45, 56, 57, 122
confidence interval   69, 93-4, 118, 122
construct validity   42, 44
consumer risk   67-9, 71-6, 84, 86, 87-9, 91, 95,
        131-3, 150-1, 156-7, 172
control group   35-6, 41, 44-6, 52-7, 108
control vs. group variation   45
correlation   53, 174, 175
costs   7, 15, 22-4, 58, 68, 69, 91, 92, 98, 145-52, 169, 170, 172
covariance   174
coverage   1, 7-10, 23, 25, 40, 68, 69, 70-5, 77-9, 80-7, 91, 93, 98-102,
        111-4, 116, 118, 120-1, 123, 125, 129, 140, 145,
        153, 164-6, 169, 170-78
cumulative probability   81-3
cybernetic   160, 164-5

D

decentralized   2, 4, 10, 24, 34, 38, 48, 71, 97, 145, 146, 149-66, 169, 170
decision rule   72-3, 75, 85, 87, 93, 119, 121, 124-5, 132, 157, 165
diffusion   45, 47, 56
DPT   11, 13-5, 98, 107, 111-6, 121, 136, 161, 174-5

E

education   4, 23, 30, 37, 42, 47, 48, 50, 52, 62, 130, 134, 136, 139, 140, 161, 166
evaluation   11, 16, 25, 39, 41, 44, 46, 59, 60, 61, 63, 68, 169, 177
Expanded Programme on Immunization   25, 30, 38, 68-70, 170-1
external validity   42, 46, 61-2